Field Guide to Psychiatric Assessment and Treatment

Socrates: *Suppose a person should come up to your friend, Eryximachus, or to his father Acumenus [physicians] and say to him: "I know how to apply drugs . . . and all that sort of thing; and knowing all this, as I do, I claim to be a doctor, and to make doctors by imparting this knowledge to others"—what do you suppose that they would say?*

Phaedrus: *They would be sure to ask him whether he also knew to whom he ought to give each kind of treatment, and when, and how much.*

Socrates: *And suppose that he were to reply: "No, I know nothing about all that; I expect the person who has learned what I have to teach to be able to do these things for himself"?*

Phaedrus: *They would say in reply that he is a madman or a pedant who imagines that he is a doctor . . .*

—Plato, *The Phaedrus,* 268b–268c

Field Guide to Psychiatric Assessment and Treatment

Mark S. Bauer, M.D.
Brown University
Department of Veterans Affairs Medical Center
Providence, Rhode Island

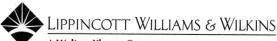

LIPPINCOTT WILLIAMS & WILKINS
A **Wolters Kluwer** Company
Philadelphia · Baltimore · New York · London
Buenos Aires · Hong Kong · Sydney · Tokyo

Acquisitions Editors: Richard Winters and Danette Knopp
Developmental Editor: Tanya Lazar
Production Editor: Emily Lerman
Manufacturing Manager: Colin J. Warnock
Cover Designer: Patricia Gast
Compositor: Circle Graphics
Printer: R. R. Donnelley, Crawfordsville

© 2003 by LIPPINCOTT WILLIAMS & WILKINS
530 Walnut Street
Philadelphia, PA 19106 USA
LWW.com

Printed in the USA

Library of Congress Cataloging-in-Publication Data

Bauer, Mark S.
    Field guide to psychiatric assessment and treatment / Mark S. Bauer.
        p. ; cm.
    Includes bibliographical references and index.
    ISBN 0-7817-3758-3 (alk. paper)
    1. Psychodiagnostics–Handbooks, manuals, etc. 2. Behavioral assessment–Handbooks, manuals, etc. I. Title.
        [DNLM: 1. Mental Disorders–diagnosis. 2. Mental Disorders–drug therapy. WM 141 B344 f2003]
    RC469.B384 2003
    616.89′075–dc21   2003040041

10   9   8   7   6   5   4   3   2   1

DEDICATION

*To the trainees and staff of the Mental Health Service
of the Providence Veterans Affairs Medical Center,
and to the individuals who come to them for care.
Without the trainees, particularly those in
Teaching Rounds each morning on Ward 3A,
this book would never have been conceptualized or written.*

Contents

Preface   xiii
How to Use This Field Guide   xv
Acknowledgments   xix

Section I. The Biopsychosocial Assessment
              and How to Get There Efficiently   1

Section II. Symptom-Driven Interviewing   15
Introduction   15

Module 1.   Depression or Fatigue.   17
Module 2.   Manic Symptoms   24
Module 3.   Anxiety/Nervousness   28
Module 4.   Psychosis (Hallucinations and Delusions).   36
Module 5.   Substance Use and Gambling   45
Module 6.   Suicidality and Assaultiveness
                     (Including Acute Management Strategies)   55
Module 7.   Change in Mental Status/Delirium   67
Module 8.   Problems with Memory or Organization   74
Module 9.   Problems with Concentration,
                     Impulsivity, and Irritability   84
Module 10.   Eating and Appearance.   86
Module 11.   Sleep Problems   91
Module 12.   Sexual Problems   100
Module 13.   Chronic Pain and Its Management
                     in "The House of Pain"   113
Module 14.   Multiple Unexplained Physical Complaints   123
Module 15.   Relationship and Personal Problems   130
Module 16.   Competency   136
Module 17.   Assessment and Management of
                     Psychotropic-Induced Movement Disorders   143
Module 18.   When the Black Dog Comes Back:
                     Thinking Through Recurrence   158

Section III. Disorders   160
Introduction   160

Mood Disorders.   164
Major Depressive Disorder   164
Dysthymic Disorder   167
Manic-Depressive (Bipolar) Disorder   169
     Type I.   169
     Type II   169
Cyclothymic Disorder   173

Anxiety Disorders   174
Panic Disorder   174

Phobias. 177
   Specific Phobia 177
   Social Phobia. 177
   Agoraphobia 177
Generalized Anxiety Disorder 180
Obsessive-Compulsive Disorder 182
Posttraumatic Stress Disorder. 184
Acute Stress Disorder 187

Substance Use Disorders and Pathological Gambling 189
Dependence 189
Abuse 189
Specific Substances: 190–195

Alcohol	Inhalants
Amphetamines	Nicotine
Caffeine	Opioids
Cannabis	Phencyclidine
Cocaine/Crack	Sedatives, Hypnotics, or Anxiolytics
Hallucinogens	Ecstasy and Related Compounds

Pathological Gambling 196

Schizophrenia and Other Psychotic Disorders 197
Schizophrenia 197
Schizoaffective Disorder. 201
Delusional Disorder. 203

Adjustment Disorders 204

Cognitive Disorders 206
Dementia 206
Attention-Deficit/Hyperactivity Disorder. 208

Somatoform and Related Disorders 210
Somatization Disorder. 210
Pain Disorder. 212
Hypochondriasis 214
Conversion Disorder 215
Factitious Disorder and Malingering Disorder. 217
Body Dysmorphic Disorder 218

Eating Disorders 220
Anorexia Nervosa 220
Bulimia Nervosa 221

Sleep Disorders 223

Sexual and Gender Identity Disorders 228

Premenstrual Dysphoric Disorder 232

Dissociative Disorders 234

Personality Disorders 236

Section IV. Treatment............................ 245
Introduction..................................... 245

Psychotherapy: Supportive Psychotherapy Techniques and
   Referral Information for Formal, Disorder-Specific
   Psychotherapies................................252–261
   Outline of Supportive Psychotherapy....................252–256
   Disorder-Specific Psychotherapies.....................257–261

Medications....................................... 262
Antidepressants.................................. 262
Tricyclics....................................... 262
   Amitriptyline................................. 262
   Clomipramine 264
   Desipramine.................................. 265
   Doxepin..................................... 267
   Imipramine 268
   Nortriptyline 270
   Protriptyline................................. 271
Selective Serotonin Reuptake Inhibitors.................. 273
   Citalopram................................... 273
   Escitalopram Oxalate 274
   Fluoxetine 275
   Fluvoxamine 276
   Paroxetine 278
   Sertraline 279
Monoamine Oxidase Inhibitors 280
   Phenelzine................................... 280
   Tranylcypromine.............................. 282
Other Antidepressants............................. 283
   Bupropion 283
   Mirtazapine 284
   Nefazodone 285
   Trazodone 286
   Venlafaxine 287

Antimanics and Putative Mood Stabilizers 288
   Carbamazepine 288
   Lamotrigine 290
   Lithium 291
   Oxcarbazepine................................ 293
   Topiramate................................... 294
   Valproate 295
   Verapamil 296

Adjuvant Mood Disorder Agents 297
   Levothyroxine (Thyroxine, L-Thyroxine) 297
   Triiodothyronine (Liothyronine) 298

Antipsychotics/Neuroleptics........................... 300
Typical Neuroleptics 300

Chlorpromazine..................................... 301
Fluphenazine 302
Haloperidol 303
Loxapine 304
Mesoridazine...................................... 305
Molindone 306
Perphenazine 307
Thioridazine...................................... 308
Thiothixene 310
Trifluoperazine 311
Atypical Neuroleptics 312
  Clozapine....................................... 312
  Olanzapine...................................... 313
  Quetiapine 314
  Risperidone 315
  Ziprasidone 316

Benzodiazepines 317
  Alprazolam 317
  Chlordiazepoxide 318
  Clonazepam..................................... 319
  Diazepam....................................... 320
  Lorazepam...................................... 321
  Oxazepam 322
  Temazepam 323
  Triazolam....................................... 323

Nonbenzodiazepine Hypnotics......................... 324
  Zaleplon.. 324
  Zolpidem 325

Other Agents Used in Anxiety Disorders................ 326
  Buspirone (Generalized Anxiety Disorder) 326
  Clonidine (PTSD) 327
  Gabapentin (Anxiety Symptoms, Pain, Mood Stabilization) .. 328
  Prazosin (PTSD) 329

Cognitive Enhancers 329
  Donepezil....................................... 330
  Galantamine..................................... 330
  Rivastigmine 331
  Tacrine... 331

Stimulants 332
  Methylphenidate 332
  Pemoline 333

Therapeutic Devices Used in Psychiatry 335
  Electroconvulsive Therapy....................... 335
  Bright Visible Spectrum Light 336
  Research Interventions 336

Appendices 337
Appendix 1: Cognitive Screening Instruments 337
Appendix 2: Alcohol and Benzodiazepine Detoxification
    Procedure: The Clinical Institute Withdrawal Assessment
    (CIWA) Protocol 339
Appendix 3: Barbiturate Detoxification and the Pentobarbital
    Challenge Test.................................... 341
Appendix 4: Opiate Detoxification Procedures 342
Appendix 5: Stimulant Detoxification Procedures 343
Appendix 6: Nicotine Detoxification Procedures. 344
Appendix 7: Biopsychosocial Approach to Sleep Complaints ... 345
Appendix 8: Abnormal Involuntary Movements Scale (AIMS).. 347
Appendix 9: Guide to Opiate Selection for Chronic Pain 349
Appendix 10: Some Self-Help Resources for Individuals
             Being Treated and Their Significant Others 350
Appendix 11: Psychotropic Drug Equivalency Tables 355
Appendix 12: Cytochrome P-450 Effects for Major
             Psychotropic Medications 358
Appendix 13: Dietary and Pharmacologic Substances Causing
             Adverse Interactions with Monoamine Oxidase
             Inhibitor (MAOI) Antidepressants 362
Appendix 14: Alternative and Complementary Agents
             Used for Psychiatric Symptoms 363
Key References: An Annotated Bibliography for Additional
  Clinically Relevant Information 365
Subject Index 373

Preface

Don't read this book. It wasn't written to be read. Much of it is not written in sentences. Full paragraphs are rarer still.

When I approached Rich Winters, at that time the Series Editor for Lippincott Williams & Wilkins' Field Guide Series, I found that we shared a similar conviction: Busy clinicians don't read books—they *use* them. In my own experience as a clinician, a book is made or broken by the clinician's ability to dip into it with a specific question, find the answer, close the book, and move on to the next clinical issue that demands attention. Well-organized tables and comprehensive lists are a godsend, and a fine index doubly so. Rich and I shared the vision of creating a psychiatric book to be used rather than read through, and Rich's record in developing the Field Guides Series stood as testament that I had found an apt partner for this project.

For whom is this book meant? Another product of our collaboration was that we merged Rich's longstanding dedication to providing specialty expertise to the primary care physician with my desire to provide a useful resource for nonspecialist clinicians working or training in the adult mental health sector. What has emerged is a book that we hope will be useful across the spectrum of clinicians who deal with adults with mental health symptoms: psychiatrists and nonpsychiatric physicians; nurses, physician assistants, social workers, and allied health specialists who encounter individuals with mental health symptoms in their work; and, of course, trainees in these fields. Physicians and other clinicians who develop and implement biopsychosocial treatment plans will find directly applicable information in all sections of this Field Guide. Social workers and allied health clinicians will find the sections on assessment, disorders, and psychotherapeutic treatment to be useful, while the section on medications will provide them with an intelligible guide to the major psychotropic medications used by those whom they treat.

Perhaps the only group of clinicians treating adults with mental health symptoms who will *not* find this book uniformly useful are the specialists working exclusively in their area of interest. I have undoubtedly gored a sacred ox or two in developing a concise generalist's manual that will be intelligible and useful in clinical practice. I hope that it is simplification, and not inaccuracy, that will pique the ire of the occasional specialist, and am particularly aware of simplifications in my own area of research, manic-depressive disorder. Perhaps, at least, such specialists will find solace in having assistance for questions outside their field of specialization.

In February 1883, in Fort Douglas, Utah, Dr. Samuel O. L. Potter penned the preface to the first edition of his *A Compend of Materia Medica: Therapeutics and Prescription Writing, with Especial Reference to the Physiological Actions of Drugs,* a pocket-sized handbook of about 200 pages covering everything from the therapeutic uses of gin to a short course in Latin for the accurate instruction of one's apothecary. Despite the intervening 120 years, I was struck by the similarity of the goals of his *Materia Medica* and those of this Field Guide—and by how persistent has been the need for comprehensive yet concise and usable reference guides for work in the field. Dr. Potter describes his volume:

> . . . brevity of statement is one of its principal features. At the same time, the essentials of the subject have been kept in view; [sic] from a desire

to make the book not only the best of its kind, but a compact compendium of the established maxims of therapeutical science, and the most advanced views concerning the physiologic actions of drugs.

One-hundred-and-twenty years notwithstanding, I could not aspire to more for this Field Guide. I hope that it will provide the busy clinician at any stage of training and experience with a useful *vade mecum,* Baedeker, Field Guide to the at-times complex world of mental health assessment and treatment. And, if you really want to read it through, I won't complain.

Peace,
Mark S. Bauer
Providence, Rhode Island
USA

How to Use This Field Guide

This Field Guide consists of six interlinked components:
- Section I: The Biopsychosocial Assessment and How to Get There Efficiently
- Section II: Symptom-Driven Interviewing
- Section III: Disorders
- Section IV: Treatments
- Appendices
- Key References: An Annotated Bibliography for Additional Clinically Relevant Information

The structure of each section allows the clinician to use the Field Guide at any of several levels of detail. It can be used as a complete interview, diagnosis, and biopsychosocial treatment planning aid by working from Section I through Section IV for any individual clinical situation. Alternatively, the clinician can refer to individual entries in each section to answer focused questions regarding any aspect of the diagnostic and treatment planning process from, for example, medical illnesses associated with depression to prevalence rates of generalized anxiety disorder in the primary care setting, to advantages or disadvantages of various treatment options for schizophrenia to drug-drug and P450 interactions for various medications. In this way the Field Guide will support the practice of clinicians and trainees across a broad range of expertise. Details of the contents and organization of each section are outlined below and then in more detail in the introduction to each section.

Section I: The Biopsychosocial Assessment and How to Get There Efficiently

This section provides an overview of the data to be gathered in a comprehensive psychiatric assessment—with knowledge that such comprehensive assessments no longer take place over days but rather, in this era of managed care, in 30 to 60 minutes.

The assessment approach is not a rehash of what is found in many texts on psychiatric interviewing, but utilizes principles of *evidence-based medicine* to assist the clinician in gathering and integrating data in the most useful and efficient manner possible (see **Section I, Panel 10**). In particular, the concepts of *sensitivity, specificity,* and *positive and negative predictive value,* typically applied to laboratory testing, are introduced here to aid in the construction of interview queries and in the integration of information on specific disorders from Section II to arrive at diagnoses as accurately and *efficiently* as possible.

At the same time, the assessment approach is firmly anchored into the Biopsychosocial Model of illness promulgated by G. L. Engel in the 1970s and in the current-day Collaborative Practice approach to assessment and treatment planning developed by Von Korff, Wagner, and others for chronic medical illness and by a number of individuals for mental illnesses as well (see **Key References** for details).

This approach throughout all sections of the Field Guide serves as an argument that an evidence-based—and, no less, a biopsychosocial—approach will be not only more *accurate* but also more *efficient* than an approach to the individual being treated that does not consider this orientation. Experience in the clinician's hands will determine the outcome of the argument.

Section II: Symptom-Driven Interviewing

This section applies the evidence-based and biopsychosocial approach to address specific presenting complaints that individuals bring to treatment. It is organized "outward" from the clinical situation—from the needs of the specific individual being assessed and treated—rather than being organized according to our technical knowledge base (e.g., Major Depressive Disorder, Manic-Depressive Disorder, Somatization Disorders, . . .).

This section is organized into modules addressing common presenting complaints (e.g., depression/fatigue, chronic pain) or clinical scenarios (e.g., management of suicidality or assaultiveness, competency assessment). The modules can be used at any of a number of levels. On a most comprehensive level, the clinician can follow the flow of diagnostic inquiry, organized into concise panels. The panels provide specific interview questions and work-up details, and the clinician can simply follow the various sequential panels to arrive at appropriate diagnoses. He or she can also consult particular panels for suggestions for specific interview queries that are based on evidence-based medicine concepts of sensitivity and specificity.

Those with greater experience can simply consult specific panels that contain tables of information frequently needed, such as mnemonics for diagnostic criteria; lists of medications and medical illnesses that can cause various symptoms; the classification and work-up for sleep disorders, sexual disorders, dementia, etc.

Regardless of the level of detail at which the modules are used, their orientation is to assist the clinician in implementing the four Core Clinical Tasks of Assessment and Treatment Planning (**Section I, Panel 1**):

- Characterize symptoms and signs.
- Build symptoms and signs into syndromes.
- Build syndromes into disorders.
- Treat the disorders

Moreover, the orientation of each module is based on the five Basic Principles of Assessment and Treatment Planning (**Section I, Panel 2**):

- A symptom does not make a syndrome.
- All behaviors have a differential diagnosis.
- Psychiatric diagnosis depends on *longitudinal* and not just *cross-sectional* data.
- Diagnosis drives treatment.
- All treatments—*all* treatments—have costs and benefits.

Section III: Disorders

This section contains an outline of each of the major adult psychiatric disorders including diagnostic criteria adapted from the American Psychiatric Association's *Diagnostic and Statistical Manual,* 4th edition (DSM-IV), as well as an outline of key clinical features and related information such as gender, cultural, and age-related issues. Prevalence rates in various settings in which these disorders might be encountered and a listing of common comorbidities assist in comprehensive screening and diagnosis of individuals according to the principles of evidence-based medicine.

Treatment planning is supported by the section for each disorder on "Treatment Considerations." This contains:

- An outline of criteria for urgent intervention
- Evidence-based medication options
- Recommendations for supportive and specialized psychotherapies

The medication and psychotherapy options listed map directly onto entries in the next section concerning treatment. Finally, the advantages and disadvantages of various treatment options are summarized in "Considerations in Choosing Among Treatments" for each disorder.

Section IV: Treatments

This section includes information on both psychotherapeutic and pharmacologic treatments. Care was taken to consult multiple references and to evaluate evidence according to the tenets of evidence-based medicine. In particular, the Cochrane Collaboration database was consulted wherever applicable, and individual studies and review data evaluated according to the evidence classification scheme of the US Agency for Health Care Policy and Research, now Agency for Healthcare Research and Quality (AHCPR/AHRQ). While the evidence classification is not explicitly listed in this small and clinically oriented book, evidence-based medicine approaches have given form to the inclusions and exclusions found herein.

The psychotherapy component of this section is comprised of two parts. The first contains a basic outline of the overall approach to supportive treatment of individuals with any mental health disorder. This approach is based on the Collaborative Practice Model, as articulated in several works found in the **Key References**. The second part of the psychotherapy component is a compilation of formal, structured psychotherapies with established controlled-trial efficacy evidence for particular diagnoses. This is not designed to teach the clinician how to do these therapies, but rather to provide them the basic information they will need in making appropriate referrals. The self-help and consumer information resources in **Appendix 10** support these psychotherapeutic efforts.

The medication component provides a summary of clinically useful information on each of the major psychotropic medications available in the U.S. today. These include on- and off-label uses, dosage and monitoring guidelines, titration and tapering schedules, side effect and toxicity profiles, contraindications and cautions, and drug interactions. Finally, each entry also contains a series of "Hints & Tips" that are based on a combination of distilled empirical data and clinical experience for those many clinical situations that have not been addressed in a formal, evidence-based manner. Devices such as electroconvulsive therapy and bright light treatment are also discussed.

Appendices

The fourteen appendices gather together clinically useful information rarely found in a single volume. These range, for example, from detoxification protocols to self-help and consumer information resources to P450 drug interactions to alternative/complementary medicine impact on traditional psychiatric treatment.

Key References: An Annotated Bibliography

A slim volume that seeks to be clinically useful on a daily basis trades comprehensiveness for conciseness and tight organization. The costs in this deal with the devil can be mitigated by providing the clinician with resources for more extensive, more specialized, or less frequently needed information. The Key

References provide such support and include for each resource what the clinician will, and won't, find in each.

A Final Note: On Language

It is beyond doubt that language affects the way we think, as well as the more readily recognized converse. Accordingly, we have taken care with the choice of language in this book, particularly the word "patient" which the clinician will find seldom if at all in this Field Guide. We have all used this useful shorthand method of referring to the individuals whom we treat as patients, and in its Latin origins there is nothing pejorative about this word, derived from *patior,* "to suffer." However, on occasion, we have undoubtedly witnessed (and, in our weaker or more fatigued moments, undoubtedly been party to) references such as "the gall bladder in bed 4" or "the diabetic in Room 617."

Somehow it seems even easier to refer to individuals with mental health symptoms as "the schizophrenic," "the manic-depressive," "the borderline," and the like. Perhaps it is because these illnesses directly alter those very aspects which make us most ourselves: our feelings, our thoughts, our behaviors.

Knowing that the language we use subtly affects our own behavior, thoughts, and feelings, the Field Guide refers mainly to the "individual being treated" rather than "the patient." In so doing we remind ourselves that those whom we treat *have* an illness, that they *are not* that illness, however powerfully it may affect every aspect of their lives.

A bit awkward? You can be the judge. The time will come when what now appear to be circumlocutions to refer to the individuals we treat will slip as easily off the tongue as some of what once appeared to be insurmountable linguistic burdens like "he or she" for simply "he," "African American" for "Negro," or "Native American" for "Indian."

Acknowledgments

This Field Guide grew out of daily Teaching Rounds on the inpatient psychiatric unit at the Veterans Affairs Medical Center in Providence, Rhode Island. Each day before clinical rounds I meet with the trainees rotating through the unit to discuss assessment, diagnosis, and treatment of the individuals they are treating on the wards. Over the months the questions posed by these psychiatry residents and medical students from Brown University, pharmacy and nursing students from the University of Rhode Island, physician assistant students from Yale, and social work interns from various programs in New England struck me as markedly similar. There appeared to be a need for similar information to assess and treat individuals with mental health problems across disciplines and across levels of training and across years. Moreover, in my consultation-liaison work with internists on the medical-surgical wards the same questions recurred. I thought it made sense to organize the information and to write it down. I thank those trainees and staff members, as well as the individuals they treat, who stimulated me to conceptualize and to write this book. I am also grateful to the nursing staff of Ward 3A who provided the climate and milieu that have made Teaching Rounds possible.

I have been blessed with a supportive group of individuals who have served as an Advisory Board since the conception of this project. Consistent with the orientation of this Field Guide, the Board is multidisciplinary, containing both trainees and seasoned clinicians, and both primary care and mental health clinicians. Their advice from the very first stages of this book including the critical issues of what to include and what not to, their proofreading of specific sections as they were developed, and their willingness to interact throughout the writing of this book have substantially improved its quality and utility. So special thanks go to the Advisory Board members: Michael Arsenault, M.D.; Dawna Blake, M.D.; Michael Mooney Bauer, P.A.-C.; Boris Royak, M.D.; and Greg Simon, M.D.

In this regard, I must also reiterate my appreciation to Richard Winters and thank Pam Sutton, Developmental Editor, who provided advice on specific formatting issues early in the development of this project.

In addition, a number of individuals helped with specific queries or provided other expert assistance at key points in the development of this book. I express my appreciation to them as well: Mark Aloia, Ph.D.; Hillel Grossman, M.D.; Evette Ludman, Ph.D.; Tom McGreevy, M.S.W.; Lorcan O'Tuama, M.D.; Nicki Pallotti, Cheryl Banick, and the staff of the Providence VA Medical Center Library; Maryann Paxson, Ph.D.; A. A. Peters, M.Div.; Katherine Phillips, M.D.; Lawrence Price, M.D.; Stephen Salloway, M.D.; Al Sirota, Ph.D.; Mark Zimmerman, M.D. They can be thanked for augmenting the quality of this book, while the blame for omissions or misstatements rests solely with me.

Very special thanks go to Tracy Wyrostek, who worked tirelessly gathering, collating, and cross-checking information throughout the development of this book. Thanks also to Murtuza Gunja who served as summer undergraduate research assistant collecting some of the medication information.

I must also acknowledge my debt to my extended family. Like many—perhaps most—American families, our family has been touched by serious mental illness. From this, I became aware that mental illnesses are real illnesses that happen to real people. This realization led in no small way to my entering the field of psychiatry in the first place, and continues to help me to order my priorities as a clinical psychiatrist and an academician.

Last, but far from least, thanks go to the "silent partners" in this endeavor: my immediate family, Beth, Nick, and Maggie. As always, they have provided the balance of support, tolerance, and diversion that have kept me going and kept me fresh.

Field Guide to Psychiatric Assessment and Treatment

SECTION I

The Biopsychosocial Assessment and How to Get There Efficiently

Orienting Notes

- Studies show that novice interviewers tend to get the same information as expert interviewers . . . in about twice the time.
- Psychiatric diagnoses are often missed, especially those that are:
  - Not the chief complaint
  - Not viewed as socially acceptable
  - Not the interviewer's focus of expertise or interest
- One (poor) way to ensure accuracy and comprehensiveness is simply to take more time interviewing.
- An alternative is to:
  - Use *evidence-based interviewing principles.*
  - Organize the interview around the *screening table of contents.*
- Be aware of three key characteristics of interview questions:
  - Open-ended versus closed-ended
  - High-sensitivity versus high specificity
  - Social valence
- A *biopsychosocial* approach (see Engel and related *Key References*) to assessment and treatment planning confers several advantages:
  - More accurate initial diagnostic assessment
  - Better alliance building
  - Long-term efficiency in treatment planning

Panel 1: The Core Clinical Tasks of Assessment and Treatment Planning

1. Characterize symptoms and signs.
2. Build symptoms and signs into syndromes.
3. Build syndromes into disorders.
4. Treat the disorders.

Panel 2: The Five Basic Principles of Assessment and Treatment Planning

1. A symptom does not make a syndrome.
2. All behaviors have a differential diagnosis.
3. Psychiatric diagnosis depends on *longitudinal* and not just *cross-sectional* data.
4. Diagnosis drives treatment.
5. All treatments—*all* treatments—have costs and benefits.

Panel 3: The Five Basic Principles of Assessment and Treatment Planning: Brief Illustrations

1. **A symptom does not make a syndrome.**
   - Depressed mood does not mean major depressive disorder. It could be:
     - Borderline personality disorder
     - Dysthymia
     - Adjustment disorder
     - Posttraumatic stress disorder, etc.
2. **All behaviors have a differential diagnosis.**
   - In addition to the implication of Principle 1, some behaviors that appear unusual to the interviewer are not symptoms at all—they may be cultural, or they may be unusual but nonpathologic variants of normal. Examples:
     - Speaking with spirits that is culturally accepted
     - Hypomanic symptoms that cause no dysfunction
     - Cross-dressing that causes the individual no distress
3. **Psychiatric diagnosis depends on *longitudinal* and not just *cross-sectional* data.**
   - Perhaps more than any other field of medicine, psychiatry depends on a longitudinal course for diagnosis. For example, symptoms of a major depressive episode (a syndrome) could be part of disorders that have different treatments:
     - Major depressive disorder, single episode
     - Major depressive disorder, recurrent
     - Bipolar disorder
     - Medical illness, medication side effect, etc.
4. **Diagnosis drives treatment.**
   - . . . as in all other fields of medicine.
   - We have increasingly broad-spectrum medications (e.g., serotonin reuptake inhibitors that have efficacy in several mood and anxiety disorders).
   - However, the longer we treat the wrong diagnosis, the more problems will arise (see *Principle 5*).
   - Furthermore, when treatments fail, management gets more complicated if you have not made an accurate diagnosis to fall back on.
5. **All treatments—*all* treatments—have costs and benefits.**
   - We, and those we treat, are lucky to have an ever-widening array of medications and psychotherapies at our disposal. Some are touted as being "safer," "more tolerable," or even "without side effects."
   - The history of psychopharmacology has always proven that such "honeymoon" claims are overblown.
   - Choosing treatments means identifying both costs and benefits. Examples:
     - The serotonin reuptake-inhibiting antidepressants do not have as significant anticholinergic or sedative side effects or arrhythmogenic toxicity in overdose as do the older tricyclics.
       - However, they cause impotence or anorgasmia quite frequently.
     - The newer atypical antipsychotics are not associated with an incidence of tardive dyskinesia as high as that found in the older typical agents.
       - However, several have greater propensity to cause weight gain and type 2 diabetes, and others have greater arrhythmogenic potential.
   - Psychotherapies are not necessarily benign either:
     - Substantial time costs
     - Substantial financial costs
     - Potential to foster dependency
     - Potential to avoid real-world issues.

Panel 4: Why *Biopsychosocial* Assessment and What's the Cost?

- Psychological and social components, in addition to biologic components, are essential for accurate assessment and treatment planning.
  - This is true not just in psychiatry, but in medicine and surgery as well (e.g., see Engel citations in *Key References*).
  - Consider treating diabetes, hyperlipidemia, or planning postoperative care:
    - Is the individual educated enough to understand instructions?
    - Does the individual have stable housing?
    - Can the individual access transportation for follow-up care?
    - Do financial or insurance limitations make it likely that prescriptions will not be filled?
    - Is there family and will they be supportive of—or a barrier to—treatment?
- But what's the *cost* of getting this information?
- Doesn't most of it come from the fearsome "social history," purported to take an hour or more, if not days?
  - Social history data sufficient for most assessments can be obtained in a few straightforward, closed-ended questions.
  - Getting relevant information at the outset is guaranteed to save time later in dealing with:
    - Alliance building
    - Compliance issues
    - Family management
  - And you'll usually end up dealing with these issues in times of crisis, so you might as well take care of them up front.

Panel 5: Components of the Biopsychosocial Assessment

The components are virtually identical to the assessment learned in the first year of medical school (with a couple of key adjustments):

- Identifying data
- Chief complaint
- History of present illness
    - Cover all manifestations of all currently active disorders back to their inception
        - Example: Don't arbitrarily cover the current manic episode here and all past mood episodes somewhere else.
    - Include here *all* active psychiatric disorders, not just those related to the chief complaint. Why?
        - Comorbidities impact on presentation, course, and treatment planning (e.g., schizophrenia with substance use disorders or anxiety disorders).
- Psychiatric review of systems (see *The Review of Systems as "Table of Contents" for the Interview, Panel 14*)
- Medical review of systems
- Medications (psychotropics, others)
- Social history (see *Panel 6*)
- Family history
    - May have impact via:
        - Nature (genetics)
        - Nurture (modeling)
    - Some examples where either nature or nurture or both may have impact:
        - Family history of substance use
        - Family history of suicide
- Physical examination
- Mental status examination (see *Panel 7*)
- Laboratories/studies
- Impression, including:
    - *Diagnostic and Statistical Manual of Mental Disorders* (DSM) System Axes I to V (see *Panel 8*)
    - Brief integrative summary including
        - Treatment priorities
        - The individual's view of the problem
        - Specific strengths/vulnerabilities of the individual being treated
- This information then feeds into a treatment plan based on the Collaborative Practice Model (see *Psychotherapy Panels 1–4* and *Key References*)

Note: This structure for the biopsychosocial assessment abolishes the "Past Psychiatric History." Although adhered to in most psychiatric texts (e.g., see the otherwise excellent Kaplan and Sadock in *Key References*), the distinction between "present" and "past" illnesses works best for acute illnesses such as appendicitis, otitis media, and the rare acute one-time psychiatric disorder. For chronic illnesses, it makes more sense to address any and *all active* problems as part of the history of present illness. The alternative (e.g., dealing with the current manic episode under history of present illness and the prior affective episodes under past medical history) makes little logical or clinical sense. The Psychiatric Review of Systems then reports past, inactive problems, as well as unsuspected current problems.

Note: Evidence of suicidality or danger to others may come up in any of several stages of the assessment. These symptoms may be part of many syndromes. It is critical that all individuals be screened for these symptoms, both current and past. See *Module 6* for details.

Panel 6: Components of the Social History

- Family of origin
  - Who was in the home?
  - Major stresses?
  - Physical/sexual abuse?

Note: See *"Normalizing Strategies"* (*Panel 13*) for tips on dealing with socially difficult issues such as childhood abuse.

  - Other trauma?
- Education
  - Years? General equivalency diploma (GED) attained? College degree or beyond? Technical school?
  - If high school not finished or GED not attained, why not?
    - External demands (e.g., family illness/business?)
    - Family neglect in a chaotic household?
    - Reform school?
  - How well does the patient read? (*Note:* Over 1 in 5 Americans have a reading level that is grade-school or below.)
- Occupation:
  - How many jobs?
  - Why were jobs left?
  - How long at longest job?
  - Unemployed periods?
  - Last work?

Note: First job is often the military. Because military experience is relatively standardized, it can tell you a lot about their capabilities:

  - Branch? Years?
  - Military occupational specialty/job? Combat?
  - Discharge rank?
  - Discharge type?
  - Is there a mismatch? For example, discharge at rank of private after 4 years signals demotion, incompetence, and/or discipline or other problems.
- Finances
  - How does he or she make ends meet?
  - Income sources besides job?
  - Current financial security?
  - Gambling problems?
- Legal problems
  - Past convictions, jail time, prison time, probations?
  - Current, including pending, court dates?
- Marital
  - Marriage(s)?
  - Kids (even if never married)?
  - If past marriage(s):
    - How ended?
    - How are relations with ex-spouse, kids now?
- Living situation
  - Own/rent/other? Homeless now—or recently?
  - Who else is there?
  - How stable is the housing? What stresses are there (e.g., drugs, alcohol)?
- How does he or she spend days
  - When feeling well?
  - Now?
- Psychosocial stressors
  - Current stressors
  - Also screen for trauma not covered in childhood, military experiences.
  - Are there weapons at home or at easy access?
- Social supports
  - Do they support health and treatment?
  - Are they counterproductive? Examples:
    - Alcoholic friends
    - Abusive spouse
    - Religious or social affiliation that does not believe in mental health treatment
- Spiritual orientation/religious affiliation
  - Helpful or not for illness management skills?
  - Helpful or not for treatment alliance?
- Cultural/Ethnic/Racial factors
  - Helpful or not for illness management skills?
  - Helpful or not for treatment alliance?
- Personal strengths
  - What are specific personal strengths?
  - How does he or she cope with symptoms?
  - How does he or she live life around the symptoms?

Panel 7: Components of the Mental Status Examination

- **Appearance** (assessment begins when, or before, the individual walks in the door)
  - Overall behavior and level of consciousness
  - Psychomotor agitation/retardation
  - Cooperation and apparent reliability
- **Orientation** (person, place, date)
- **Perception** (e.g., hallucinations, illusions)
- **Thought form** (speech, language, formal thought disorder)
- **Thought content** (e.g., delusions, obsessions, preoccupations, poverty of content)

Note: See *Module 4* for categorization of pathologic perception, thought form, and thought content.

- **Mood/affect**
  - Mood is a *symptom:* what the individual reports.
  - Affect is a *sign:* what the interviewer observes.
  - Are they congruent? Are they appropriate to content/situation?
- **Attention and memory**

Note: See *Module 8* for assessment of memory and organizational problems. See Mini-Mental State Examination for a standardized assessment of attention and memory in the *Appendix 1*.

- **Judgment**

Note: Inference of judgment from how individuals are handling their life and their symptoms is usually more informative than time-honored, but overrated, what-if queries such as "What would you do if you found a letter with an address and a stamp on it lying in the street?" Don't waste your time on those.

Panel 8: Notes on the DSM System for Diagnosis

- The DSM is the official nomenclature system of the American Psychiatric Association.
- It serves as the basis of diagnosis throughout most of modern mental health practice and is highly coordinated with the International Classification of Diseases system.
- Although it is the *lingua franca* of psychiatric diagnosis, it is a far from perfect system.
- Positives:
  - It provides explicit, reproducible criteria for diagnosis.
  - The diagnoses are for the most part empirically based.
  - The diagnoses are for the most part not based on unprovable theories.
- Negatives:
  - It provides a *categorical* system—either an individual has a diagnosis or does not: reality is, in many cases, likely *dimensional,* or graded.
  - Its empirical bases are not consistently strong.
  - In its efforts to work without theory it has left some gaps, such as the wide array of behavior formerly labeled as "neurotic" and now awkwardly handled across several disorders, if at all. See, for example, *Module 15* on personal/relationship problems and *Module 12* on sexual problems.
- Nonetheless, it is important to master the DSM criteria:
  - Think of learning the DSM categories as playing scales and basic pieces in music.
  - Once the basic categories are mastered, the diagnostician can begin to improvise.
  - But first know the categories cold!

Panel 9: The Classic "Open-Ended Question": *Pros* and *Cons*

- Classically, teaching interviewing has focused on the sacrosanct open-ended questions. This is reasonable because open-ended questions . . .
  - Support comprehensiveness in the interview because they allow individuals to determine what's important to them.
  - Build the treatment alliance by showing concern for what's on the individual's mind.
- However, the downside to open-ended questioning is:
  - It doesn't guarantee identifying the most important clinical syndromes because nonprofessionals do not think like clinicians.
  - Exclusively open-ended interviews take forever. And if an interview takes forever:
    - The interviewer gets tired and loses energy and focus.
    - The interviewer gets backed up and preoccupied with all the other duties awaiting them . . . and sometimes even gets cranky.
    - The individual being interviewed gets fatigued and sometimes lost in the interview.
- *Evidence-based interviewing principles* provide an alternate method to organize the interview.

Panel 10: Evidence-Based Interviewing Principles: Background

- For the past 15 to 20 years, general internal medicine, and to a degree primary care, have embraced a series of methods and concepts gathered under the rubric of "evidence-based medicine" to guide practice.
- Mental health practice is about 10 years behind general medicine, but the same methods and concepts have proven quite helpful in mental health (e.g., in developing clinical practice guidelines for various psychiatric disorders).
- The area of evidence-based medicine known as *decision sciences* is of particular relevance to psychiatric interviewing.
- Decision sciences have been concerned primarily with developing optimal testing strategies to detect and rule out specific diseases. For example:
  - Optimal screening for hypothyroidism in women at risk
  - Preventing contamination of the blood supply with human immunodeficiency virus (HIV)
  - Detection of colorectal cancer in middle-aged men
- Key concepts in testing (explained qualitatively):
  - *Sensitivity:* High sensitivity tests are those that "cast a wide net"—that is, tests that won't miss a diagnosis, even at the risk of identifying some false-positive results.
    - High-sensitivity tests are used when there's a high cost to missing a diagnosis—that is, when you don't want to miss a diagnosis under any circumstances.
    - Example: Thyroid-stimulating hormone set at a cut-off of 5 IU/L or above won't miss many people with hypothyroidism—even if it mistakenly identifies some people who aren't truly hypothyroid.
  - *Specificity:* High-specificity tests are those that "apply a winnowing fan" to "separate the wheat from the chaff" to make sure no people who don't have the disease of interest are not falsely identified.
    - High-specificity tests are used when you don't want to misidentify anyone by mistake as having the disease—for example, when the costs of misdiagnosis or costs of treatment are high.
    - Example: HIV screening

Note: There's always a trade-off between sensitivity and specificity: know when to use which type of question.

  - *Predictive value positive:* Given a positive test result, the likelihood that an individual has the disease. This depends on:
    - Test sensitivity and specificity
    - Prevalence of the disease in the population
  - *Predictive value negative:* Given a negative test result, the likelihood that an individual doesn't have the disease. This depends on:
    - Test sensitivity and specificity
    - Prevalence of the disease in the population
- Optimal testing strategies typically use multiple tests in sequence:
  - First, screen with a *high-sensitivity* test.
  - Second, test screen-positive individuals with a *high-specificity* test to confirm or rule out the diagnosis.

Note: For more technical review of decision sciences concepts and evidence-based medicine in general, consult decision sciences citations in the *Key References*.

Panel 11: Evidence-Based Interviewing Principles: Specific Interviewing Strategies

- "Tests? What's that got to do with psychiatric interviewing?"
  - Think of each interviewing question as a test for a specific condition.
- Use **high-sensitivity questions** to screen for specific psychiatric disorders.
  - If a high-sensitivity (screening) question about a particular group of conditions yields a negative response, don't waste your time: move on to the next set of diagnoses.

Note: Of course, if your lead screening questions are *not* high sensitivity, you can't be so confident that a negative response rules out a disorder, and you'll have to ask a bunch more questions.

- Use **high-specificity questions** to follow up, to confirm, or to rule out the suspected diagnosis.
  - Pursue aggressively using queries based on DSM criteria until you're certain whether or not the individual meets criteria for a suspected diagnosis.

Note: High-sensitivity/-specificity questions are not necessarily open ended—and, in fact, usually are not.
Note: To aid in interviewing, throughout *Section II, Symptom-Driven Assessment Section*:

- High-sensitivity questions are marked with a wide net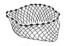

- High-specificity questions are marked with a winnowing fan to separate the wheat from the chaff

Panel 12: Evidence-Based Interviewing Principles: An Example

Example: Screening for Psychosis

- In *Module 4,* several high-sensitivity (screening) questions for psychosis are provided:

> "Sometimes when people . . . [supply major complaint, e.g., "feel depressed," "are under a lot of stress"] . . . they hear voices or sounds that are not there. I wonder if this has ever happened to you?"
>
> "Sometimes when people . . . they:
> . . . become concerned that people they don't know are out to do them harm."
> . . . become suspicious of people they aren't usually concerned about."
> . . . feel like people they don't know are out to get them."
> . . . Does that ever happen to you?"

Note: The "Sometimes people . . ." construction is discussed further in *Panel 13.*

- For reasons explained in *Module 4,* high-sensitivity questions focus on *auditory hallucinations* and *paranoia.* This is because these are the most common types of, respectively, hallucinations and delusions.
- If the responses to these high-sensitivity screening questions are negative, few individuals with psychosis will be missed.
- There is little utility in continuing to ask questions about less common manifestations of psychosis, such as:
  - "Do you ever feel that TV news anchors are talking about you when they report the news?"
  - "Do you ever feel that people are snatching thoughts from your head while you are thinking?"
- These latter queries are high-specificity questions and may be used, if responses to high-sensitivity screening questions are positive, to confirm the diagnosis.
- Otherwise, don't bother with high-specificity questions—time is a-wasting, and you have more to cover!

Note: As you will see in *Module 4,* psychosis is a syndrome, not a disorder. To identify the disorder of which psychosis is a part (e.g., "Is this psychotic syndrome part of schizophrenia, delirium, manic-depressive disorder", etc.), similar sensitivity/specificity strategies are used.

Panel 13: Another Critical Aspect of Interview Questions: *Social Valence*

- As noted above, interview questions can be:
  - Open-ended or closed-ended
  - High-sensitivity or high-specificity
  - A third critical characteristic of interview questions is the *social acceptability* or *social valence* of the area that they investigate.
- Certain areas are "sensitive" or negatively socially valenced—perhaps even more so in mental health than in other fields of medicine.
- Questions on these negatively valenced areas include the obvious, for example:
  - "How much do you drink?"
  - "How is your sex life?"
  - An example from an old lawyer quip tries to skirt around the negative valence, and in doing so illustrates social valence quite effectively: "When did you stop beating your wife?"
- However, as clinicians, we often forget that certain other areas that we need to cover in the psychiatric interview are also quite embarrassing or stigmatizing. Examples of questions on these more subtle areas include:
  - "Did you ever think about ending your life?"
  - "Do you ever hear voices?"
  - "Are you having problems with your memory?"
- Two *"normalizing strategies"* can help get more accurate data:
  - First, **do not bring up sensitive issues until well into the interview,** after:
    - You have established a reasonable treatment alliance, in part by demonstrating your interested, skillful, and comprehensive approach in the individual and his or her problems, and
    - The individual understands that the information he or she gives is not simply for your personal interest, but will determine the course of the next question, and the next, and so on (i.e., you have demonstrated that you are listening to the individual and you change your behavior based on what he or she says).
    - How not to do it: "Hello, my name is Dr. Bauer. I understand that you have been having nightmares and are nervous during the day. Were you ever sexually abused as a child?"
    - A better way: After having screened for posttraumatic stress disorder symptoms using high-sensitivity questions, investigate for the specific traumas, explaining the reason for the line of questioning.
  - Second, **prefacing questions** can often reduce negative social valence.
    - People typically don't like to talk with anyone about their mental symptoms.
    - So they often suspect that they are the only ones in the world to have a particular symptom (this may be hard to appreciate since we, as clinicians, may deal with such symptoms day in and day out).
    - Simply informing the individual that this or that symptom is not unheard of or unique reduces the negative valence enough that the individual can provide a forthright answer. Examples:
    - "Sometimes when people are quite depressed, they hear voices when there's no one there. Has that ever happened to you?"
    - "Sometimes when people feel as you do, they tend to drink more than is good for them. I wonder if that has ever been the case with you?"

Note: If the individual is too embarrassed to respond to negatively socially valenced queries, the *sensitivity* of your questioning will clearly be compromised. Normalizing strategies can protect the sensitivity of your screening queries.

Panel 14: Structuring the Interview. I: The Review of Systems as "Table of Contents" for the Interview

- Using the sensitivity/specificity approach to structuring your interview leads naturally into an overall flow that makes it unlikely anything will be missed:
  - Screen using high-sensitivity queries.
  - If positive, pursue with high-specificity queries to rule out or confirm the condition.
  - If negative, move on to the next topic.

  Note: In brief, colloquial terms:
  - Screen negative: Knock the dust from your shoes and move on to the next town.
  - Screen positive: Hang on like a pit bull until you know for sure.
- To ensure a comprehensive **review of systems** for psychiatric disorders, consider yourself as moving down a table of contents that includes all relevant psychiatric conditions. For example:
  - The table of contents from the DSM-IV
  - The **Symptom Modules** that follow in this book
  - Some other scheme that covers psychiatric conditions comprehensively

  Note: Recall that diagnoses are typically missed because information is missed. A comprehensive mental table of contents will reduce that chance. The more interviews you do, the more the table of contents will be ingrained in your memory.

Panel 15: Structuring the Interview. II: A Strategy for Starting Off

- Classically, in medicine, we start off the interview with the chief complaint.
- It may work better to make the chief complaint the *second* area to address.
- Begin the interview with a few key pieces of social history.
  - "Where do you live? With whom?"
  - "Are you currently working? What do you do?" If not currently working: "When was the last time you worked?"
  - "How do you make ends meet?"
  - "How do you spend your days when you're feeling well? How about now?"
- Why? Two reasons:
  - Alliance building
  - Evidence-based diagnostic acumen
- Alliance building:
  - Being a patient can be a dehumanizing experience. We're all warned in our early clinical interviewing training against falling into the rut of referring to "the gallbladder in 607," "the diabetic in bed 5," "the schizophrenic in seclusion." Nonetheless, our duties tend to make us pathology-focused.
  - A few basic inquiries about the person's life behind the pathology conveys subtly but effectively to the individual: "I accept that you are more than your chief complaint."
  - Not only does this help to build the treatment alliance, it confers a sense of dignity that is curative in its own right.
- Evidence-based diagnostic acumen:
  - In *Panel 10*, we noted that *predictive value positive/negative* outcomes depend not only on the characteristics of the question, but also on the *prevalence,* or frequency, of a condition in a given population.
  - If we know more about the population from which an individual comes, we'll be *more suspicious* of certain disorders, *less suspicious* of others.
  - Example:
    - Chief complaint of "I just flew in from Oregon to save New England because God sent me" in a 35-year-old man who has never worked, lives in a rooming house, and leads a life devoid of hobbies and social interaction raises suspicions of schizophrenia. However:
    - Chief complaint of "I just flew in from Oregon to save New England because God sent me" in a 35-year-old man who is a lawyer, married, raising a 5-year-old son and a 4-year-old daughter, and spends his free time coaching soccer, playing golf with his friends, and taking tango lessons with his wife lowers suspicions of schizophrenia and raises suspicions of mania, toxic psychosis, and several other diagnoses.
- Conceptually, these few bits of social history obtained initially give us the outline of the individual's *life narrative*—the structure on which we will hang the chief complaint and other Review of Systems data.

Panel 16: A Final Note on Prevalence and Predictive Value: Of Zebras and Horses

- In *Panel 15,* we noted that the *life narrative*—technically, key demographics—can help us know what to suspect more or less strongly.
- In each entry of *Section III, Disorders,* additional data help us to know what to suspect more or less strongly—again based on evidence-based principles. These include:
  - Demographics of specific disorders, including age of onset, gender distribution, and course factors
  - Prevalence rates of the disorder in various populations
- These prevalence, or frequency, rates for various populations are provided where available for the various settings in which the clinician may find himself or herself:
  - General population/community work
  - Primary care
  - Outpatient mental health clinic
  - Inpatient psychiatry unit
- Examples:
  - New-onset voices in a 50-year-old are less likely to be schizophrenia than several other diagnoses such as bipolar disorder, delirium, etc.
  - Refusal to eat in a 65-year-old man is less likely to be anorexia nervosa than depression, dementia, etc.
  - Although excessive use of alcohol is sometimes the chief complaint in a general outpatient mental health clinic, it is *five times more likely to be identified only during the Review of Systems as a secondary complaint.*

Note: Hence, the critical importance of the Review of Systems!

Note: The old clinical saw, "When you hear hoofbeats in Wyoming, think horses, not zebras," predates the formal development of evidence-based medicine, but captures the essence of decision sciences quite nicely!

SECTION II

Symptom-Driven Assessment

INTRODUCTION

This symptom-driven assessment section provides entry into the *Field Guide* in order to support the four core tasks of psychiatric assessment and treatment planning (**Section I, Panel 1**):

1. Characterize symptoms and signs.
2. Build symptoms and signs into syndromes.
3. Build syndromes into disorders.
4. Treat the disorders.

Unlike many guides to psychiatric assessment and treatment, the *Field Guide* is not organized around areas of knowledge. Rather, it is organized around symptoms: one might say that it is built "outward" from the individual seeking treatment to the established knowledge base rather than the reverse. It is symptom-oriented, as is the process of assessment.

This section is built upon the core principles and procedures outlined in **Section I**. In particular, the first three of the **five Principles of Assessment and Treatment Planning** (**Section I, Panels 2 and 3**) guide the specific organization of this section and the interview process that derives from it:

- A symptom does not make a syndrome.
- All behaviors have a differential diagnosis.
- Psychiatric diagnosis depends on *longitudinal,* as well as *cross-sectional* data.

This section contains 18 **Modules** that are each organized around a common presenting complaint such as depression, anxiety, or sexual problems, or around a specific clinical need such as competency evaluation or the unanticipated recurrence of symptoms previously successfully treated. The clinician can use the modules at any of three levels of detail:

- Clinicians who are particularly experienced with a particular type of symptom and only need a reminder or memory jog, or need to cross-check to ensure completeness of their differential diagnosis, can simply refer to the **Orienting Notes** and **Differential Diagnosis panels** that begin each module. From there, they can move directly into the relevant entry in **Section III: Disorders.**
- Clinicians also can follow the sequential flow of the panels to step through a diagnostic decision algorithm to arrive at the relevant diagnostic possibilities. The outcome of this algorithmic path will be one or several possible disorders to consider, and the clinician is referred from the module panels to the relevant disorder entry in **Section III: Disorders.**
- Clinician also can turn to specific panels for specific assistance. For instance:
  - Each module contains several verbatim diagnostic queries based on evidence-based interviewing to assist the clinician in evaluating a particular set of symptoms.
  - Modules also contain several summary panels that tabulate frequently used clinical information (e.g., mnemonics for the hard-to-remember criteria for various disorders; medications that cause a particular symptom; laboratory and imaging workup for dementia).

Note in particular that the diagnostic decision algorithms are structured around the principles of evidence-based interviewing, particularly the concepts of *sensitivity, specificity,* and *positive and negative predictive value* (**Section I,**

Panels 10–12). As outlined in **Section I, Panel 11,** the clinician is urged to proceed as follows:
- First, screen for possible syndromes and disorders using high-sensitivity queries and . . .
- Then, if screening queries are positive, follow-up using high-specificity queries to confirm, revise, or rule out the suspected diagnoses.

To do this, the clinician can use specific high-sensitivity probes for screening and high-specificity probes for diagnostic confirmation that are provided throughout the modules:
- High-sensitivity probes are marked by the symbol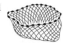

- High-specificity probes are marked by the symbol

Furthermore, the clinician can refer iteratively to the disorder entries in **Section III** to consult the prevalence and demographic data provided. This allows the clinician to improve diagnostic acumen by considering predictive values based on the prevalence rates of the various disorders which they suspect may underlie the symptoms. The old clinical truism noted in **Section I, Panel 16** states the issue in a colloquial, but no less accurate, manner: When you hear hoofbeats in Wyoming, it's likely to be horses and not zebras. To give yet another example: Given the demographic and prevalence information in the disorder entries in **Section III,** one can determine that new-onset conviction that one has a nose that looks like a monkey's in a 59-year-old man in a hospital emergency room is more likely to be attributable to a psychotic or delirious disorder than to body dysmorphic disorder.

The clinician is urged to use these modules *iteratively* as potential comorbidities are identified. He or she may loop back and forth across the symptom modules as needed until all symptoms are assigned to relevant syndromes and disorders.

Note:
Finally, clinician, do not be hesitant to take this book into the interview with you and refer to it as you like! Less experienced clinicians are especially hesitant to consult references during the interview, as they feel that it appears to advertise to the individual being interviewed one's inexperience, insecurity, and general clinical ineptitude. Not so with most people you will interview: what matters most to them is that you listen to them and that you do what it takes to give them the best possible care.

M o d u l e   1

Depression or Fatigue

Orienting Notes

- Depression is a common presenting complaint for several disorders
- Alternate presentation is loss of "zest" for life:
  - Decreased energy, fatigue
  - Loss of interest or pleasure in typical activities
- Comorbidities are common.

Differential Diagnosis

Primary Mood Disorders

- Major depressive disorder (see *Disorders Section,* page 164)
  - Single episode
  - Recurrent
- Manic-depressive (bipolar) disorders (see *Disorders Section,* page 169)
- Dysthymia (see *Disorders Section,* page 167)
- Cyclothymia (see *Disorders Section,* page 173)

Other Disorders

- Adjustment disorder (see *Disorders Section,* page 204)
- Posttraumatic stress disorder (PTSD) (see *Disorders Section,* page 184)
- Generalized anxiety disorder (see *Disorders Section,* page 180)
- Substance use disorders (see *Disorders Section,* page 189)
- Medical illness (see *Panel 5*)
- Medication side effect (see *Panel 6*)

 Panel 1: Depression Screen

"Have you been depressed/blue/sad/down most of the time for the last couple of weeks?"

"Have you (lost interest in/stopped doing) things you usually like to do for the last couple of weeks?"

- If either of these questions are answered "Yes," continue to **Panel 2, Stress.**
- Otherwise, explore further to determine if other symptoms are present, and review other Modules for other possible alternative problems.

Panel 2: Stress

"Did anything seem to bring it on, like stress in your life or physical changes like illness or medication changes?"

- If stress appeared to bring on or worsen the depression/fatigue, continue to **Panel 3, Stress Differential Diagnosis.**
- If no stress brought on the depression/fatigue, continue to **Panel 7, Major Depressive Episode: "SPACES-G"**

Panel 3: Stress Differential Diagnosis

> *Note: Stress-associated depression does not necessarily mean symptoms will not respond to medications. Assess stress as below.*
> **Bereavement?**
> Loss of a loved one within the past 2 months.
> Go to *Panel 4*
> **Physical Change?**
- Medical illness
- Medication change/cessation
- Substance use/cessation
  Psychosocial stressor?

- If the depression/fatigue is associated with loss of a loved one, go to **Panel 4, Bereavement.**
- If the depression/fatigue is associated with a medical illness, go to **Panel 5, Common Medical Illnesses that Can Cause Depressive Symptoms**
- If the depression fatigue is associated with a recent change in medication, go to **Panel 6, Medication Change/Cessation and Depressive Symptoms**
- If the depression/fatigue is associated with use of substances (or their cessation), go to **Module 5, Substance Use and Gambling.**
- Adjustment disorder is diagnosed when symptoms of depression are linked to a specific psychosocial stressor but do not meet criteria for other mood disorders. If so, go to **Adjustment Disorders** (see page 204).

Panel 4: Bereavement

Bereavement is normal if *without:*

- Excess guilt
- Thoughts of death or suicide
- Marked psychomotor slowing
- Marked impairment in daily function
- Psychosis

- If any of the above are present, this is a concerning sign for complicated bereavement, with possible major depressive episode that needs treatment. If so, go to **Panel 7, Major Depressive Episode: "SPACES-G."**
- If none of the above is present, this may be considered normal bereavement. Watchful waiting is indicated, continuing to monitor for complications. Referral for pastoral counseling or psychotherapy may be appropriate.

Panel 5: Common Medical Illnesses that Can Cause Depressive Symptoms

Neurologic disorders
  Stroke
  Head trauma
  Dementia
  Brain tumors
  Infection (including HIV, syphilis)
  Multiple sclerosis
  Parkinson disease
  Huntington disease

Endocrine disorders
  Addison disease
  Cushing disease
  Hypothyroidism
  Hyperthyroidism

Hypoparathyroidism
Hyperparathyroidism

Cancers
  Pancreatic

Metabolic disorders
  B_{12}, folate deficiencies

Menstrual cycle–related factors
  Premenstrual phase of cycle
  Menopause
  Postpartum status (see **Panel 9**)

Other
  Systemic lupus erythematosis
  Fibromyalgia/chronic fatigue

- If any of the above is present, the first line of intervention is to identify and correct the underlying medical disorder. If residual depressive symptoms continue, further evaluation for a major depressive episode may be warranted; if so, go to **Panel 7, Major Depressive Episode: "SPACES-G."**
- Note that *any* medical disease may cause significant loss of function or self-esteem and, secondarily, clinically significant major depression that requires concurrent treatment. If so, go to **Panel 7, Major Depressive Episode: "SPACES-G."**

- As with medical illnesses, if a medication is suspected as the inciting factor for depression/fatigue, it should be discontinued or switched to another medication if at all possible.
- If the medication must be continued (e.g., steroids for asthma or rheumatoid arthritis; interferon for hepatitis C), then continued evaluation and cotreatment of depression may be necessary. If so, continue to **Panel 7.**
- If substance use is suspected, as noted above, go to **Module 5, Substance Use and Gambling.**

 Panel 7: Major Depressive Episode: "SPACES-G"

For individuals who have screened as positive for either of the **Panel 1** queries, the presence of four or more symptoms of the SPACES-G items is consistent with a major depressive episode:

Sleep: decreased[a,b,c]/increased
Psychomotor: agitation[a,b]/retardation
Appetite/weight: increased/decreased
Concentration: decreased[a,b]
Energy: decreased[a]
Suicide/death preoccupation (go also to *Module 6, Suicidality/Assaultiveness*)
Guilt, excessive

[a]Also criterion for generalized anxiety disorder; refer to page 180.
[b]Also criterion for PTSD; refer to page 184.
[c]Insomnia can be initial, middle, or terminal (early awakening).

• Continue to **Panel 8, Mania Screen.**

Panel 8: Mania Screen

"Ever have times when you felt the *opposite* of depressed? Like you were on top of the world, but *too* good?"

". . . Times when you had too much energy and didn't *need* to sleep for more than a few hours a night?"

". . . Times when you felt high on drugs, like amphetamines or too much caffeine, but weren't taking drugs?"

"When? For how long?"

• If any of screening questions are endorsed as occurring for 4 days or more, go to **Module 2, Manic Symptoms.**
• If results of mania screen are negative and four or more **"SPACES-G"** symptoms have been identified, you have diagnosed a major depressive episode as part of major depressive disorder. Go to **Major Depressive Disorder, Disorders Section** page 164.
  • *Note: For further diagnostic subtypes, go to Panel 9.*
• If results of mania screen are negative and fewer than four **"SPACES-G"** symptoms have been identified, go to **Panel 11, Note on Dysthymia and Subsyndromal Depression.**

Panel 9: Depressive Episode/Disorder Specifiers

Specifier	Definition	Treatment Implications?
Chronic	>2 years	Long-term treatment
Melancholic	Go to *Panel 10*	Tricyclic/MAO inhibitor anti-depressants
Atypical	Go to *Panel 10*	MAO inhibitors or selective serotonin reuptake inhibitors
Postpartum	Within 4 weeks of giving birth	Treatment as needed plus recurrence watch during next childbirth
Psychotic	See *Module 7, Delirium*	ECT or neuroleptics plus antidepressants
Catatonic	See *Module 7, Change in Mental Status/ Delirium*	ECT or benzodiazepines
Seasonal pattern	Onset/offset at particular season without regular stressor; no other episodes for ≥2 years	Bright visible spectrum light

- Continue to **Panel 10, Melancholic/Atypical Episode Definition.**

Panel 10: Melancholic/Atypical Episode Definition

Symptom	Melancholia	Atypical
Variability of mood or reactivity to good events	Lost	Intact
Sleep	Terminal insomnia	Increased
Weight/appetite	Decreased	Increased
Quality of depression	Distinct mood: never experienced outside of depression	Physical: "leaden paralysis"
Self-concept	Excessive guilt	Interpersonal rejection sensitivity (long-standing)
Diurnal variation of mood	Worse in morning	—
Psychomotor	Agitation/retardation	—

Panel 11: Note on Dysthymia and Subsyndromal Depression

- If depressive symptoms have lasted "years" even if fewer than four SPACES-G symptoms have been identified, go to *Dysthymia, Disorders Section,* page 167.
- Mild depressive symptoms (sometimes called "minor depression:) are not uncommon. Treatment is not clear unless chronic (dysthymia).
- A form of "recurrent brief depression" has also been described, with bouts of 3 to 4 days of the full depressive syndrome occurring frequently. Antidepressant treatment may help.

Module 2

Manic Symptoms

Orienting Notes

- Mania is an episodic change of behavior characterized by heightened activation/activity and a change in mood.
- Mood in mania is predominantly and abnormally:
  - Elevated or
  - Expansive or
  - Irritable
- Behavior and mood changes are typically episodic (weeks to several months) and are not chronic personality features.
- Hypomania is a milder form of mania.
- (Hypo)mania typically occurs as part of manic-depressive (bipolar) disorder, but may be part of other disorders.
- Comorbidities, especially substance use disorders, are common.

Differential Diagnosis

- Manic-depressive (bipolar) disorder, type I (with mania) (see *Disorders Section,* page 169)
- Manic-depressive (bipolar) disorder, type II (with hypomania) (see *Disorders Section,* page 169)
- Cyclothymia (see *Disorders Section,* page 173)
- Schizophrenia (see *Disorders Section,* page 197)
- Substance use disorders (see *Disorders Section,* page 189)
- Pathologic gambling (mania) (see *Module 5,* page 45)
- Attention deficit disorder (see *Disorders Section,* page 208)
- Medical illnesses (see *Panel 6*)
- Medication side effects (see *Panel 5*)

Panel 1: Mania Screen

"Ever have times when you felt the *opposite* of depressed? Like you were on top of the world, but *too* good?"

". . . Times when you had too much energy and didn't *need* to sleep for more than a few hours a night?"

". . . Times when you felt high on drugs, like amphetamines or too much caffeine, but weren't taking drugs?"

"When? For how long?"

- If any of these questions are answered, "Yes," continue to **Panel 2, Mood in Mania.**

Panel 2: Mood in Mania

Mood in mania is abnormally elevated, expansive, or irritable:

- **Elevated** means unrealistically happy, unwarranted by or oblivious to actual circumstances.
- **Irritable** has all the connotations of its lay use: argumentative, hostile, or easily upset or angered.
- **Expansive** is difficult to define (and may not strictly speaking be a "mood") but can be characterized by a view of the world that assumes that the individual plays an important, central role. Characteristics include marked enthusiasm, dominating conversations, assuming others will listen as they set the agenda for an interaction. The phrases in common parlance "larger than life" and "large and in charge" come to mind.

"Did any physical changes seem to bring this on, like substance use, illness, or medication change?"

- If these symptoms are not associated with physical changes, go to **Panel 3, Manic/Hypomanic Episode: "TRENDAR."**
- If these symptoms are associated with substance use or a medication change, go to **Panel 5, Medications that Can Cause Manic Symptoms.**
- If these symptoms are associated with the onset or worsening of a medical illness, go to **Panel 6, Medical Conditions that Can Cause Manic Symptoms.**

 Panel 3: Manic/Hypomanic Episode: "TRENDAR"

Talkative
Racing thoughts
Esteem (self-esteem unrealistically high)
Need for sleep decreased (*need,* not just sleep time)
Distractibility
Activities/agitation (too many projects or motor agitation)
Risky business (activities with high probability of trouble, e.g., sexual promiscuity, gambling, physical risk taking)

For how long?

- If these symptoms have lasted at least 4 days and mood is predominantly euphoric or expansive with three or more **"TRENDAR"** symptoms identified, go to **Panel 4, Mania or Hypomania?**

- If these symptoms have lasted at least 4 days and mood is predominantly irritable with four or more **"TRENDAR"** symptoms identified, go to **Panel 4, Mania or Hypomania?**
- If these symptoms have lasted fewer than 4 days or if fewer than three or four symptoms have been identified, go to **Panel 7, Note on Cyclothymia and Subsyndromal or Fluctuating Manic Symptoms.**

Panel 4: Mania or Hypomania?

Note: Mania = Hypomania + one of the following:

- *Psychotic symptoms* (Go to *Module 4, Psychosis*)
- *Hospitalization*
- Such severe symptoms that the individual *cannot fulfill basic occupational duties or social role function.* Examples:
  - Deserting usual roles for impulsive cross-country travel
  - Endangerment of self/others because of symptoms
  - Incapacitation as mother, father, spouse, worker

- If the episode meets criteria for hypomania, the diagnosis is probably manic-depressive disorder type II.
- If the episode meets the criteria for mania, the diagnosis is probably manic-depressive disorder type I.
- In either event, go to **Manic-Depressive Disorder, Disorders Section,** page 164.

Panel 5: Medications that Can Cause Manic Symptoms

Antidepressants
    Pharmacologic antidepressants
    Bright visible spectrum light treatment
    Electroconvulsant therapy

Adrenergic agents
    Decongestants
    Bronchodilators
    Stimulants

Drugs of abuse
    Amphetamines
    Cocaine

Anabolic steroids
Alcohol
    Stimulants
Dopaminergic agents
    Levodopa
    Disulfiram
Other agents
    Isoniazid
    Corticosteroids
    Theophylline

If due to drugs of abuse, go to *Module 5, Substance Use and Gambling.*

- If a medication is suspected as the inciting factor for manic symptoms, it should be discontinued or switched to another medication if at all possible.
- If the medication must be continued (e.g., steroids for asthma or rheumatoid arthritis; dopaminergic agents for Parkinson disease), then continued evalua-

tion and cotreatment of manic symptoms may be necessary. If so, go to **Manic-Depressive (Bipolar) Disorder, Disorders Section,** page 169.
- On occasion, individuals may be so severely impaired that they require symptomatic treatment for manic symptoms even if a reversible cause is being corrected. If so, go to **Manic-Depressive (Bipolar) Disorder, Disorders Section,** page 169.

**Panel 6: Medical Conditions
that Can Cause Manic Symptoms**

Neurologic Disorders

Stroke
Head trauma
Dementia
Brain tumors
Infection (including human immunodeficiency virus, syphilis)
Multiple sclerosis
Huntington disease

Endocrine

Hyperthyroidism (in those with preexisting manic-depressive disorder)
Postpartum status

- If any of the above is present, the first line of intervention is to identify and address the underlying medical issue.
- On occasion, individuals may be so severely impaired that they require symptomatic treatment for manic symptoms even if a reversible cause is being corrected. If so, go to **Manic-Depressive (Bipolar) Disorder, Disorders Section,** page 169.

**Panel 7: Note on Cyclothymia and Subsyndromal
or Fluctuating Manic Symptoms**

- If a single bout of brief or subsyndromal manic symptoms occurs, watchful waiting or reevaluation of differential diagnosis for other syndromes may be in order.
- If recurrent bouts of mild manic symptoms occur that may alternate with depressive symptoms over months or years, go to **Cyclothymia, Disorders Section,** page 173.

Module 3

Anxiety/Nervousness

Orienting Notes

- Some people do not understand "anxious" as "nervous" (they think of being anxious as "anticipating": "I'm anxious to start my vacation"), so be sure to use language that you both understand the same way.
- Anxiety can be *chronic* or *episodic,* and this helps differentiate among the disorders.
- Anxiety can be associated with a specific *stress* or not, and this also helps differentiate among the disorders.
- Anxiety is common in other disorders, such as major depressive disorder, so careful differential diagnosis is necessary.
- Comorbidities are common and may be the major presenting feature, with anxiety "hidden" but driving or complicating other disorders—especially substance use disorders.

Differential Diagnosis

- Primary Anxiety Disorders:
  - Panic disorder with or without agoraphobia (see *Disorders Section,* page 174)
  - Generalized anxiety disorder (GAD) (see *Disorders Section,* page 180)
  - PTSD (see *Disorders Section,* page 184)
  - Social phobia (see *Disorders Section,* page 177)
  - Simple phobia (see *Disorders Section,* page 177)
  - Obsessive-compulsive disorder (OCD) (see *Disorders Section,* page 182)
  - Acute stress disorder (see *Disorders Section,* page 187)
- Other Disorders:
  - Adjustment disorder (see *Disorders Section,* page 204)
  - Major depressive disorder (see *Disorders Section,* page 164)
  - (Hypo)mania in manic-depressive (bipolar) disorders (see *Disorders Section,* page 169)
  - Substance use disorders (see *Disorders Section,* page 189)
    - Use of stimulants
    - Withdrawal from alcohol, sedatives
  - Somatization disorder (see *Disorders Section,* page 210)
  - Medical illness (see *Panel 10*)
  - Medication side effects (see *Panel 11*)

**Panel 1: "Do You Consider Yourself
a Nervous or Anxious Person?"**

Responses will typically be of three overall types:

A. "Always, all of the time."	B. "Only since ____"	C. "Only at times; only when ____ happens"
Main differential diagnostic possibilities:	**Main differential diagnostic possibilities:**	**Main differential diagnostic possibilities:**
Primary anxiety disorders: GAD PTSD OCD	Primary anxiety disorders: PTSD Acute stress disorder	Primary anxiety disorders: Panic ± agoraphobia PTSD Social/specific phobia
Other disorders: Somatization disorder Substance use disorders	Other disorders: Major depressive disorder (Hypo)mania Substance use disorders Adjustment disorder Medical illness Medication side effect	Other disorders: Substance use disorders

- Go to **Panel 2.**

Panel 2: The Next Steps in Screening

- Notice that responses sort themselves into
  - Chronic (**A**) versus episodic [discrete onset, longer periods (**B**) or paroxysmal (**C**)]
  - Anxiety disorder versus other disorder
  - Trauma-associated anxiety versus not; trauma-associated anxiety can follow any of the three patterns
- Screening for trauma is an important next step, and you will combine information from Panels 1 and 3 to proceed.

- Go to **Panel 3.**

Panel 3: Screening for Trauma

- Trauma is quite common in modern societies.
- Not all persons who experience significant trauma have psychiatric symptoms.
- However, trauma frequently does have far-reaching and long-lasting behavioral consequences.
- Trauma is defined by DSM-IV as an event that "involved actual or threatened death or serious injury, or a threat to the physical integrity of self or others."
- Trauma can be sustained by the person or witnessed by the person.
- Examples of common trauma are:
  - Childhood abuse (physical or sexual, once or repeated).
  - Military combat.
  - Civilian involvement in political conflicts (e.g., detention, torture, collateral damage). Screening for detention and torture is of particular concern in immigrant populations.
  - Assaults experienced or witnessed as an adult or child (e.g., rape, robbery).
  - Motor vehicle, other accidents, or natural disasters.

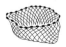

"Sometimes people are anxious/nervous because of serious/traumatic/disturbing things that happened in the past. They just can't put the events out of their mind. I wonder if this has happened with you?"

Note: People often have difficulty talking about trauma (see Panel 4, Hints on Screening for Trauma).

- Continue to **Panel 4.**

Panel 4: Hints on Screening for Trauma

- Some people have great difficulty talking about traumatic events—talking stirs up many disturbing memories and symptoms, or they may have blocked out aspects of the event.
- Other people cannot stop talking about the event once they get started.
- In the service of screening for a disorder, it is helpful at this stage of the interview to focus on *symptoms* rather than the event—the event can be handled, for now, as a "black box" of sorts.
- Specifics of the event can then be elucidated at a later stage. Primary care providers may leave further probing for mental health consultants, while mental health practitioners will certainly want more information on specific aspects of the trauma when it will be a focus of treatment.
- The following may be helpful to establish the "black box" approach:

"We don't need to talk now about the actual events if that would be disturbing for you. But it will help to know more about the symptoms you're having these days—how these events are still alive for you."

- If responses are positive for trauma, go to **Panel 5.**
- If responses are negative for trauma
  - and response type A, go to **Panel 6.**
  - and response type B, go to **Panel 7.**
  - and response type C, go to **Panel 8.**

Panel 5: Trauma-Associated Anxiety Disorders

- Trauma-associated anxiety disorders are of two main types: PTSD or the more recently recognized acute stress disorder.
- Symptoms of each are similar, and of three main types:
  - Reexperiencing the event, for example:
    - Recurrent nightmares of the event.
    - "Flashbacks" in which the person is fully awake but feels as if the trauma is occurring again in real time. Sometimes this can be a single sensation (smell, feel, vision), and sometimes it is described as a multisensory "home movie."
    - Intense discomfort or other symptoms when exposed to stimuli associated with the trauma.
  - Avoidance of stimuli related to the trauma or overall numbing of emotions, for example:
    - Avoiding activities, places, people that bring up memories of the event
    - Inability to recall aspects of the event
    - Overall detachment from others, emotional numbing
  - Hyperarousal, for example:
    - Chronic insomnia
    - Chronic irritability
    - Hypervigilance of the environment and easy startle

- Symptoms of PTSD may last for (or in rare cases, may begin) years after the trauma. If so, go to **Posttraumatic Stress Disorder, Disorders Section,** page 184.
- Symptoms of acute stress disorder by definition occur within 4 weeks of the trauma. If so, go to **Acute Stress Disorder, Disorders Section,** page 187.

 Panel 6: Response Type A: Nontrauma Anxiety Disorders with Chronic Symptoms

- The simplest approach to chronic anxiety is to rule out underlying causes first, and then pursue a primary anxiety disorder diagnosis if no other cause can be found:
- If anxiety is associated with use of substances (or their cessation), go to *Module 5, Substance Use and Gambling*
- If physical ailments are the main focus of concern, and the concern is unrealistic, and there is little or no anxiety about other issues, go to *Module 14, Multiple Unexplained Physical Complaints.*

- If no trauma has been identified and no other cause can be found, go to **Panel 9.**

 Panel 7: Response Type B: Nontrauma Anxiety Disorders with Discrete Onset, Longer Periods

- Primary anxiety disorders may have a discrete onset, as may other psychiatric disorders. If the symptom pattern does have a discrete onset and offset, it is important to look for other disorders that may cause the symptoms.
- As in Panel 6, rule out other causes first, and if none are found, consider a primary anxiety disorder:
- If anxiety is associated primarily with periods of depression, go to *Module 1, Depression or Fatigue,* or with manic symptoms, go to *Module 2, Manic Symptoms.*
- If anxiety is associated with the use of substances (or their cessation), go to *Module 5, Substance Use and Gambling.*
- Adjustment disorder is diagnosed when symptoms of anxiety are linked to a specific stressor but do not meet criteria for other anxiety disorders. If so, go to *Adjustment Disorders,* page 204.
- If anxiety is associated with a medical illness, go to *Panel 10: Common Medical Illnesses that Can Cause Anxiety/Nervousness.*
- If anxiety is associated with a recent change in medication, go to *Panel 11, Medication Change/Cessation and Anxiety.*

- If no trauma has been identified and another cause can be found, re-review for chronic anxiety disorders and go to **Panel 9.**

Panel 8: Response Type C: Nontrauma Anxiety Disorders with Paroxysmal Episodes

- As in Panels 6 and 7, rule out other causes and if none are found, consider a primary anxiety disorder.
- If anxiety is associated with the use of substances (or their cessation), go to *Module 5, Substance Use and Gambling.*

• If no precipitating substance use can be found, go to **Panel 12.**

Panel 9: Generalized Anxiety Disorder and Obsessive-Compulsive Disorder

- GAD is characterized by chronic, excessive worry about several life issues
- Worry is accompanied by cognitive and physical symptoms
- The mnemonic **CRIMES** may help:
  - **C**oncentration problems
  - **R**estlessness or feeling keyed up
  - **I**rritability
  - **M**uscle tension
  - **E**asy fatigue
  - **S**leep disturbance (insomnia or fitful sleep)
- If a person endorses several of these symptoms and other causes are ruled out, go to *Disorders Section, Generalized Anxiety Disorder,* page 180.
- OCD is characterized by intrusive thoughts (obsessions) and/or a drive to perform repetitive behaviors that the person cannot easily resist (compulsions).
  - Examples of common obsessions are counting, praying, and a preoccupation with cleanliness.
  - Examples of compulsions are hand washing, ordering clothes or items at home, and excessive attention to detail in tasks such as driving and parking.
- OCD symptoms waste an hour or more each day or interfere with role function.
- If a person endorses several of these symptoms and other causes are ruled out, go to *Disorders Section, Obsessive-Compulsive Disorder,* page 182.

Note: Many people we encounter may be characterized as "obsessive" or "compulsive" for their personality style; these tend to be chronic, fixed, pervasive characteristics. In contrast, OCD symptoms are typically paroxysmal, intrusive, and disabling. For the former, see ***Disorders Section, Personality Disorders,*** page 236.

**Panel 10: Common Medical Illnesses
that Can Cause Anxiety/Nervousness**

Neurologic
  Multiple sclerosis
  Cerebrovascular disease
  Postconcussive syndromes
  Traumatic brain injury

Pulmonary
  Asthma
  Chronic obstructive pulmonary
    disease
  Restrictive lung disease
  Pulmonary edema

Cardiac
  Myocardial infarction
  Congestive heart failure
  Mitral valve prolapse
  Premature ventricular
    contractions

Endocrine
  Hypoglycemia
  Hyperthyroidism
  Hyperparathyroidism
  Cushing disease
  Addison disease
  Pheochromocytoma
  Carcinoid syndrome

Menstrual cycle-related issues
  Premenstrual phase of cycle
  Menopause

Other
  Systemic lupus erythematosis
  Vitamin B_{12} deficiency
  Folate deficiency

- If any of the above is present, the first line of intervention is to identify and correct the underlying medical disorder.
- Note that *any* medical disease may cause significant loss of function, increased stress, and secondary anxiety that is clinically significant. If so, go to **Disorders Section, Adjustment Disorders,** page 204.

Panel 11: Medication Change/Cessation and Anxiety

Stimulants
  Decongestants
  Diet medications
  Caffeine

Psychotropic Medications
  Antidepressants (especially stimulating
    agents)
  Cessation of antidepressants
  High potency neuroleptics

Drugs of abuse
  Amphetamines
  Cocaine
  Hallucinogens
  Other stimulants

Neurologic medications
  L-dopa
  Sumatriptan

Hormones
  Estrogens
Other agents
  Metoclopramide
  Metronidazole
  HMG-CoA reductase
    inhibitors ("statins")

Cessation of:
  Alcohol
  Barbiturates
  Benzodiazepines
  Opiates
  Other sedatives

• If substance use is suspected, go to **Module 5, Substance Use and Gambling.**

 Panel 12: Social/Specific Phobia, Panic Disorder

• Specific phobia is characterized by intense anxiety in the presence of a discrete stimulus.
  • Individuals usually readily identify the stimulus, e.g., heights, closed spaces, water, insects, etc.
  • Anticipatory anxiety and avoidance are also common.
  • Panic attacks (see below) may occur, or anxiety may be less specific in pattern.
• Social phobia may be considered a subtype of specific phobia in which an individual experiences marked anxiety or panic in performance situations or when meeting new people. Again, individuals typically readily identify this.
• If so, go to *Disorders Section, Specific Phobia,* page 177, or *Social Phobia,* page 177.

Panic Disorder With or Without Agoraphobia

• Panic disorder is defined by recurrent panic attacks plus worry or avoidance regarding having another attack.
• This can be complicated by generalized reduction of one's ability to go out of the house or into situations where they may not be able to escape during a panic attack. This is known as agoraphobia. Rarely, agoraphobia can occur alone.
• Panic attacks have a discrete course, including crescendo onset in minutes and typical duration of less than an hour, although they can last longer.
• Symptoms are predominantly autonomic (contrast with GAD symptoms, **Panel 9,** which are more general).
• A mnemonic may help (with apologies for license with the spelling)—**Go FAST—SPEDe!:**
  • **F**ears one will **Go** crazy or die
  • **F**aintness
  • **A**bdominal distress: nausea/vomiting
  • **S**weating
  • **T**remors
  • **S**hortness of breath, chest pain
  • **P**alpitations
  • Par**E**sthesias (numbness, tingling in extremities or periorally)
  • **De**realization/depersonalization (a physical sense of being separated from the environment or of unreality of the environment)
• If a person endorses several of these symptoms, go to *Disorders Section, Panic Disorder With or Without Agoraphobia,* page 174.

Module 4

Psychosis (Hallucinations and Delusions)

Orienting Notes

- Psychosis is a syndrome. Individuals are considered *psychotic* according to the DSM system if they have specific symptoms:
  - Hallucinations
  - Delusions
  - Thought disorder as evidenced by disorganized speech
  - Disorganized or catatonic behavior
- *Hallucinations* are single modality sensory perceptions without an external object (see *Panel 1*).
- *Delusions* are fixed, false beliefs (see *Panel 2*).
- *Thought disorder* can be of various types (see *Panel 3*).
- Individuals with psychosis can be disorganized in behavior, but they are typically alert and do not have waxing and waning consciousness (see *Panel 4*).
- Psychosis can occur in a variety of *disorders,* some life-threatening, that have very different treatments.
- Differential diagnosis is therefore of great importance.

Differential Diagnosis

- Psychosis is a *syndrome,* not a *disorder.*
- Sometimes individuals have symptoms that are unusual or bizarre, but not truly psychotic.
- Disorders that may have truly psychotic syndromes and those that may have unusual nonpsychotic symptoms are listed separately below.

Disorders that May Have Psychotic Symptoms

- Schizophrenia (see *Disorders Section,* page 197)
- Delusional disorder (see *Disorders Section,* page 203)
- Manic-depressive (bipolar) disorder type I, manic or depressive episode (see *Disorders Section,* page 169)
- Manic-depressive (bipolar) disorder type II, depressive episode (see *Disorders Section,* page 169)
- Major depressive disorder (see *Disorders Section,* page 164)
- Delirium (see *Module 7*)
- Dementia (see *Disorders Section,* page 206)
- Medical illness (see *Panel 8*)
- Medication side effect (see *Panel 9*)
- Rare and thematically consistent delusion in:
  - Obsessive compulsive disorder (OCD) (see *Disorders Section,* page 182)
  - Body dysmorphic disorder (see *Disorders Section,* page 218)

Disorders that May Have Nonpsychotic Bizarre-Appearing Symptoms

- Manic-depressive (bipolar) disorder, type I, manic episode (see *Disorders Section,* page 169)
- OCD (see *Disorders Section,* page 182)
- Posttraumatic stress disorder (PTSD) (see *Disorders Section,* page 184)
- Simple phobia (see *Disorders Section,* page 177)
- Dissociative disorders (see *Disorders Section,* page 234)
- Eating disorders (see *Disorders Section,* page 220)
- Body dysmorphic disorder (see *Disorders Section,* page 218)
- Schizoid or schizotypal personality disorder (see *Disorders Section,* page 237)
- Avoidant personality disorder (see *Disorders Section,* page 239)
- Personality disorders that employ primitive defense mechanisms such as projection (see *Disorders Section,* page 236)
- Movement disorders (see *Module 17*)
- Disorders that may have depersonalization/derealization (see *Panel 1*), for example, anxiety or mood disorders
- Disorders that may have excessive self-consciousness, for example, anxiety or mood disorders
- Seizure disorder with preictal aura

Other Nonpsychotic Findings that May Come to Clinical Attention

- Hypnogogic/hypnopompic hallucinations (while falling asleep or waking)
- Beliefs based on cultural, religious, or other existential value systems
- Culture-bound syndromes that present with bizarre-appearing behavior or beliefs
- Idiosyncratic personal beliefs not fixed or not falsifiable.
- Overvalued personal beliefs that are not fixed or not falsifiable.

- Separating psychotic from nonpsychotic symptoms requires clarification of terms. In **Panels 1 to 3,** varieties of perception, belief, thought pattern, and behavioral disorganization that may come to clinical attention are outlined.
- An algorithm to identify or rule out a psychotic syndrome follows in subsequent panels.

Panel 1: Some Definitions—Perceptions

- *Hallucinations:* Single modality sensory perceptions without an external object.
  - May be in any sensory modality.
- *Illusions:* Single modality sensory misperceptions of an external object.
  - May or may not be psychotic depending on the fixity of belief in the reality of the sensation.
  - Example: "I saw the face of Jesus in the leaves of the tree."
- *Flashbacks:* Sensory perceptions of past experience.
  - May be in any sensory modality.
  - Example: "I felt I was being penetrated again like when I was raped."
  - May be multisensory, a "home movie" experience.
  - May entail loss of contact with current reality.
  - Example: "I thought I was back in Vietnam: I heard the choppers, I smelled napalm. I hit the deck and crawled under what I later found out was a park bench."
- *Dissociation:* A splitting of consciousness and/or behavior.
  - Typically behavior is appropriate to environmental demands.
  - *Amnesia:* Inability to recall important personal facts.
  - *Fugue:* Behavior atypical for a person, often with travel, plus inability to recall important personal facts.
  - *Identity (multiple personality):* Two or more distinct personalities in the same person, often with limited awareness or memory of each other's activities.
- *Depersonalization/derealization:* A sense of being detached or separate from one's body or one's environment.
  - Usually described as uncomfortable and unnerving.
  - However, behavior is typically normal and others are not aware of symptoms.
  - Example: "I thought I was floating above the room watching myself converse." "I felt like someone else was moving my mouth, my arms, my legs." "I felt like I was looking at the world through a long tube."
- *Religious or culturally sanctioned experiences*
  - Must be accepted by culture or group of which the individual is a member.
  - Example: Speaking with spirits, hearing God's voice.
  - Some culture-bound syndromes with perceptual changes, although atypical in dominant Western culture, are not necessarily psychotic when considered in cultural context.

Panel 2: Some Definitions—Beliefs

- *Delusions:* Fixed, false beliefs.
  - Fact-based, not values.
    Example (assuming these are not true!): "The Department of Homeland Security is after me." "I am Jesus." "I am the Son of God and I know this because I can . . ." "I can fly." "My insides are rotting with cancer." "This hospitalization will cost me my life's savings because managed care won't pay."
- *Ideas of reference:* A subtype of delusion based on misinterpretation of actual fact.
  Example: "When the news anchor was talking about people being obese, I know she was directing those comments to me personally."
- *Overvalued ideas:* Opinion- and value-based perceptions of the world that may be atypical or inaccurate.
  - Not considered psychotic, although they may be misguided.
    Example: "You can't trust people that work for you. They're always out to take your job." "I know you're thinking I'm ugly; you can probably hardly stand to be in the room with me."
  - Individuals may know or suspect that their strongly held belief may not be true.
  - May still represent symptoms that require treatment.
    Example: "I know I'm only 99 pounds, but I'm so fat—everyone can see that."
- *Religious, cultural, or existential values*
  - Culturally sanctioned or accepted beliefs or values are not psychotic.
    Example: "I know I will go to hell because I had that abortion." "My grandmother foretells the future. She does it for lots of people I know."
  - Sometimes these beliefs are not widely accepted and are unusual but may still be considered cultural, depending on context (e.g., being abducted by aliens).
  - Some culture-bound syndromes with unusual beliefs, although atypical in dominant Western culture, are not necessarily psychotic when considered in cultural context.

Panel 3: Some Definitions—
Thought Pattern Characteristics

- *Thought-disordered* implies a psychotic level of disorganization of thinking.
  - Characteristics typically representing psychotic levels of disorganization are noted by *boldface print.*
- *Pressured speech:* Increased speed of verbal productivity; may or may not be loud.
  - Nonspecific; characteristic of (hypo)mania, many anxiety states, and may be personality style.
- *Flight of ideas:* Quick but logical progression from topic to topic.
  - Typical of (hypo)mania.
- *Circumstantiality:* Circuitous way to reason or recount from topic A to topic B, with many intervening statements that may be of minimal relevance but still maintain the logical flow.
  - Nonspecific, as for the above items.
- *Tangentiality:* Reasoning or recounting circumstantially from topic A but never making it to topic B.
  - Clearly pathologic but nonspecific
- *Loose associations:* Loss of logical link between topics.
  - Example: "My best friend lives down the block. Donuts are fattening."
- *Derailment:* A less precise term denoting loose associations or sometimes other disruptions in flow of speech or thought.
- *Clang associations:* Association of words or topics by their sound rather than their conceptual content.
  - Example: "My mother lives down the block. Clock, clocks, clocks—they're always ticking. What a licking my mother gave me!"
- *Echolalia:* Repeating the word or phrase just used by the interviewer or by the individual himself or herself.
  - Often accompanied by stereotypic or negativistic behavior
  - *Note: Negativistic behavior* refers to simple motor behaviors contrary to verbal or physical requests/cues (e.g., moving the individual's arm to the left is countered by movement to the right).
  - Often a feature of delirium such as catatonia (see *Module 7, Change in Mental Status/Delirium*).
- *Word salad:* Words used in nonsensical combinations; incoherence.
- *Neologisms:* Combinations of word sounds used as made-up words without sense.
- *Thought blocking or thought withdrawal:* Cessation of speech about which the individual relates that "All my thinking stopped."
  - Not all stoppage of speech is blocking. May also be due to ruminations, lack of attention, or even flight of ideas.
- *Thought insertion:* Subjective experience that thoughts are being put into one's head by an outside force or person.
- *Response to internal stimuli:* Disruption in speech or attention that the individual relates to distraction by hallucinations.
- *Mutism:* Total, extended cessation of speech.
- *Perseveration:* Obsessive repetition of same topic.
  - Repetition of same word is *echolalia.*
- *Poverty of content:* Paucity of conceptual content or concrete detail despite ample verbal productivity.
  - Considered psychotic if it lacks content to the degree that virtually no information is conveyed during extended speech.
- *Concreteness:* Lack of abstraction to a conceptual level; often assessed in formal examination through proverb interpretation.
  - Very nonspecific and probably overvalued by psychiatrists and psychologists as a diagnostic aid.
  - Can be present in many situations ranging from psychosis to depression to limited intellect.
  - Proverbs are all culture-bound. Individuals from different cultures frequently do not interpret proverbs according to the expectations of the reference culture, or cannot make sense of them.

Panel 4: Data Gathering for Psychosis Assessment

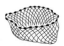

Observation, in addition to subjective report, plays an important role in assessment of psychosis.

• A key aspect of differential diagnosis is observation of unusual or bizarre behavior during the interview, e.g., response to internal stimuli or repetitive or stereotyped motions.

Most individuals with psychosis due to a psychiatric disorder have normal attention and vigilance, without waxing and waning consciousness.

• In fact, many individuals with psychosis are hypervigilant regarding their environment:
  • They may notice (and question) the color of your shoes, noises outside the window, whoever passing in the hallway.
• If an individual has waxing and waning consciousness, it is delirium and may be an acute medical emergency; see *Module 7, Change in Mental Status/Delirium*).
  • Although *catatonia* is listed in many textbooks as a psychotic symptom or a subtype of schizophrenia, *it is a type of delirium.*
  • Catatonia is the most frequently found medical disorder, not schizophrenia. Therefore, we will address catatonia in *Module 7*.

• If the individual is without waxing and waning consciousness, continue to **Panel 5.**
• If waxing and waning consciousness, go to **Module 7, Change in Mental Status/Delirium**.

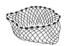

Panel 5: Interviewing Probes for Psychosis

If psychosis is suspected from observation (e.g., a person with obviously bizarre or unusual behavior or appearance), open-ended interviewing initially can be helpful in eliciting psychotic symptoms. Allowing the person to describe his or her concerns will provide a speech sample from which thought disorder may be assessed.

Screening question for persons who don't present as obviously odd or bizarre should be high sensitivity queries:

- Auditory hallucinations (voices) are the most common sensory modality for hallucinations.
- Paranoid delusions are probably the most common delusion. They are not always readily apparent because of the individual's fear and reticence to trust. Grandiose delusions are usually more readily disclosed.
- Sense psychotic symptoms have a negative social valence, and individuals may be ashamed to discuss them. Normalizing with lead-in statements can sometimes be helpful, as illustrated below.

"Sometimes when people . . . [supply major complaint, e.g., "feel depressed," "are under a lot of stress"] . . . they hear voices or sounds that are not there. I wonder if this has ever happened to you?"

"Sometimes when people . . . they:
. . . become concerned that people they don't know are out to do them harm."
. . . become suspicious of people they aren't usually concerned about."
. . . feel like people they don't know are out to get them. I wonder if this has ever happened to you?"

- Beware the word "paranoid," whether you or the person being evaluated uses it: they may not understand the word in the technical psychiatric sense.

- If results of the observational and interrogative assessment are negative, continue with review of systems in other modules.
- If positive, continue to **Panel 6.**

Panel 6: Stress

"Did anything seem to bring it on, like stress in your life or physical changes like illness or medication changes?"

Note: Clearly, in severe cases, collateral information from family and medical records will need to be consulted.

- If stress appeared to bring on or worsen the psychosis, continue to **Panel 7, Stress Differential Diagnosis.**
- If no stress brought on the psychosis, continue to **Panel 10.**

Panel 7: Stress Differential Diagnosis
Physical Change?

- Medical illness
- Medication change/cessation
- Substance use/cessation

Psychosocial Stressor?

- If the psychosis is associated with a medical illness, go to **Panel 8, Common Medical Illnesses that Can Cause Psychosis.**
- If the psychosis is associated with a recent change in medication, go to **Panel 9, Medication Change/Cessation and Psychosis.**
- If the psychosis is associated with use of substances (or their cessation), go to **Module 5, Substance Use and Gambling.**
- Brief reactive psychosis is diagnosed when symptoms of psychosis are acute and are linked to a specific psychosocial stressor but do not meet criteria for other psychotic disorders. If so, it is treated until symptoms resolve as for **Schizophrenia and Other Psychotic Disorders,** page 197.

Panel 8: Common Medical Illnesses that Can Cause Psychosis

Delirium of any cause

Neurologic disorders
  Stroke
  Head trauma
  Dementia
  Brain tumors
  Infection (including HIV, syphilis)
  Multiple sclerosis
  Parkinson disease
  Huntington disease

Endocrine
  Addison disease
  Cushing disease
  Severe hypothyroidism
    (myxedematous madness)
Other
  Systemic lupus erythematosis
  Hepatic encephalopathy

Panel 9: Medication Change/Cessation and Psychosis

CNS-active drugs
  L-Dopa
  Selegiline
  Other dopaminergic compounds
  Stimulants
  Anticholinergics (in elderly or
    neurologically compromised
    patients)
  Antidepressants

Hormones
  Corticosteroids
  Anabolic steroids

Ulcer medications
  Cimetadine
  Ranitidine

Other medications
  Angiotensin-converting enzyme
    inhibitors

Fluoroquinolone antibiotics
  Acyclovir
  Cyclobenzaprine
  Cycloserine

Drugs of abuse
  Alcohol
  Amphetamines
  Caffeine in very high doses
  Cannabis
  Cocaine
  Codeine
  Ecstacy and related drugs
  Ketamine
  Phencyclidine

Cessation of:
  Alcohol
  Barbiturates

Panel 10: Psychosis Without Clear Precipitant

- At this point, the differential diagnosis turns on whether or not the psychotic symptoms are part of another psychiatric disorder.
  - Review of Systems should probe for disorders in the *Differential Diagnosis Panel* above.
- If no psychiatric or medical disorder is identified, go to *Disorders Section, Schizophrenia and Other Psychotic Disorders,* page 197.

Module 5

Substance Use and Gambling

Orienting Notes

- Substance use and gambling are both treated here since both involve addictive behaviors that may cause social, financial, and legal difficulties.
  - For assessment of gambling behavior, see *Panel 11*.
- Substance dependence is a *behavioral* disorder: A person may be dependent with no physiologic signs or symptoms.
- Substance dependence and abuse represent a spectrum of severity.
- Substance use disorders have high rates of comorbidity with:
  - Other psychiatric disorders
  - Secondary medical disorders
- Three phases of substance use may cause psychiatric symptoms:
  - Intoxication
  - Withdrawal
  - Sequelae of long-term use

- However, symptoms of a primary psychiatric disorder may be erroneously ascribed to substance use, particularly by persons not clinically trained.

  Note: See *Appendices 2 to 6* for relevant detoxification protocols.

Differential Diagnosis

- Differential diagnosis in evaluating substance use focuses on detecting other disorders that might be missed or mistaken for effects of substance use alone.
- When one substance is identified, always consider ***multiple*** substances.
- Intoxication with stimulants, alcohol, hallucinogens:
  - Acute head trauma
  - Withdrawal from sedatives or alcohol
  - Purposeful overdose with medications or substances (see *Module 6*)
  - Neurologic disorders
  - Delirium from other causes (see *Module 7*)
  - Psychotic disorders (see *Module 4*)
  - (Hypo)mania in manic-depressive (bipolar) disorders (see *Disorders Section,* pg 169)
- Intoxication with sedatives (e.g., benzodiazepines, barbiturates):
  - Acute head trauma
  - Purposeful overdose with medications or substances (see *Module 6*)
  - Neurologic disorders
  - Delirium from other causes
- Withdrawal from stimulants, alcohol:
  - Major depression and dysthymia (see *Module 1*)
  - Adjustment disorder due to social sequelae of substance use
- Withdrawal from sedatives, alcohol:
  - See above, intoxication with stimulants, alcohol, hallucinogens.

Panel 1: Tasks in Characterizing Substance Use Disorders

- Identify the substance used (*Panel 3*).
- Delineate extent of use (*Panel 3*).
- Identify phase of use (*Panels 4 and 5*).
- Identify/delineate phase iteratively until all substance use is identified.
- Identify complications (*Panels 6 and 7*).
- Identify comorbidities (*Panels 8 and 9*).

Note: These tasks require the use of *all* phases of the biopsychosocial assessment described in *Section I:* history of present illness, psychiatric review of systems, medical review of systems, social history, and family history.

- Continue to **Panel 2.**

Panel 2: Screening for Substances Used

- Strategies such as the **CAGE** questions for alcohol have good screening characteristics and may be adapted for other substances:

  C: Ever felt you should **C**ut down on your drinking?

  A: People ever **A**nnoy you by criticizing your drinking?

  G: Ever feel bad or **G**uilty about your drinking?

  E: Ever need an **E**ye-opener in the morning to steady your nerves or to get rid of a hangover?

- Individuals with substance use disorders are not necessarily the habitual liars they are often made out to be. However, they often minimize
  - their use of substances
  - its impact on their lives
- Therefore, collateral information from informants and medical records should be used whenever possible.

Note: The variety and popularity of substance used, particularly by teens and young adults, is constantly changing. The web site for Partnership for a Drug-Free America is a particularly useful source of current information. It is frequently updated and contains a précis on most substances of abuse (including jargon names, which can be helpful in interviewing): *www.drugfreeamerica.org.*

- Continue to **Panel 3.**

Panel 3: Delineate Extent of Use

- What substances are used?
- How much? How often? Chronically or episodically?
- Route: Oral? Intravenously (i.v.) injected? Smoked? Inhaled?
- Triggers? Stressors?
- History of withdrawal symptoms?
  - For alcohol, benzodiazepines, and barbiturates
    - Delirium or hallucinations during withdrawal?
    - Seizures during withdrawal?
- Hallucinations or blackouts during intoxication?
- Treatment history:
  - Number of detoxifications? Inpatient/outpatient?
  - Number of rehabilitation programs? Inpatient/outpatient?
  - Aftercare and self-help involvement? Active sponsor?
- Longest period clean and sober?
  - When?
  - How achieved?
  - How did it end?
  - What was life like when clean and sober?
- Family history: genetic or modeling factors?
- Social supports stimulate or impede substance use?

Note: Several instruments are available to assist in delineating substance use and sequelae. See instruments in the *Key References* for resources to help in evaluating and choosing such instruments.

- Continue to **Panel 4.**

Panel 4: Current Phase of Use

- People present for care in various phases of substance use/sequelae.
- Propensity for abuse, dependence, or long-term physical sequelae varies from substance to substance, and is tabulated in *Disorders Section, Substance Use Disorders,* page 189.

  Phases:

- *Current abstinence* (may or may not need ongoing support/assessment)
- *Current episodic use*
- *Intoxication*
  - Management of acute intoxication involves protection of the individual and others. See *Module 6, Suicidality and Assaultiveness.*
  - Intoxication with one substance doesn't rule out withdrawal from another.
  - Alcohol withdrawal can begin for above legal levels of intoxication.
- *Withdrawal* (for common specific withdrawal syndromes, go to *Panel 10*)
  - Withdrawal from alcohol and sedatives can be life-threatening. See *Treatment Section, Detoxification Protocols.*
  - Discomfort from opiate or nicotine withdrawal can be mitigated somewhat. See *Treatment Section, Detoxification Protocols.*
  - Withdrawal from other substances is primarily supportive.
- *Residual symptoms* from past long-term use
  - Neurologic
  - Other physical
  - Social

- If any current or recent use, or withdrawal, has occurred, go to **Panel 5.**
- If only residual symptoms from long-term past use are present, go to **Panel 6.**

Panel 5: Dependence or Abuse?

- Abuse and dependence are considered part of the same behavioral spectrum.
- Recall that dependence may be *behavioral* only, without *physiologic* symptoms of tolerance or withdrawal.
- For dependence, the DSM system requires the concurrent presence of at least three of the following:
    - *Tolerance:* Increased amounts for same effect, or less effect with same amount.
    - *Withdrawal:* Characteristic syndrome, or using to prevent withdrawal (for common specific withdrawal syndromes, go to *Panel 10*).
    - Use more or for longer time than intended.
    - Desire or failed attempts to control use.
    - Much time to obtain or use substance.
    - Role function or activities compromised.
    - Use continues despite awareness that use is causing physical or mental problems.
- For abuse, the DSM system requires the presence of at least one of the following:
    - Role function or activities compromised
    - Recurrent use when physically hazardous
    - Recurrent legal problems
    - Continued use despite recurrent social problems due to use

- Continue to **Panel 6.**

Panel 6: Psychiatric Complications of Substance Use

- Current substance use or withdrawal can result in a wide variety of psychiatric symptoms, including mood, anxiety, and psychotic syndromes.
    - Psychiatric symptoms likely due to substance use are considered by the DSM system "substance-induced" (secondary) syndromes.
    - Nonetheless, they may require concurrent treatment based on clinical judgment (e.g., severe depressive or anxiety symptoms after alcohol withdrawal).
- Past long-term use of some substances can cause enduring neuropsychiatric sequelae that require treatment:
    - Alcohol, some stimulants, inhalants: Dementia or cognitive problems
    - Hallucinogens: Persistent reexperiencing (flashbacks)
    - See also Substance Use Disorders in *Section III*.

Note: Common independent (*primary*) psychiatric comorbidities are summarized in *Panel 8*.

- Continue to **Panel 7.**

 **Panel 7: Social Sequelae
of Substance Use Disorders**

A thorough social history is necessary for assessment and for planning treatment.

- Impact and social morbidity
- Specific vulnerabilities, triggers
- Potential sources of strength

Specific foci:

- Occupational
  - Work and military history: Impairment, jobs lost? Longest job ever?
  - Current/last job: performance?
  - Current income sources?
- Housing: Stability? Other users? Transportation to treatment?
- Marital:
  - Spouse: Living situation? Physical abuse? Co-user?
  - Children: Abuse? Neglect? Children who use?
- Legal:
  - Driving while intoxicated, disorderly conduct, assaults, dealing?
  - Jail time? Prison time? Probation? Pending court dates?
- Social activities
  - Time spent using, social cues, important co-users?
  - Any alternate leisure activity maintained?
- Social support system that:
  - Promotes substance use
  - Supports sobriety or provides social alternatives
- Religious/spiritual sources of strength

- Continue to **Panel 8.**

Panel 8: Identify Common Independent Psychiatric Comorbidities

Common psychiatric comorbidities across all substance use disorders include:

Substance-Related
- Use of other substances
- Concurrent intoxication and withdrawal from multiple substances
- Alcohol withdrawal despite residual symptoms of intoxication and legally elevated blood alcohol level.

Other Psychiatric
- Mood disorders (see *Modules 1 and 2, Depression or Fatigue and Manic Symptoms*)
- Anxiety disorders (see *Module 3, Anxiety/Nervousness*).
- Adjustment disorders due to social impact of substance use (see *Disorders Section, Adjustment Disorders*).
- Schizophrenia and related psychotic disorders (see *Module 4, Psychosis*)
- Dementia and related cognitive disorders (see *Module 8, Problems with Memory or Organization*).

- Continue to **Panel 9.**

Panel 9: Identify Medical Comorbidities and Complications of Acute/Chronic Use

A thorough medical Review of Systems is required. Some complications are life threatening acutely.

Intravenous

- Bacterial endocarditis
- HIV/AIDS
- Hepatitis B or C
- Tuberculosis
- Cellulitis
- Track marks: disfiguring, lack of venous access

Inhaled or Smoked

- Nasal irritation and perforated nasal septum
- Asthma, chronic pulmonary disease

Specific Agents: Tobacco

- Oral and pulmonary cancers

Specific Agents: Opiates

- Decreased libido, erectile dysfunction
- Menstrual irregularities

Specific Agents: Stimulants

- Seizures
- Cardiac arrhythmias

Specific Agents: Alcohol

- Neurologic: delirium, acute head trauma, dementia, cerebellar atrophy, peripheral neuropathy, withdrawal seizures
- Skin: petechiae, spider angiomata, palmar erythema
- Endocrine: decreased androgens and:
  - Men: testicular atrophy, gynecomastia
  - Women: decreased fertility, amenorrhea
- Metabolic: vitamin B_{12}/folate deficiency, thiamine deficiency (Wernicke-Korsakoff syndrome), hyponatremia, hyperglycemia, obesity, hypoalbuminemia
- Eyes, ears, nose, and throat: oral cancers
- Pulmonary: aspiration pneumonia during intoxication
- Cardiac: dilated cardiomyopathy, hypertension, and atrial fibrillation in binges or withdrawal
- Gastrointestinal: esophageal varices,[a] erosive esophagitis,[a] gastritis and duodenal ulcers,[a] cirrhosis,[a,b] ascites, splenomegaly and platelet sequestration,[a] hepatic cancers, decreased protein synthesis and drug-binding capacity,[b] decreased vitamin K synthesis
- Hematologic: macrocytic anemia, anemia due to blood loss, leucopenia, thrombocytopenia[a]
- Musculoskeletal: trauma during intoxication or drug procurement, myopathy, increased creatine phosphokinase, osteopenia, Dupuytren contractures

[a]Contributes to increased risk of acute hemorrhage.
[b]Contributes to increased risk of medication toxicity.

- Continue to **Panel 10.**

Panel 10: Synopsis of Common Specific Withdrawal Syndromes

Note: See *Appendices 2 to 6* for relevant detoxification protocols.

Alcohol, Benzodiazepines, Barbiturates

- Autonomic hyperactivity
  - Increased pulse
  - Increased blood pressure
  - Sweating
  - Tremors
- Insomnia
- Nausea, vomiting
- Anxiety/agitation
- Seizures
- Hallucinations
- Delirium tremens (DTs) is a delirium characterized by:
  - Hallucinations (tactile > visual > auditory)
  - Severe autonomic hyperactivity
  - Fever
  - Possible circulatory collapse and death
- Course:
  - Alcohol
    - Onset: 4 to 12 hours
    - Duration: 2 to 5 days
  - Benzodiazepines and barbiturates: depends on half-life of substance used and is quite variable
    - Onset: several hours to 3 days
    - Duration: 2 to 7 days

Note: Delirium/DTs is not uncommon in alcohol or barbiturate withdrawal and is a medical emergency (see *Module 7*).

Note: In cases of multiple withdrawal, barbiturates will cover benzodiazepine and alcohol withdrawal, but benzodiazepines will *not* cover barbiturate withdrawal. See *Appendices 2 and 3* for relevant *detoxification protocols* and specific strategies.

Stimulants

- Fatigue
- Insomnia/hypersomnia, nightmares
- Psychomotor retardation/agitation
- Increased appetite and weight gain
- Depression/anxiety/irritability
- Course:
  - Onset: 6 hours to 1 day
  - Duration: 2 to 5 days

Opiates

- Nausea, vomiting
- Muscle aches
- Runny nose, tearing
- Autonomic hyperactivity:
  - Dilated pupils
  - Sweating
  - Tremors
  - Diarrhea
- Insomnia
- Yawning
- Depression/anxiety/irritability
- Course depends on half-life of substance used and is quite variable.
  - Onset: 6 hours to 2 to 4 days for methadone
  - Duration: 3 to 7 days, longer for methadone
  - Methadone can have weeks of nonspecific dysphoria beyond physiological symptoms

Nicotine

- Depression/anxiety/irritability
- Insomnia
- Poor concentration
- Restlessness
- Increased appetite and weight gain
- Pulse decrease by up to 12 beats/min
- Course:
  - Onset: hours
  - Duration: days to several weeks for acute symptoms

Note: It is not uncommon with any substance to have months of craving and nonspecific dysphoria. Relapse risk is, of course, particularly high during this time.

Panel 11: Gambling

- Gambling is considered pathologic according to the DSM system if there is social dysfunction or personal suffering. Pathologic gambling is diagnosed with the presence of five or more of the following:
  - Preoccupied with gambling-related activities
  - Increasing amounts to achieve desired thrill
  - Unsuccessful attempts to cut down
  - Restless/irritable when cutting down
  - Gambling to escape problems or to relieve bad mood
  - Frequent returns to gambling to recoup losses
  - Lying about gambling
  - Illegal acts to finance gambling
  - Jeopardized/lost role function because of gambling
  - Reliance on gambling to repay debts from gambling
- As with substance use, accurate assessment requires corroborating information from others and/or medical records.
- An important item in the differential diagnosis of pathologic gambling is (hypo)mania during bipolar disorder (see *Module 2, Manic Symptoms*).
  - Treatment is psychosocial, with structured clinical programs and/or self-help groups. See *Appendix 10* for resources.

Module 6

Suicidality and Assaultiveness
(Including Acute Management Strategies)

Orienting Notes

- Suicidality and assaultiveness are both addressed here because each involves danger to person and because their assessment and acute management use similar approaches.
- Clinicians are not very accurate in predicting future violence to self or others, even in those who have committed such acts in the past.
- Terminology and underlying concepts regarding suicide are inconsistent: "gesture," "attempt," "passive suicidality," "ideation," "lethality" are all used imprecisely.
- However, careful evaluation can improve both assessment and treatment planning.
- Assessment of suicidality and assaultiveness runs through each of the components of the Biopsychosocial Assessment outlined in **Section I.**
- Acute management focuses on maximizing the probability that the individual and others will be safe. This may involve:
  - Acute medical assessment and stabilization
  - Voluntary or involuntary hospitalization
  - Deescalating the crisis and close outpatient follow-up
  - Collaborative care with family or friends providing close observation
  - Legal intervention for assaultiveness not due to a psychiatric condition

Differential Diagnosis

Suicidality is a particular concern in:

- Depressive disorders (see *Module 1*)
- Manic-depressive (bipolar) disorders (in depression or [hypo]mania) (see *Disorders Section,* page 169)
- Schizophrenia and related psychotic disorders (see *Module 4*)
- PTSD (see *Disorders Section,* page 184)
- Delirium (see *Module 7*)
- Dementia (see *Disorders Section,* page 206)
- Substance use disorders (see *Module 5*) with:
  - Intoxication
  - Withdrawal
  - Long-term social dysfunction
- Adjustment disorder with recent loss, including bereavement (see *Disorders Section,* page 204)
- Borderline personality disorder (see *Disorders Section,* page 238)
- Antisocial personality disorder (see *Disorders Section,* page 237)
- Anorexia nervosa (see *Disorders Section,* page 220)
- Chronic medical illness
- Chronic pain (see *Module 13*)

Assaultiveness is a particular concern in:

- (Hypo)mania in manic-depressive (bipolar) disorders (see *Disorders Section,* page 169)
- Schizophrenia and related psychotic disorders (see *Module 4*)
- PTSD (see *Disorders Section,* page 184)
- Delirium (see *Module 7*)
- Dementia (see *Module 8*)
- Substance use disorders (see *Module 5*) with:
  - Intoxication
  - Withdrawal
  - Long-term social dysfunction
- Antisocial personality disorder (see *Disorder Section,* page 237)

Report of suicidal or assaultive ideation also may be due to:

- Factitious disorder (see *Disorder Section,* page 217)
- Malingering (see *Disorder Section,* page 217)

Panel 1: Assessment of Suicidality and Assaultiveness

- As with substance use disorders, accurate assessment often requires information from collateral sources such as friends, family, and medical records.
- Straightforward queries are appropriate when assessing a current episode.
- Straightforward queries about prior actions should be part of every psychiatric Review of Systems.

Note: Asking about suicide will *not* put the idea in someone's head. On the contrary, it is usually a relief to the individual to finally share this shameful and disturbing thought that he or she has sometimes been living with for days or weeks.

- As with psychotic disorders, delirium, and dementia, assessment includes observation from the moment the interview begins, in addition to specific interview queries.
  - Disorganized behavior, psychomotor agitation, or responding to internal stimuli suggests the inability to control impulses.
  - Intoxication increases the risk for suicidality.
  - Intoxication, especially with alcohol or stimulants, greatly increases the risk for assaultiveness.
  - Psychomotor retardation may be due to severe depression.
  - *But:* in cases of psychosis or delirium, psychomotor retardation may portend explosive behavior about to occur.

Note: No clinician practices good medicine when scared.

- Concerns may be:
  - Personal physical safety
  - Safety of the individual or of others
  - Fear of losing a patient
  - Legal and peer review repercussions
- Get support. Get consultation. Early.
- See also *Panel 14.*

- Continue to **Panel 2.**

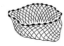

Panel 2: Information Comes from All Components of the Biopsychosocial Assessment

All components of the biopsychosocial assessment contribute important diagnostic and treatment planning information.

- Demographics
  - Age
  - Gender
- History of Present Illness
  - Description of the intent/act
  - Currently active psychiatric disorders
- Psychiatric Review of Systems
  - Other psychiatric disorders that may contribute
- Medical Review of Systems
  - Chronic illnesses
  - New diagnosis or downturn
  - Chronic pain
- Social History
  - Marital status
  - Occupational status
  - Recent losses
  - Social acceptance of suicidality/assaultiveness
  - Counterbalancing supports and strengths
    - Support from family, friends
    - Desire to protect loved ones from repercussions
    - Personal coping skills
    - Religious/spiritual factors
- Family History
  - Genetic predisposition
  - Modeling

Note: specific risk factors are detailed in *Panel 6.*

- Continue to **Panel 3.**

Panel 3: Assessing the Suicidal or Assaultive Intent or Act

- Current intent:
  - Planning to date
    - What, when, where, how?
    - Who's been told?
    - Collateral behaviors; for example, giving away possessions?
    - Procuring means?
  - How easy is access to weapons?
  - For assaultiveness: specific target? See *Panel 13.*
- Recent act:
  - What was done?
  - How did the person end up in a clinical assessment: Did he or she tell someone? Did he or she come on their own? Did someone else bring him or her?
  - What (if anything) stayed his or her hand?
- Any prior acts or ideation?

- Continue to **Panel 4.**

Panel 4: The Anti-"Gesture" Panel

- The word *gesture* to describe low-intent, low-lethality suicidal behavior is meaningless, or worse.
  - It conveys a sense of trivializing an act that typically is caused by substantial psychic pain and lack of coping skills:
    - Who wouldn't rather be reading, visiting friends, or watching a ball game than, for example, taking 10 Tylenol and calling 911?
  - It tends to cloud our thinking about *this* person, *this* act, at *this* time.
  - There is good evidence that "gestures" do not protect against subsequent serious suicide attempts. For example:
    - Studies indicate that a prior gesture does *not* mean that the next act won't be high intent and high lethality.

- Continue to **Panel 5.**

Panel 5: Intent and Lethality

- It is useful to assess intent and lethality separately.
  - Often they are associated, that is, acts or plans that are high intent may be high lethality, and those of low intent may be low lethality
  - However, some low-intent acts are highly lethal, and some low-lethality acts derive from high intent that may strike again.
- Intent and lethality have different implications for treatment planning.
  - High intent: Manage high risk of recurrence regardless of lethality.
  - High lethality: Medically stabilize and educate, regardless of intent.
- Therefore, consider suicidal or assaultive acts and plans on Cartesian coordinates of *intent × lethality:*

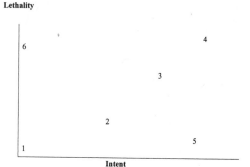

Examples of suicidal acts:

1. Man takes 5 aspirin in front of his wife after an argument and calls 911.
2. Woman cuts her wrists while home alone, considers alternatives, and runs to her neighbor's house.
3. Man waits until no one is home, makes noose and ties it to an attic rafter; he considers alternatives, walks downstairs, and comes to the hospital.
4. Woman takes full bottle of benzodiazepine washed down with liquor in a car in the woods and is found by a passing hiker.
5. Man takes his daily dose of coumadin, drinks a pint of vodka, superficially cuts wrists, and lies down in bed to bleed to death in his sleep.
6. Adolescent girl takes a bottle of Tylenol and yells for her parents who then call 911; she later relates, "I didn't really want to kill myself; otherwise, I'd have taken aspirin."

- Continue to **Panel 6.**

Panel 6: Risk Factors for Suicide and Assaultiveness

- Recall that we are not good predictors of future violence to self or others.
- Given report of intent or plan, knowledge of relevant risk factors may improve our positive predictive value (See *Section I, Panel 10*).
- However, absence of risk factors does *not* imply absence of risk—we are dealing here with probabilities, not certainty.

Suicide Risk Factors

- Demographics:
  - Age over 45
  - Male
  - Caucasian
- Psychiatric disorders:
  - See **Differential Diagnosis Panel** above
  - Some notes on prevalence of suicide/attempts:
    - Mood disorders: up to 10%
    - Bipolar disorder: 2.5 attempts/year per 100 individuals
    - Alcohol dependence: up to 10%
    - Schizophrenia: up to 10%
    - Borderline personality disorder: up to 10%
- Medical disorders:
  - Chronic illness
  - New diagnosis or recent downturn
  - Chronic pain
  - Delirium
- Social history factors
  - Recent loss—tangible *or* symbolic
  - Unemployed
  - Separated, divorced, widowed
  - History of abuse
- Family history of attempts

Assault Risk Factors

- Demographics:
  - Age 15 to 24
  - Male
- Psychiatric disorders:
  - Psychosis
  - Mania
  - Substance intoxication or withdrawal
  - Antisocial personality disorder
- Social history factors
  - Recent loss—tangible *or* symbolic
  - Low socioeconomic status
  - History of abuse
  - Violent culture
- Family history of violence

Note: Although psychosis and mania are risk factors for violence, in the community most individuals with serious mental illnesses are more often victims than victimizers.

• Continue to **Panel 7.**

Panel 7: Simplified Mnemonic for Major Risk Factors for Suicide

Gender
Age
Loss
Attempts in past
Medical illness
Anxiety/mood disorders
Psychosis
Substance use disorders

- Continue to **Panel 8** for acute management strategies.

Panel 8: Acute Management of Suicidal or Assaultive Acts or Plans

- Get available information about the individual before meeting him or her.
- Establish safe surroundings:
  - Know the panic/alert system.
  - Plan egress for the assaultive individual and for yourself.
- *Job #1 is to develop a therapeutic alliance:*
  - Instills hope
  - Implies alternatives to harm to self/others
  - Supports self-esteem
- Do not confront assaultive individuals:
  - Be low-key at all times.
  - Set limits empathically, reasonably.
- Offer alternatives/choices wherever possible.
- Reorient the individual to reality frequently if needed.
- Offer medications where appropriate.
- Determine inpatient versus outpatient management (see *Panel 9*).
- Know physical restraint procedures and your place on the team.
- If office-based, have emergency contact procedure ready (e.g., 911 call).

Note: In the case of threat of assault to a specific other, "duty to warn" may apply (see *Panel 13*).

- Continue to **Panel 9.**

Panel 9: Managing the Suicidal Act That Has Occurred

- Address medical necessities
  - Emergent medical evaluation
  - Supportive care (e.g., i.v. fluids)
  - Monitoring (e.g., telemetry)
  - Removal of substance in overdose
    - Charcoal and gastric lavage
    - Lactulose
    - Dialysis

  Note: Overdose toxicity of common psychotropic medications is found in each entry in *Section IV, Treatment.*

- Implement psychiatric support (in descending order of intensity):
  - Restraint/seclusion
  - One-on-one inpatient observation (ensure direct hand-off to observer)
  - Involuntary/voluntary psychiatric admission (see *Panel 10*)
  - Crisis observation bed
  - Return home with close clinical follow-up (see *Panel 11*)
    - Community diversion program
    - Observation by friends/family
    - Alone
  - Medications for active psychiatric disorders (dispense sublethal prescriptions for individuals treated in outpatient settings)

- Continue to **Panel 10.**

Panel 10: Involuntary Commitment

- Almost all states and countries allow involuntary detainment for imminent danger to self or others.
  - Immediate and short-term detainment for evaluation is usually delegated by legal authorities to *clinicians.*
  - Subsequent detainment for treatment is typically a *legal* matter decided in the courts.
- However, rules and procedures vary greatly even from state to state.
  - Grounds for establishing danger to self or others may vary.
  - Clinical and subsequent civil procedures often idiosyncratic can be labyrinthine.
- Therefore, know your local requirements before you have to use them at 3 AM!

- Continue to **Panel 11.**

Panel 11: Stay or Go Home?

Perhaps the most difficult decision in managing an individual with suicidal thoughts is whether or not to admit him or her to the hospital.

Benefits:

- Observation increases likelihood of immediate safety.
- Hospital milieu often provides support and relief.

Costs:

- Involuntary admission may compromise treatment alliance and long-term management.
- Voluntary or involuntary admission may lead to regression in some individuals.
- Admission may be costly to the individual in terms of:
  - Financial burden
  - Stigma
  - Disruption of support/coping strategies (family, work roles)

The decision is often made on the basis of a "contract for safety." Continue to *Panel 12.*

Panel 12: The "Contract for Safety"

- An individual is frequently triaged to outpatient care if they can contract for safety.
- The contract for safety usually refers to an individual's ability to tell the clinician that he or she won't harm himself or herself or anyone else until the next clinical contact.
  - As typically used, it is more of a *promise* by the individual than a *contract* that involves both parties.
  - Even having a written "contract" confers no legal benefit in malpractice proceedings.
- Time is better spent:
  - Establishing a supportive treatment alliance.
  - Delineating a reasonable, concrete follow-up plan that includes:
    - When the individual will next be seen clinically
    - By whom the individual will be seen (introduce them if possible)
    - Method of telephone access if in crisis in the interim
    - Method of walk-in access if in crisis in the interim
    - Method of transportation in crisis if necessary
  - Documenting efforts and plans in the medical record
  - Optimally, involving a significant other in monitoring and access procedures

Note: Involving significant others in assessment and treatment planning not only improves assessment and treatment, but also usually reduces risk of malpractice litigation.

- Continue to **Panel 13.**

Panel 13: Breaking Confidentiality and Duty to Warn

- Confidentiality between clinician and individual in treatment is a core clinical value.
- Confidentiality can be violated only in certain specific circumstances.
- In the situation of acute danger to self, violation of confidentiality to obtain potentially life-saving information is usually warranted.
- In situations of danger to others, the doctrine of "duty to warn" may also apply.
  - Established by the initial Tarasoff decision, a clinician has a duty to warn another individual who is the object of an expressed threat.
  - A second Tarasoff decision ruled that a clinician also has a "duty to protect" by taking appropriate protective action.
- Duty to warn applies when a *specific*, *credible* threat is made against a *specific*, *identifiable* individual. Examples:
  - "I'm gonna shoot that contractor who botched my job." This represents potential for duty to warn.
  - "If anyone tries to mess with my girlfriend, I'll kill 'em." This is hypothetical, but clearly warrants more explanation.
- Preventing a credible threat (e.g., through voluntary or involuntary hospitalization) may make duty to warn no longer applicable.
- If the threat is resolved (e.g., through voluntary or involuntary hospitalization) duty to warn no longer applies.

- Continue to **Panel 14.**

Panel 14: Debriefing after a Suicide or Assault

If you treat individuals with serious mental illnesses, sooner or later it *will* happen: despite your best efforts, one of the individuals you are treating will complete a suicide or a serious assault. Maybe it will even be an overdose that includes a prescription you've just written or will happen just after you've seen the individual.

- Typical reactions:
  - Usually, the first reaction is to be scared for yourself. This is normal.
  - Fear comes from factors that are:
    - External: possible legal, peer-review repercussions
    - Internal: self-doubt about professional capabilities
  - Anger at the individual percolates through.
  - Self-doubt, self-deprecation, and shame typically lurk around the edges.
- Coping strategies:
  - Discuss the incident and your reactions with supportive colleagues—don't bear it alone.
  - If you have a supervisor, use him or her to review the case and your reactions.
  - Evaluate the legal issues and get appropriate support—this addresses a great source of anxiety.
  - Keep the "continuous quality improvement (**CQI**)" mindset:
    - In any situation, there are opportunities for improvement.
    - With 20:20 hindsight, how would you have done things differently?
  - Within the limits of confidentiality, get support from your own significant others.
  - Give yourself a break!
  - In the case of suicide, participate if appropriate in the grieving process with the individual's significant others (e.g., send condolences, attend the wake or funeral, arrange a follow-up visit with the survivors).
- A note on peer-review processes:
  - Peer review processes vary greatly in structure and demeanor, depending on:
    - Specific personalities involved
    - Institutional priorities and demands
  - Some are friendly, some less so.
  - Some are judgmental, some are constructive.
  - Even the friendliest and most constructive process is intimidating and anxiety provoking.
  - Coping strategies:
    - Come well prepared to discuss the case and alternative strategies
    - Keep a calm demeanor.
    - Keep the CQI mindset—peer review committees almost always speak CQIese.

Module 7

Change in Mental Status/Delirium

Orienting Notes

- Delirium is a disturbance of *vigilance*.
  - Other terms:
    - Reduced "awareness," "alertness" regarding the surrounding environment
      - "Waxing/waning mental status"
      - "Change in mental status"
  - May be stupor, disorganized agitation, or may alternate between the two
  - May be dramatic or, when superimposed on dementia, a subtle "change in mental status"
- The key task is to identify and treat reversible causes:
  - Medical illnesses
  - Medication side effects
  - Psychiatric illnesses
- Common in dementia
- Associated with high morbidity
- Two deliria that often come to psychiatric attention:
  - Catatonia (see *Panels 5 and 6*)
  - Neuroleptic malignant syndrome (NMS) (see *Panels 7 and 8*).

Differential Diagnosis

- Dementia (see *Module 8 and Panel 2 below*)
- Psychosis (see *Module 4 and Panel 2 below*)
- Dissociation (see *Module 4*)

Panel 1: Adapted DSM System Definition of Delirium

- Disturbance of consciousness (reduced clarity of awareness of environment) with reduced ability to focus, sustain, or shift attention. Examples:
  - Stuporous
  - Too lethargic to attend to environment
  - Inability to attend to environmental cues, demands
  - Purposeless, agitated activity
- Change in cognition such as memory, orientation, or language, or perceptual disturbance not accounted for by dementia.
- Develops over hours to days and tends to fluctuate.

• Continue to **Panel 2.**

 Panel 2: Differentiating Delirium, Dementia, and Psychosis

The three syndromes often overlap. The key task is to identify a delirium that may have a reversible cause. The table helps in their clinical differentiation.

	Delirium	Dementia	Acute Psychosis
Onset	Acute	Subacute/ chronic	Acute/subacute
Vigilance	Decreased	No change until end- stage	Hypervigilance
Gross cognitive Decline (see *Module 8*)	Yes	Yes	No
Hallucinations or delusions	Maybe	Maybe	Yes
Course	Fluctuating	Persistent	Persistent
Outcome	Acute with treatment	Chronic	Either
Medication- induced	Yes	No	Rarely
Due to medical condition	Yes	Yes	Rarely if psychosis alone

• Continue to **Panel 3.**

Panel 3: Common Medical/Psychiatric Conditions that May Cause Delirium

Underlying Cause	Diagnostic Assessment[a]
Trauma	
Subarachnoid hemorrhage	Noncontrast CT, MRI
Subdural hemorrhage	Noncontrast CT, MRI
Cerebrovascular	
Transient ischemic attack	Carotid doppler
Acute large vessel thrombosis/ hemorrhage	Noncontrast CT at 48 hr, MRI
Multiple lacunar infarcts	MRI
Anoxic encephalopathy	Noncontrast CT,
Hypertensive encephalopathy	Blood pressure
Cardiovascular	
Myocardial infarction	EKG, cardiac enzymes
Congestive heart failure	Chest radiography
Pulmonary embolus	VQ scan
Endocardial embolus	Echocardiogram
Neoplasm	
Primary CNS	Contrast CT, MRI
Metastasis	Contrast CT, MRI
Metabolic	
Hypoxia	Arterial blood gas
Hypoglycemia	Serum glucose level
Dehydration	Serum electrolytes
Electrolyte imbalances	Serum electrolytes
Hepatic failure	Liver function tests, ammonia
Renal failure	BUN, creatinine
B_{12}/folate deficiency	Serum levels (CBC may be normal)
Thiamine deficiency (Wernicke encephalopathy if acute)	Clinical examination (nystagmus, lateral gaze paralysis, ataxia), noncontrast CT, MRI
Nicotinic acid (niacin) deficiency	Clinical examination (*d*ementia, *d*ermatitis, *d*iarrhea), serum levels
Endocrine	
Diabetic ketoacidosis	Serum glucose, electrolytes, arterial blood gas
Diabetic hyperglycemic hyperosmolar nonketotic coma	Serum glucose, electrolytes
Hypothyroidism/hyperthyroidism	Thyroid function tests
Addison disease	Dexamethasone suppression test, CRF stimulation test, adrenal CT, pituitary MRI
Cushing disease	ACTH stimulation test, adrenal CT
Infections	
Urinary tract infection in elderly	Urinalysis, urine culture
Meningitis	Lumbar puncture
CNS emboli	Contrast CT, MRI
Encephalitides	Noncontrast CT, EEG, biopsy
Syphilis	RPR or VDRL followed by FTA-ABS or MHA-TP
Acquired immunodeficiency syndrome	HIV serology, T-cell counts
Sepsis	CBC, Blood cultures
Autoimmune	
Multiple sclerosis	MRI
Systemic lupus erythematosis	ANA and antibody pattern
Temporal arteritis	ESR, temporal artery biopsy
Other	
Hyperthermia/hypothermia	Core body temperature
Severe pseudodementia	See *Module 8*

[a]It is assumed that a history and physical examination will identify key events (e.g., overdose, heavy metal exposure) or disorders (e.g., hypothyroidism, lupus); if specific, classic findings are present on clinical examination, they are so noted.

- Continue to **Panel 4.**

Panel 4: Common Medications that May Cause Delirium at Therapeutic Doses

Analgesics
  Codeine
  Opiates
  Meperidine
Antiarrhythmics
  Lidocaine
  Procainamide
Antibiotics
  Acyclovir
  Interferon
  Fluoroquinolones
  Isoniazid
  Rifampin
Anticholinergics
Anticonvulsants
  Barbiturates
  Benzodiazepines
  Topiramate
Antihistamines (H_1 and H_2 blockers)
Antihypertensives
  Methyldopa
  Angiotensin-converting enzyme inhibitors
  Calcium channel blockers
Antiinflammatory agents
  Indomethacin

Antineoplastic agents
Antiulcer
  Cimetadine
  Ranitidine
Hormones/vitamins
  Anabolic steroids
  Corticosteroids
  Hypervitaminosis A/D
Muscle relaxants
  Cyclobenzaprine
Stimulants/sympathomimetics
Other CNS-active agents, especially:
  Antidepressants
  Disulfiram
  Dopaminergic agents
  Electroconvulsive therapy
  Ergotamines
  Hallucinogens
  Neuroleptics (with or without NMS, see *Panels 7 and 8*)
Withdrawal from:
  Alcohol
  Barbiturates
  Benzodiazepines

- Continue to **Panel 5.**

Panel 5: Catatonia: Diagnosis

- Catatonia is a delirium.
- It is a syndrome that can occur in many medical or psychiatric disorders, not just schizophrenia.
  - Prevalence in: medical disorder > affective disorder > schizophrenia.
  - Critical issue: identify and treat reversible causes.
- Adapted DSM system definition requires the presence of at least two of the following:
  - Motoric immobility or catalepsy (see ***Note***) or stupor
  - Excessive and purposeless motor activity
  - Negativism (motiveless resistance to passive movement, or moving the opposite way in response to passive movement or verbal instruction) or mutism
  - Stereotyped behavior or assumption of inappropriate or bizarre posture
- Catatonia may alternate dramatically between stupor and excitement.
  - The stupor may be converted to excitement with mild noxious stimuli or touch, and may result in injury to individual or examiner—approach the stuporous catatonic with care.
  - Even in stupor, the individual typically is aware of the environment and will remember some of what happened—approach the stuporous catatonic with respect.
- However, catatonia has a spectrum of severity and not all symptoms may be present at all times.

Note: There has been some confusion in describing the motor immobility of catatonia. Catatonic individuals can often be placed into bizarre postures, which they hold indefinitely—for example, twisting arms over head, bending legs in typically uncomfortable positions. The examiner feels the limbs to be like a warm candle being bent. The classic name for this is *flexibilitas cerea,* now called *catalepsy,* or sometimes by the somewhat less precise translation of the Latin, *waxy flexibility*—all are synonyms. The "waxy" feel without the posturing has sometimes, somewhat generously, been called waxy flexibility as well. Note that the unfortunately similar term *cataplexy* describes a totally different phenomenon: the sudden loss of all muscle tone associated with narcolepsy, not catatonia (see *Module 11, Panel 1*).

- Continue to **Panel 6.**

Panel 6: Catatonia: Management

- Identify and correct underlying medical disorder.
- Supportive treatment (milieu, restraint, hydration, nutrition, self-protection especially in excited phase).
- Discontinue neuroleptics, which perpetuate the syndrome.
- Syndrome lysis as soon as possible.
- Two major methods of lysis:
  - Intravenous/intramuscular lorazepam followed by oral maintenance
    - 2 mg i.v. with repeat at 30 minutes if necessary often results in prompt awakening.
    - Intramuscular administration can be used, but response is slower.
    - Partial initial response is not uncommon, and full response may take several days of high dose lorazepam.
    - Relapse after awakening with parenteral lorazepam is typical unless maintained on oral lorazepam.
    - Typical oral maintenance dose 4 to 10 mg/day lorazepam.
  - Electroconvulsive therapy if no response to lorazepam.
  - 75% to 80% will respond, assuming medical disorder corrected.
- Conundrum: When to restart neuroleptics in schizophrenia with catatonia?
  - No clear answer.
  - Empiric approach:
    - When catatonia resolves on maintenance lorazepam, slowly reintroduce neuroleptic.
    - Cotreat with high doses of lorazepam plus neuroleptic for several weeks.
    - Slowly taper lorazepam.
    - If catatonia recurs, reinstitute high-dose lorazepam and/or taper neuroleptic and repeat taper attempt after 1 to 2 weeks of further stability.

- Continue to **Panel 7.**

Panel 7: Neuroleptic Malignant Syndrome: Diagnosis

- NMS is a delirium associated with use of neuroleptics (any type).
- Prevalence: some studies show rates as high as 1% to 2% of psychiatric/medical admissions on neuroleptics.
- Identical syndrome can rarely be seen without neuroleptics: "Malignant catatonia."
- No universal definition; components of syndrome:
  - Delirium
  - Hyperthermia without other cause
  - "Lead pipe" rigidity leading to muscle breakdown, increased serum creatine phosphokinase (CPK), myoglobinuria, and possible renal failure
  - Extrapyramidal symptoms: cogwheeling, dystonia, chorea
  - Autonomic instability: hypertension, tachycardia, diaphoresis, sialorrhea
- Associated laboratory findings:
  - Increased CPK (1,000–10,000 units/L not uncommon)
  - Leukocytosis
  - Myoglobinuria, proteinuria
  - Secondarily increased blood urea nitrogen (BUN), creatinine
- Complications:
  - May be lethal
  - Circulatory collapse
  - Acute renal failure
  - Accidental self-harm due to delirium

- Continue to **Panel 8.**

Panel 8: Neuroleptic Malignant Syndrome: Management

- Identify and correct underlying medical disorder.
- Supportive treatment (cooling, hydration, self-protection, nutrition, prevent aspiration).
- Discontinue neuroleptics, which perpetuate the syndrome.
- Lysis if syndrome does not resolve with treatment of underlying disorder and supportive treatment.
- Syndrome lysis:
  - Bromocriptine (dopamine agonist) 2.5 to 5 mg orally or via nasogastric tube three times daily and increase by 2.5 mg per dose each day until response or dose reaches 60 mg/day.
  - Dantrolene (muscle relaxant): 25 mg twice daily and increase by 50 mg/day for response up to 400 mg/day.
  - Dantrolene i.v.: 2 to 3 mg/kg four times daily up to 10 mg/kg/day

Module 8

Problems with Memory or Organization

Orienting Notes

- It is useful to consider together three overlapping groups of pathologic cognitive problems: delirium, dementia, and executive function deficits.
- *Delirium* is typically reversible and may represent an acute medical emergency (see *Module 7*).
- Some cognitive problems/*dementias* are treatable by treating the underlying cause (e.g., vitamin B_{12} deficiency, medication side effect).
- Some *dementias* are modifiable by treating their neuropsychiatric basis (e.g., Alzheimer disease).
- *Executive function* deficits occur in a wide range of psychiatric disorders:
  - They impact greatly on treatment adherence.
  - They correlate highly with functional abilities.
  - They are frequently not identified.
  - Recognition will improve treatment planning and compliance.
- The major tasks in the biopsychosocial assessment of dementia are:
  - Identify treatable/modifiable forms/factors.
  - Assess impact on the individual and their caregivers.

Differential Diagnosis

Conditions sometimes mistaken for dementia:

- Delirium (see *Module 7*)
- Psychosis (see *Module 4*)
- Depression (see *Module 1*)
- Amnestic disorders (see *Panel 6*)
- Traumatic brain injury (see *Panel 6*)
- Executive function deficits as part of other disorders (see *Panel 11*)
- Normal aging

Note: Dementia also may be complicated by delirium, psychosis, and/or depression (see *Panel 10*).

- For assessment and subtypes of dementia, continue to **Panel 1.**

Panel 1: Definition of Dementia

- Dementia is defined by clinical criteria
  - Not by imaging or other studies
  - Not by a simple number on a rating scale
- However, imaging and quantitative rating scales may be important in assessment.
- DSM-based criteria for dementia consist of chronic:
  - Memory impairment (learning or retrieval) and
  - One or more of the following:
    - Aphasia (deficits in language)
    - Apraxia (deficits in motor tasks despite normal motor function)
    - Agnosia (deficits in object identification despite normal sensation)
    - Disturbances in executive function
- *Executive function deficits* are deficits in planning, organizing, sequencing, abstracting, or inhibiting behavior
  - Executive ability is required for complex tasks necessary for treatment participation, such as maintaining medication supply, following multistep medication regimens, planning and scheduling appointments, and arranging transportation.
  - They are nonspecific and occur in many mental disorders.
  - They are often unrecognized and are not identified by measures of gross cognitive function [e.g., the Mini-Mental State Examination (MMSE) see *Appendix 1*.].

- To assess multimodal cognitive dysfunction, continue to **Panel 2.**
- To assess suspected executive dysfunction, go to **Panel 11.**

Panel 2: Overview of Biopsychosocial Assessment of Cognitive Problems

- Characterizing the deficits: see *Panels 3 and 4.*
- Co-occurring symptoms: see *Panel 5.*
- Assessing impact on function: see *Panel 6.*
- Assessing impact on caregivers: see *Panel 7.*
- Types of dementia: see *Panel 8.*
- Identifying reversible causes: see *Panel 9.*
- Common comorbidities: see *Panel 10.*

- Continue to **Panel 3.**

Panel 3: Characterizing the Deficits

- Criterion-based assessment is the core of diagnosis.
  - As for psychosis, delirium, and substance use, important information may need to be gathered from collateral sources, including significant others and medical records.
- For each deficit, characterize:
  - How long has the deficit been apparent?
  - How is it manifest in terms of specific symptoms?
  - What is its impact on function?

Notes on Presentation
- Onset usually subacute/chronic
- Abrupt onset or waxing/waning consciousness requires prompt workup for delirium (see *Module 7*).
- Course must be chronic.
- Often comes to first clinical attention because of:
  - Environmental reasons (e.g., "I changed jobs and just couldn't keep an eye on her all night." "We moved and he just seemed to fall apart." "I got sick and he went out and was gone for 2 days until the police found him wandering around.") or
  - Co-occurring symptoms ("We've been married 45 years and now she thinks I'm having an affair.")
- Assessing specific cognitive criteria:
  - Memory, aphasia, apraxia, agnosia: go to *Panel 4.*
  - Executive function: go to *Panel 11.*
  - These four domains—memory, aphasia, apraxia, and agnosia—are not easily reparable clinically; tasks in daily living typically draw on multiple domains.
- Once dementia is diagnosed, a rough clinical guide to severity scaling using the MMSE is:
  - MMSE score 15 to 24 out of 30: mild-moderate dementia
  - MMSE fewer than 15 out of 30: severe dementia
  - Typical decline: 2 to 4 points per year

  Note: MMSE reference and a screening examination for executive function deficits can be found in *Appendix 1.*

- Imaging and laboratory studies
  - Do *not* correlate well with severity of cognitive or functional deficits.
  - *Are* important to identify reversible causes and to subtype the dementia.

- Continue to **Panel 4.**

Panel 4: Assessing Specific Criteria for Dementia

Domain	Report of Individual or Significant Other	Clinical Examination
Memory		
Short-term	Day/date, car keys lost, things on stove	MMSE: orientation, object recall
Long-term	Wandering, birthdays, major events	Presidents, geographical QQ's
Aphasia		
Receptive	Following instructions, stories	Following instructions including MMSE reading item
Expressive	Frustration in self-expression, naming, "talking around" items or subjects, unusual word use (paraphrasia), paucity of speech	Open-ended questions for fluency, content MMSE speaking, writing items
Apraxia	Inability to use common household objects, fix simple objects, cook, dress	Inability to sequence meaningful motor movements (e.g., MMSE 3-stage command); inability to use common objects [e.g., "Show me how to . . . blow out a match . . . comb your hair . . . use a hammer" (with pantomime object)]
Agnosia	Inability to recognize faces, voices of family members, identify famous people, name common objects	MMSE naming items, recognizing photographs of famous people

• Continue to **Panel 5.**

Panel 5: Assessing Co-occurring Symptoms

- Other symptoms commonly occur as part of the dementia syndrome:
  - Apathy/neglect
  - Agitation
  - Depression
  - Anxiety
  - Irritability
  - Impulsivity
  - Psychosis
- May warrant symptomatic treatment
- May represent comorbid disorders (see *Panel 10*)

- Continue to **Panel 6.**

Panel 6: Assessing Severity of Functional Impact

- Information often needs to come from caregivers.
- Domains of social history may reveal functional deficits:
  - Occupational function decline
  - Marital strife
  - Mismanagement of finances
  - Impulsivity leading to legal encounters, social embarrassment
  - Withdrawal from social roles and relationships
  - Impoverishment of leisure time activities
  - Increased need for support in activities of daily living

- Continue to **Panel 7.**

Panel 7: Assessing Severity of Impact on Caregivers

- Caregiver burden is a major source of personal and societal cost.
- Caregivers frequently need treatment for depressive, anxiety, and adjustment disorders.
- Assessing burden follows from sequelae of social history items (see *Panel 6*).
- Perhaps the most operationally complex and emotionally difficult aspect of treatment planning derives from caregiver burden: to seek or not to seek institutional placement?
- Considerations:
  - Availability of intermediate in-home supports
  - Matching needs to institutional level (e.g., assisted living for couple vs. nursing home for individual)
  - Practicalities of finance
  - Insurance, Medicare, Medicaid procedures and resources
  - Social/functional burdens on spouse now left alone
  - Personal value conflicts, guilt, blame from other family members
  - Conflicts, bickering over possessions among other family members

Note: The decision to seek Medicaid funding for nursing home placement initiates a somewhat arcane bureaucratic process that varies from state to state since Medicaid is a state-administered program. Families are best advised to seek legal advice from a lawyer with expertise in this area. Resources can often be identified through the local chapter of the American Association of Retired Persons (AARP) or similar organization.

- Continue to **Panel 8.**

Panel 8: Major Types of Dementia, Their Workup, and Interventions

Type	Major Clinical Findings	Clinical Imaging Studies	Modifiable/ Treatable?
Alzheimer[a]	Gradual onset of global cognitive deficits (see *Panels 4, 5, 11*) without focal motor findings	Noncontrast CT or MRI for atrophy especially with coronal sections through the hippocampus	Cognitive enhancing agents
Vascular[a] Large vessel or lacunar Cortical or subcortical	Acute, stair-step, or chronic decline of global cognitive deficits often with focal motor findings based on site of infarcts	Noncontrast CT for suspected large vessel (≥48 hr post-CVA) MRI for suspected lacunar or subcortical	Reduce risk factors, e.g., hypertension, vascular disease
Parkinson	Characteristic motor findings, dementia in 20%–40%, may have psychosis	Noncontrast CT for atrophy	Dopaminergic agents for motor signs, clozapine for psychosis
Lewy body	Features of both Alzheimer and Parkinson diseases with prominent visual hallucinations, fluctuating arousal, delirium, possible REM sleep behavior disorder	Noncontrast CT for atrophy	Minimize neuroleptics and use cognitive enhancers, clonazepam for REM sleep behavioral symptoms
Frontotemporal (e.g., Pick)	Impulsivity, apathy, personality changes may be more prominent than cognitive changes	Noncontrast CT for atrophy, predominantly in frontal and temporal lobes	—
Dementia due to specific medical causes	See *Panel 9*		
Amnestic disorders	Not strictly dementia since other functions spared; may represent mild form of or early Alzheimer disease	Noncontrast CT for atrophy	Cognitive enhancing agents
Traumatic brain injury	Not strictly dementia since other functions may be spared; may involve only personality change, impulsivity, mood lability	Trauma history, neuropsychologic testing assist in diagnosis; noncontrast CT or MRI for atrophy, scarring	Variable; treatment is aimed at symptom reduction, rehabilitative

[a]Mixed vascular–Alzheimer-related dementia is common.

• Continue to **Panel 9**.

Panel 9: Common Reversible/Modifiable Causes of Cognitive Problems (See also *Module 7*)

Underlying Cause	Diagnostic Assessment[a]
Anatomic	
Tumor	Contrast CT, MRI
Trauma	Noncontrast CT, neuropychologic assessment
Normal pressure hydrocephalus	Clinical examination (dementia, urinary incontinence, ataxia), ventricular flow studies
Infectious	
Syphilis	RPR or VDRL followed by FTA-ABS or MHA-TP
Acquired immunodeficiency syndrome	HIV serology, T-cell counts
Embolic	Contrast CT, MRI
Encephalitis	Noncontrast CT, EEG, biopsy
Cardiovascular (see also *Panel 8*)	
Acute large vessel thrombosis/ hemorrhage	MRI
Embolism	Contrast CT, MRI
Anoxic encephalopathy	Noncontrast CT
Genetic	
Huntington disease	Family history
Wilson disease	Slit-lamp examination, serum ceruloplasm
Metabolic	
B_{12}/folate deficiencies	Serum levels (CBC may be normal)
Thiamine deficiency (Korsakoff syndrome; see also Wernicke encephalopathy, *Module 7*).	Clinical examination (nystagmus, lateral gaze paralysis, ataxia), MRI
Nicotinic acid (niacin) deficiency (pellagra)	Clinical examination (*d*ementia, *d*ermatitis, *d*iarrhea), serum levels
Hypothyroidism	Thyroid function tests
Cushing disease	Dexamethasone suppression test, CRF stimulation test, adrenal CT, pituitary MRI
Addison disease	ACTH stimulation test, adrenal CT
Autoimmune	
Multiple sclerosis	MRI with contrast for white matter lesions
Systemic lupus erythematosis	ANA and antibody pattern
Temporal arteritis	ESR, temporal artery biopsy
Toxins	
Irradiation	MRI with contrast for white matter lesions
Chronic medication overdose	Serum, urine levels
Heavy metals (arsenic, lead, manganese, mercury, thallium)	Serum, nail, hair, urine levels
Dialysis (aluminum)	
Carbon monoxide	
Major depressive disorder	See *Panel 10*

[a]It is assumed that a history and physical will identify key events (e.g., overdose, heavy metal exposure) or disorders (e.g., hypothyroidism, lupus); if specific, classic findings are present on clinical exam, they are so noted.

- Continue to **Panel 10.**

Panel 10: Assessing Comorbidities

- In addition to co-occurring symptoms, full-blown comorbidities may develop:
  - Delirium (see *Module 7*)
  - Major depressive disorder (see *Module 1*)
  - Adjustment disorders (see *Disorders Section,* page 204)
  - Substance use disorders (see *Module 5*)
- Major depressive disorder superimposed on mild cognitive deficits or dementia can produce a syndrome called *pseudodementia.*
  - Preexisting cognitive deficits can become far worse.
  - The syndrome is fully reversible with adequate antidepressant treatment.

Note: Although cognitive slowing can be part of a major depressive episode, a major depressive episode does not typically produce pronounced cognitive decline without preexisting deficits. Other causes must be sought.

Panel 11: Assessing Executive Function

Note: Executive function deficits are not limited to dementia. They can occur in individuals with any mental illness and can have a wide-ranging impact both on treatment compliance and on function.

- Executive functions include planning, organizing, sequencing, abstracting, and inhibiting behavior.
- The MMSE and other measures of global cognitive function are not sufficiently sensitive to detect executive deficits.
  - The MMSE is weighted heavily toward responding to structured queries (e.g., "What day is it?" "What is this?").
  - Executive tasks often require generation *de novo* of behaviors from a repertoire, or sorting and imposition of order on a variety of relevant and irrelevant stimuli.
- These latter tasks are typical of those required (e.g., by treatment adherence). For example:
  - Develop methods to remember medication schedule.
  - Have foresight to realize when medications are running low.
  - Plan the scheduling, finances, telephone contact, and transportation to prevent lapse in prescriptions.
  - Executive function must also be relatively intact to allow independent living.
- Clinically feasible methods for assessing executive function also can be divided into report of the individual or significant other and the clinical examination.
- Report of executive deficits will frequently come from significant others.
  - Problems in organization, task completion, activities of daily living (e.g., managing finances, planning, and budgeting) are often deficient.
  - The clinician should become suspicious with frequent bouts of unexplained noncompliance with treatment.
  - The "deer in the headlights" look when the clinician is explaining a treatment plan should also be a clue that an individual's executive function may not be up to the tasks required—and they will rarely say, "I don't understand" or "You've lost me there."
- Screening can be done in less than 5 minutes by the primary care or mental health professional, or with extended batteries by specially trained professionals.
  - A screening examination based on the Executive Function Interview (EXIT) can be found in *Appendix 1*.
  - Specialized testing by a neuropsychologist can provide detailed assessment.
- Another valuable assessment typically conducted by occupational therapists is the Kohlman Evaluation of Living Skills (KELS assessment). This is particularly useful in assessing the need for living structure (e.g., independent living vs. assisted living vs. nursing home). This brief evaluation consists of a series of ecologically valid tasks that cover:
  - Self-care (e.g., dressing and hygiene)
  - Safety and health (e.g., recognizing dangerous household situations, calling 911)
  - Money management (e.g., making change, budget for month sheet)
  - Transportation/telephone (e.g., use of a phone book, bus schedule)
  - Work/leisure activities

Module 9

Problems with Concentration, Impulsivity, and Irritability

Orienting Notes

- Problems with concentration/attention, impulsivity, and irritability are handled together because:
  - They are common complaints and are often the focus of requests for treatment, but:
    - They can be frustratingly nonspecific and can be part of many syndromes, and
    - They commonly co-occur.
- Their co-occurrence in some disorders may help to focus the differential diagnosis.
- The tabular summary below can guide differential diagnosis in conjunction with other relevant modules.
- Note that key issues in assessment are:
  - How severely disordered is behavior? Irritability that involves physical fights is clearly of more acute concern than irritability that is limited to subjective feelings.
  - Can collateral sources of information, such as significant others and medical records provide better diagnostic data, especially with regard to severity?

Differential Diagnosis

Disorder	Decreased Concentration	Impulsivity	Irritability
Adjustment disorder	+		±
Anorexia nervosa	—	Thematic	—
Bulimia	—	Thematic	—
Attention deficit disorder	+	+	—
Delirium	+	+	—
Dementia	+	±	±
Dissociative disorders	+	±	—
Dysthymia	+	—	—
Factitious disorder/ malingering	—	±	±
Generalized anxiety disorder	+	—	±
Major depressive episode	+	±	*a*
Manic/mixed episode	+	+	+
Obsessive-compulsive disorder	—	Thematic	—
Panic disorder	—	—	*a*
Phobia, social	—	Thematic	—
Phobia, specific	—	Thematic	—
Posttraumatic/acute stress disorder	+	+	+
Premenstrual dysphoric disorder	+	±	+
Somatoform disorder	—	—	Thematic
Substance use disorders: intoxication	+	+	+
Substance use disorders: withdrawal	+	+	+
Substance use disorders: long-term sequelae	+	±	±

*a*It is not unusual to see marked irritability in men with major depressive episode, and not unheard of to see panic attacks in men with a predominantly irritable rather than anxious presentation.

+, typically reported; ±, sometimes reported; —, not typically seen at greater than chance rates. Thematic, impulsivity related to theme of the disorder (e.g., impulsivity around eating in eating disorders).

Module 10

Eating and Appearance

Orienting Notes

- Anorexia nervosa and bulimia are classified as eating disorders in the *Diagnostic and Statistical Manual of Mental Disorders* (DSM) system, whereas body dysmorphic disorder is classified with the somatoform disorders. However they are all addressed in this module because:
    - They share the common core feature of unrealistic concern regarding appearance.
    - Presenting complaints for each tend to focus on dissatisfaction with appearance and need to be differentiated.
- Keep in mind that developed societies put a high premium on appearance, so that discontent with appearance is frequently encountered in primary care and mental health practices; not all situations fulfill criteria for a DSM-based diagnosis.
- Keep in mind that developed societies have a high prevalence of obesity. Dealing with obesity may or may not involve eating disorder behaviors.
- Keep in mind that many psychotropic medications induce weight gain and secondary concerns with appearance.
- Whatever the source of obesity, prevention is easier than remediation.

Differential Diagnosis

- Psychotic disorders (see *Module 4*).
- Major depressive disorder (see *Disorders Section,* page 164)
- Somatization disorder (see *Disorders Section,* page 210)
- Phobia, social or specific (see *Disorders Section,* page 177)
- Obsessive-compulsive disorder (see *Disorders Section,* page 182)
- Borderline personality disorder (see *Disorders Section,* page 238)
- Avoidant personality disorder (see *Disorders Section,* page 239)
- Medical disorders causing anorexia/vomiting
- Obesity with repeated failed attempts at weight reduction
- Obesity with pathologic compensation
- Subpathologic or "neurotic" concern over appearance

Panel 1: Screening for Disorders of Eating and Appearance

"Do you have particular concerns about your appearance? For instance, your weight or other features of how you look?"

- Additional probes may be necessary to characterize the concern.
- Concerns are considered pathologic if they are *unrealistic*.
- Unrealistic concerns (i.e., loss of insight) rarely may reach delusional proportions.
  - Symptoms are better understood on a dimensional, graded basis than on a categorical either/or basis.
  - Symptomatic treatment of psychotic symptoms may be necessary if dysfunction is substantial.
- *Thematic* and *circumscribed* delusions may sometimes be seen in severe anorexia nervosa or body dysmorphic disorder.
  - Additional psychotic diagnoses are not usually given in this situation.
  - However, symptomatic treatment with antipsychotic medications is sometimes necessary.

- If response is "Yes," continue to **Panel 2.**
- If No, consider other items in the **Differential Diagnosis.**
- If clear psychotic symptoms are present, go to **Module 4.**

Panel 2: Determining the Focus of Concern

Note: For *Panels 2* through *4*, several items are followed by letters in parentheses [e.g., "(**A-A**)," "(**B-D**)," etc.]. These notations assist the reader by mapping on the item to the corresponding diagnostic criterion for anorexia nervosa or bulimia. The first letter refers to the disorder (**A**norexia or **B**ulimia) and the second to the specific criterion (**A** through **D**). Each criterion must be met for either disorder.

- Unrealistic weight concerns? Including:
  - Too heavy or intense fear of gaining weight though underweight (**A-B**)
  - Disturbed body perception (e.g., weight, or shape of specific part such as thighs, buttocks) (**A-C**)
  - Self-esteem overly tied to weight (**B-D**)
- Unrealistic concern about appearance of other specific physical attribute?

- If Yes to first query, continue to **Panel 3.**
- If Yes to second query, go to **Panel 6.**

 Panel 3: Evaluation of Physical Status

- Low body weight? (**A-A**)
  - Clinical judgment must be used.
  - Suggested guidelines:
    - Weight 85% below normal
    - Body mass index less than 17.5 kg/m^2
- No menses for at least three consecutive cycles? (**A-D**)

- Continue to **Panel 4.**

 Panel 4: Binging and Compensation

- Binging? (**B-A**)
  - Eating larger amounts of food than normal in a single episode (e.g., 2 hours)
  - Feeling of lack of control during the episode
- Compensation? (**B-B, A-A**)
  - Purging
    - Self-induced vomiting
    - Laxatives
    - Enemas
    - Diuretics
  - Nonpurging compensation
    - Excessive exercise
    - Fasting
- Frequency of twice per week or more for at least 3 months (**B-C**)

- If individual meets criteria **A-A** through **A-D,** diagnosis is anorexia nervosa.
- If individual meets criteria **B-A** through **B-D,** diagnosis is bulimia.
- If individual meets some but not all criteria but symptoms are a focus of concern, consider behavior on the eating disorder spectrum [official DSM system diagnosis would be "Eating Disorder Not Otherwise Specified (NOS)"].
- For any of these three outcomes, continue to **Panel 4.**
- If concern is limited to perception of a discrete body part such as thighs or buttocks in **Panel 2** (**A-C**) without meeting other criteria, go to **Panel 6.**

Panel 5: Physical and Laboratory Evaluation

- Each of the eating disorders can lead to high medical morbidity.
- Comprehensive physical evaluation is required.
- Most of the morbidity derives from restriction of protein and calorie intake and resultant weight loss.
- Findings that may occur with purging alone (i.e., regardless of body weight and nutritional status) are marked with a **P**.

Physical Examination and Review of Systems Findings

- General
  - Dehydration, cachexia
- Vital signs
  - Hypothermia
  - Bradycardia
  - Hypotension
- Head, eyes, ears, nose, and throat
  - Eroded dental enamel (**P**)
  - Hypertrophy of salivary glands
- Skin
  - Lanugo (fine hair/fuzz over body, common in newborns)
  - Petechiae
  - Dry, scaly skin
  - Carotenemic (yellowish) skin tone
- Pulmonary
  - Aspiration pneumonia/pneumonitis (**P**)
- Cardiovascular
  - Mitral valve prolapse
  - Tachyarrhythmias
  - Symptoms of congestive heart failure due to ipecac-induced cardiomyopathy (**P**)
- Gastrointestinal
  - Erosive esophagitis (**P**)
  - Esophageal tears (**P**)
- Musculoskeletal
  - Peripheral edema
  - Ipecac-induced myopathy (**P**)

Laboratory Finding

- Electrolytes
  - Alkalosis (**P**)
  - Hypokalemia (**P**)
  - Decreased Mg, Ca, PO_4
- Renal function
  - Prerenal azotemia (increased BUN/creatinine)
  - Decreased urine specific gravity
- Endocrine
  - Decreased estrogen (women) or testosterone (men)
  - Decreased luteinizing hormone/follicle-stimulating hormone (women)
  - Decreased triiodothyronine (T_3), increased reverse T_3, normal thyroxine
- Cardiac
  - Electrocardiography: increased QT and prominent U waves due to hypokalemia (**P**)
  - Ventricular tachyarrhythmias
  - Mitral valve prolapse
  - Ipecac-induced cardiomyopathy (**P**)
- Metabolic
  - Decreased vitamin B_{12}, folate
  - Decreased bone mineral density

Note: Cardiac arrhythmias are of great concern because they may lead to sudden death.

- Address medical issues and:
  - If anorexia nervosa, go to *Disorders Section,* page 220.
  - If bulimia, go to *Disorders Section,* page 221.
  - If eating disorder NOS, go to the disorder that most closely matches symptom profile.

Panel 6: Body Dysmorphic Disorder

- Body dysmorphic disorder is defined as a preoccupation with an imagined physical anomaly, or overestimation of disfigurement due to a minor anomaly.
- Other disorders (e.g., eating disorders, psychotic disorders) take precedence in terms of the DSM diagnostic hierarchy.
- Go to *Disorders Section,* page 218.

Module 11

Sleep Problems

Orienting Notes

- Sleep disorders can be divided into disorders of:
  - Amount or timing (*Dyssomnias*)
  - Events during sleep (*Parasomnias*)
- Sleep disorders are classified by several systems, including:
  - International Classification of Sleep Disorders (comprehensive, specialty oriented)
  - DSM-IV (adequate for nonspecialist clinical needs, which we will follow here)
- "I don't sleep well . . . I don't feel rested after I wake up . . ." are among the most common reasons for seeking clinical care.
- Sleep complaints contribute greatly to subjective quality of life.
- Primary sleep disorders are not uncommon.
- Sleep disturbances are also common in psychiatric and medical illnesses.
- Therefore, rule out causes of secondary sleep disturbance (see *Differential Diagnosis* and *Panels 4* and *5*) before making diagnosis of primary sleep disorder.

Differential Diagnosis

Note: Characteristic sleep findings in these psychiatric disorders are summarized in *Panel 5*.

- Major depressive disorder (see *Disorders Section,* page 164)
- Dysthymia (see *Disorders Section,* page 167)
- Mania (see *Module 2*)
- GAD (see *Disorders Section,* page 180)
- PTSD (see *Disorders Section,* page 184)
- Panic disorder or nocturnal panic attacks (see *Disorders Section,* page 174)
- Adjustment disorder/bereavement (see *Disorders Section,* page 204)
- Substance use disorders (see *Module 5*)
  - Intoxication
  - Withdrawal
- Dementia (see *Disorders Section,* page 206)
- Delirium (see *Module 7*)
- Psychosis (see *Module 4*)
- Anorexia nervosa (see *Disorders Section,* page 220)
- Medical illness or conditions (see *Panel 4*)
- Medication side effect (see *Panel 6*)
- Use of caffeine, nicotine
- Normal aging (see *Panel 3*)

Panel 1: Some Definitions

Key Sleep Architecture Terms

- *Stage 1 sleep:* Transition between wake and sleep, about 5% of sleep time.
- *Stage 2 sleep:* Next stage in deepening, has "K-complexes" on sleep electroencephalography, about 50% to 70% of sleep time and increases with age.
- *Stages 3 and 4 sleep:* Deeper sleep, without dreams, 20% to 25% of sleep time in teens and declines with age.
- *Delta sleep:* Stages 3 and 4; night terrors occur here.
- *Non-REM sleep:* Stages 1 to 4.
- *REM sleep:* Rapid eye movement sleep; dreaming occurs here.

Key Parasomnia Terms

- *Cataplexy:* Sudden, brief loss of muscle tone often triggered; nothing to do with *catalepsy* (see *Module 7, Panel 5*).
- *Hypnagogic/hypnopompic hallucinations:* Hallucination going, respectively, into and out of sleep; typical in narcolepsy. Also common, nonspecific, and nonpathologic—and responds to simple education and reassurance.
- *Sleep paralysis:* Brief periods of paralysis going into or out of sleep, typical of narcolepsy

Key Circadian Rhythm Terms

- *Circadian rhythm:* Daily (*circa diem*) variation in amplitude of a function or occurrence of an event.
  - Most human physiologic functions have a circadian rhythm (e.g., hormonal secretion, blood pressure, sleep/wake cycle).
- *Period:* Cycle length.
  - Most human circadian rhythms are just longer than 24 hours.
- *Phase:* Timing of a circadian event (e.g., sleep onset/offset, hormonal secretion peak).
  - Those who tend to go to sleep late and arise late are sometimes called "*owls.*"
  - Those who go to sleep early and arise early are sometimes called "*larks.*"
  - They are, respectively, relatively phase-*delayed* and phase-*advanced* with respect to the majority.
  - Their circadian periods are, respectively, relatively longer and shorter than those of the majority.
- *Zeitgeber:* "Time-giver"—external cues that set the phase of circadian rhythms. Major zeitgebers in humans are:
  - Social rhythms
  - Bright light

- Continue to **Panel 2.**

Panel 2: Sleep Symptom Probes

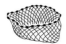

"How is your sleep? Do you have any problems trying to sleep? Do you feel rested during the day?"

- Sleep problems may be only one symptom of more extensive, treatable psychiatric illnesses:
  - Individuals often don't think in syndromes like clinicians do—e.g., they may not even know the words depression and anxiety.
  - Often sleep complaints are the most evident or most troubling to the individual; therefore, it is of great importance to screen individuals with sleep problems with a good medical (*Panels 4* and *6*) and psychiatric (*Panel 5*) review of systems.

Note: A number of self-reports such as the Pittsburgh Sleep Quality Index may be useful as a self-report screening tools. See the Instruments entries in *Key References.*

Characterizing sleep problems:

- Problems in timing or amount?
- Problems with events during sleep (e.g., nightmares, panic, sleepwalking)?
- How long a problem?
- How often?
- Link to any factors (e.g., psychosocial stress, psychiatric symptoms, medical symptoms, medications, shifting zeitgebers like shift work or time zone changes)?
- Ever before?
- Sleep routine nightly (may gather prospective diary data)
- Extent of daytime dysfunction?
- Medical review of systems (*Panels 4 and 6*)
- Psychiatric review of systems (*Panel 5*)

- If dyssomnia (amount/timing problem):
  - Continue to **Panel 3** if individual is over 60.
  - Otherwise go to **Panel 4.**
If parasomnia (event problem), go to **Panel 4.**

Panel 3: Features of Sleep in Aging

Over Age 65

- Total sleep time actually increases.
  - Number of long-sleepers (>9 hours) increases.
  - Number of nappers increases.
- However, number of short-sleepers (<5 hours) also increases.
- 35% report sleep symptoms and secondary daytime problems.
- 9% report chronic insomnia lasting more than 6 months.
- More initial insomnia.
- More easily aroused from sleep.
- Sleep onset/offset phase advances.
- Stages 1 and 2 increase.
- Stages 3 and 4 decrease.
- More medical problems.
- More pain.
- More medications.

- Continue to **Panel 4.**

Panel 4: Medical Conditions Associated with Sleep Symptoms

D = dyssomnias including frequent awakenings.
P = parasomnias.

Neurologic

Cluster headaches (D)
Degenerative neurologic disorders (D)
Huntington disease (D)
Hypothalamic lesions (D)
Migraine (D)
Neuropathic pain (D)
Parkinson disease [D, P (REM sleep behavior disorder)]
Seizure disorder [P (nocturnal seizures)]
Stroke (D)
Traumatic brain injury (D)

Cardiovascular

Angina (D)
Congestive heart failure (D)

Pulmonary

Asthma (D)
Central sleep apnea (D)
Chronic obstructive pulmonary disease (D)
Obstructive sleep apnea (D)

Gastrointestinal

Gastroesophageal reflux disease (D)
Peptic ulcer disease (D)

Genitourinary

Nocturia (D)
Uremia [D, P (restless legs syndrome)]

Endocrine

Diabetes, especially hypoglycemia [D, P (nightmares, panic, delirium)]
Hyperthyroidism (D)
Hypoglycemia [D, P (nightmares, panic, delirium)]
Obesity (D)
Perimenopause (D)
Pregnancy [D, P (restless legs syndrome)]
Premenstrual phase of menstrual cycle (D)

Musculoskeletal

Fibromyalgia (D)
Rheumatoid arthritis [D, P (restless legs syndrome)]

Other Conditions

Hospitalization or other noxious environment (D)
Pain, acute or chronic (D)
Sleep deprivation (D)

• Continue to **Panel 5.**

Panel 5: Sleep Symptoms in Selected Psychiatric Disorders

Disorder	Typical Sleep Symptom
Mood disorders	
Major depressive episode	Initial/middle/terminal insomnia
	Diurnal variation of mood (worse in morning)
(Hypo)manic episode	Decreased *need* for sleep
Anxiety disorders	
Generalized anxiety disorder	Initial insomnia
Panic disorder	Nocturnal panic attacks
Posttraumatic stress disorder	"Nightmares" in REM sleep and night terrors in delta sleep
Cognitive disorders	
Delirium	Loss of circadian sleep–wake cycle
Dementia	Loss of circadian sleep–wake cycle, "sundowning" (disorientation, disruptive behavior, psychosis in late afternoon through morning)
Substance abuse	
Intoxication with stimulants/ sedatives	Decreased/increased sleep
Withdrawal from stimulants/ sedatives	Increased/decreased sleep
Psychosis	Insomnia
Eating disorders	Insomnia
Anorexia nervosa	

• Continue to **Panel 6.**

Panel 6: Medications Associated with Sleep Symptoms

Note: Primary finding is insomnia unless otherwise noted.

- Alcohol
  - Use (hastens sleep onset, insomnia later in the night)
  - Withdrawal
- Antiasthmatics (β agonists, theophylline)
- Antidepressants (stimulating)
  - Abrupt withdrawal of any antidepressants
  - Serotonin reuptake inhibitors can cause vivid dreaming
- Antipsychotics (high potency)
  - Akathisia
  - Parkinsonian symptoms
- Baclofen
- Barbiturate withdrawal
- Benzodiazepines
  - Tolerance
  - Nocturnal rebound insomnia with short-acting agents
  - Withdrawal
- Caffeine
- Carisoprodol withdrawal (metabolized to meprobamate)
- Cimetidine
- Clonidine
- Decongestants
- Diphenhydramine
  - Paradoxic insomnia not infrequent
- Diuretics
  - Nocturia leading to insomnia
- Dopamine agonists
- Nicotine
- Opiates
  - Use
  - Withdrawal
- Steroids (corticosteroids, anabolic steroids)
- Stimulants

- Continue to **Panel 7.**

Panel 7: Primary Sleep Disorders of *Timing/Amount* (Dyssomnias)

Disorder	Key Clinical Features	Workup
Primary insomnia	Problems initiating or maintaining sleep or not feeling rested after sleep	Clinical diagnosis; diagnosis of exclusion
Primary hyper-somnia	Prolonged sleep episodes or daytime sleep not explainable by other disorders	Requires sleep EEG to document true hypersomnia, not just daytime fatigue
Narcolepsy	Classic tetrad: Daytime sleepiness Cataplexy Sleep paralysis Hypnogogic/pompic hallucinations May have familial pattern	Clinical diagnosis
Breathing-related sleep disorders (may include mixed features):	Daytime sleepiness in all; hypnotics may worsen	Each requires sleep EEG for diagnosis
Obstructive sleep apnea	Obesity, snoring are common	
Central sleep apnea[a]	Not typically obese or snorers	
Obesity hypoventi-lation syndrome (*pickwickian syndrome*)	Obesity, reduced air exchange and respiratory drive	
Circadian rhythm sleep disorder (or sleep–wake schedule disorder)	Chronic insomnia or exces-sive daytime sleepiness due mismatch between personal circadian cycle and zeitgebers (e.g., shift work, recurrent time zone shifts)	Clinical diagnosis; rarely caused by extreme variant of personal circadian period (e.g., extreme "lark" or "owl" pattern), occasionally with total blindness

[a]Central sleep apnea is of two types:

• Central (or primary or chronic) alveolar hypoventilation is a disorder of central respiratory drive and is chronic (*Ondine's curse*),

• Temporary central sleep apneas have normal central respiratory drive and are due to temporarily or paroxysmaly low CO_2 levels with corresponding decreases in respiratory drive that result in erratic Cheyne-Stokes respiratory pattern. Examples include the normal transition from wake to sleep (elderly may have problems with this), congestive heart failure, and hypoxia from various sources with compensatory paroxysmal hyperventilation and reduction in CO_2 and respiratory drive.

• Continue to **Disorders Section, Sleep Disorders,** or
• Continue to **Appendix 7, Biopsychosocial Management of Insomnia.**

Panel 8: Primary Sleep Disorders of *Event* (Parasomnias)

Disorder	Key Clinical Features	Workup
Nightmare disorder	Awakening repeatedly from terrifying dreams, followed by full awakening and rapid reorientation to reality, dreams typically remembered	Clinical diagnosis; occurs during REM sleep and primarily in second half of sleep period; rare in adults
Sleep terror disorder	Repeated abrupt awakening with intense panic and autonomic arousal, difficulty in reorientation, amnesia for event	Clinical diagnosis; occurs during delta sleep and primarily in first half of sleep period; rare in adults
Sleepwalking disorder	Repeated sonambulation, unresponsiveness to environment, amnesia for event	Clinical diagnosis; occurs during delta sleep and primarily in first half of sleep period
REM sleep behavior disorder[a]	Sonambulation or other activities that appear to be acting out of dream material; likely due to loss of REM-related muscle atonia	Clinical diagnosis; occurs during REM sleep and primarily in second half of sleep period
Periodic limb movements in sleep (or nocturnal myoclonus)[a]	Leg or foot jerks every 20–40 seconds accompanied by insomnia, akathisia in lower limbs (*restless legs syndrome[b]*), hot/cold feet, daytime sleepiness	Clinical diagnosis; sleep EEG can substantiate; partner often reports and individual not aware of movements, just insomnia and sleepiness; common in middle age

[a]The DSM system would classify this under "Parasomnia Not Otherwise Specified"
[b]*Restless legs syndrome* consists of nocturnal akathisia limited to lower limbs, also causing insomnia; almost all individuals with nocturnal myoclonus have restless legs syndrome, but not vice versa.

- Continue to **Disorders Section, Sleep Disorders,** or
- Continue to **Appendix 7, Biopsychosocial Management of Insomnia**

Module 12

Sexual Problems

Orienting Notes

- The DSM system categorizes sexual problems according to a large and complicated classification scheme.
- However, the underlying logic is straightforward and based on symptom description.
- Attention to a few characteristics can guide the clinician quickly through the daunting array.
- Think of sexual disorders as grouped into three main categories:
  - Disorders of *drive* (DSM Sexual Dysfunctions)
  - Disorders of *direction* (DSM Paraphilias)
  - Disorders of *match* (DSM Gender Identity Disorders)
- It is of great importance to identify other treatable psychiatric disorders presenting as apparently isolated sexual complaints:
  - Depressive disorders (see *Module 1*)
  - Anxiety disorders (see *Module 3*)
  - Personality disorders (see *Module 15*)
  - Adjustment disorders (see *Module 15*)
  - Neuroses (see *Module 15*).

Differential Diagnosis

- Depressive disorders (see *Module 1*)
- Anxiety disorders (see *Module 3*)
- Personality disorders (see *Module 15*)
- Adjustment disorders (see *Module 15*)
- Neuroses (see *Module 15*).
- Medical illnesses (see *Panel 5*)
- Medication side effects (see *Panel 6*)

Panel 1: Categorizing Sexual Problems

Consider sexual problems as belonging to one of three categories:

- Disorders of *drive* (DSM Sexual Dysfunctions)
  - Low desire or impaired performance
  - Pain with performance
- Disorders of *direction* (DSM Paraphilias)
  - Urges or behaviors directed toward inappropriate objects
- Disorders of *match* (DSM Gender Identity Disorder)
  - Symptoms or dysfunction due to desire to be, or behave as, the opposite sex

- Continue to **Panel 2.**

Panel 2: Normal Sexual Response:

- Normal sexual intercourse stages (Masters and Johnson):
  - Excitement (arousal)
  - Plateau (maximal preorgasm arousal)
  - Orgasm
  - Refractory period
- Normal sexual intercourse stages (Helen Singer Kaplan):
  - Desire
  - Excitement (arousal)
  - Orgasm
- In aging:
  - Men: slower to erection, longer refractory period
  - Women: less vaginal lubrication

- Continue to **Panel 3.**

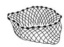

Panel 3: Screening for Sexual Problems

- Questions about sexual function are highly socially valenced (see *Section I, Biopsychosocial Assessment, Panel 13*).
  - If a presenting complaint, be aware that the specific queries needed to make a diagnosis may cause discomfort in the individual—even if they want help with the problem.
  - If not a presenting complaint, address relevant sexual issues once a reasonable treatment alliance has been established.
  - Remember to use *normalizing strategies* in your questioning.
- Some screening queries:
  - "Are you satisfied with your sex life?"
  - "Are sexual difficulties causing any problems in your life?"
- To further characterize dysfunction:
  - Problems with desire?
  - Problems with performance?
    - Erection/lubrication?
      - For men: ever awake with an erection?
    - Orgasm: Too late? Too early?
    - Pain?
  - Since when?
  - Any precipitants (e.g., medications, illnesses, surgery, depression, life changes)?
  - How often?
  - Under what circumstances?
  - Your partner's reaction?
    - What is your interpretation of what they feel and do?
    - Now, what is the reality?
  - Your reaction?
  - Secondary fall-out in relationship?
- If screen-positive for possible paraphilia or gender identity disorder:
  - Has this caused social problems?
  - Has this caused legal problems?
- Have you seen anyone for treatment (clinical, pastoral, other)?
- What have you tried on your own (herbs, devices, other people's medications, etc.)?

- If primarily a disorder of drive, continue to **Panel 4.**
- If primarily a disorder of direction, go to **Panel 8.**
- If primarily a disorder of match, go to **Panel 9.**

Panel 4: Sexual Drive Problems: Primary or Secondary or "Pseudo-Primary"?

- The clinician's first task is to rule out psychiatric and medical disorders that cause sexual problems, particularly in Disorders of Drive (i.e., *desire* or *performance*).
- Sexual problems may be the presenting "tip of the iceberg" of more extensive, treatable psychiatric illnesses:
  - Individuals often don't think in "syndromes" like clinicians do; for example, they may not even know the words *depression* or *anxiety*.
  - Presenting symptoms—sexual or otherwise—are those that are most evident, or most troubling, to the individual.
  - Therefore, it is of great importance to screen individuals who present with sexual complaints with a good medical (*Panels 5* and *6*) and psychiatric Review of Systems.
- Most common among psychiatric disorders with sexual drive reductions are:
  - Depressive disorders (*Module 1*)
  - Anxiety disorders (*Module 3*)
  - Neuroses and interpersonal conflicts (*Module 15*)

Note: As discussed in *Module 15*, the term *neurosis* was expurgated from the DSM system for a number of reasons. The DSM also does not handle interpersonal relationship problems very well. These decisions have led to both benefits and detriments. One detriment is that findings that are obvious symptoms of underlying intrapsychic or interpersonal difficulties are elevated to the status of "disorder" and disconnected from the other clinically relevant findings, and likely mechanisms. This is especially true of sexual findings, because according to the DSM system, a "primary" sexual disorder is diagnosed, even if the symptoms are due to intrapsychic or interpersonal problems. *With sexual symptoms, always look for more extensive intrapsychic or interpersonal findings.* See also *Module 15*.

- Any medical illness can cause sexual problems by virtue of:
  - Fatigue.
  - Anxiety.
  - Medications that reduce sexual drive or performance.
  - Occasionally, specific medical illnesses may have reduced sexual drive or performance as a symptom.

- To screen for underlying psychiatric disorders, use the relevant high-sensitivity screening questions from the appropriate **Modules.**
- To rule out medical illnesses that may present as isolated disorders of sexual drive, go to **Panel 5.**
- To identify medications that may reduce sexual drive or performance, go to **Panel 6.**
- If the sexual findings appear to be part of broader intrapsychic or interpersonal problems, go to **Module 15.**
- Otherwise, go to **Panel 7.**

103

Panel 5: Medical Illnesses that May Present as Disorders of Sexual Drive

Cardiac

- Abdominal aortic aneurysm
- Congestive heart failure

  Gastrointestinal

- Cirrhosis (hypogonadism)
- Postsurgical
- Radiation therapy

Genitourinary

- Women:
  - Vaginitis
  - Endometriosis
  - Polycystic ovary disease
  - Pelvic inflammatory disease
- Men:
  - Varicocele
  - Prostatectomy
- Either:
  - Cystectomy
  - Retroperitoneal resection

Neurologic

- Epilepsy (especially temporal lobe)
- Multiple sclerosis
- Parkinson disease
- Peripheral neuropathies
- Spinal cord injury
- Spinal disk disease
- Stroke

Hematologic

- Sickle cell disease

Endocrine

- Addison disease
- Diabetes
- Hypogonadism
- Hypo/hyperthyroidism

Metabolic

- Malnutrition
- Lead poisoning
- Heavy metal toxicity
- Herbicide exposure

- Continue to **Panel 6.**

Panel 6: Medications that May Reduce Sexual Drive

Cardiovascular
Beta-blockers
Clonidine
Digoxin
Hydrochlorthiazide
Methyldopa
Spironolactone
Endocrine
Estrogen (in men)
Progesterone
Gastrointestinal
Cimetadine
Neurologic and Pain Management Agents
Anticonvulsants
Carisoprodol
Dopaminergic drugs
Opiates
Psychotropics
Anticonvulsants
Barbiturates
Benzodiazepines
Carisoprodol
Lithium
Monoamine oxidase inhibitors
Neuroleptics (***Note:*** Thioridazine, mesoridazine: retrograde ejaculation)
Opiates
Serotonin reuptake inhibitors (***Note:*** Extremely common!)
Tricyclic antidepressants (***Note:*** Trazodone may cause priapism.)
Drugs of Abuse
Alcohol
Barbiturates
Cannabis
Cocaine
Opiates

- Continue to **Panel 7.**

Panel 7: Characterizing Primary Disorders of Sexual *Drive* (Sexual Dysfunctions)

- Sexual desire disorders
  - Hypoactive sexual desire disorder
    - Key characteristic: low drive, desire, fantasy—accounting for current age, social situation
  - Sexual aversion disorder
    - Key characteristic: avoidance of/aversion to genital contact with a sex partner
- Sexual arousal disorders
  - Female sexual arousal disorder
    - Key characteristic: inability to maintain adequate *physical* response during intercourse (e.g., swelling, lubrication)
  - Male erectile disorder
    - Key characteristic: analogue of female sexual arousal disorder—that is, inability to maintain adequate *physical* response during intercourse (i.e., erection)

Note: Of the sources of male impotence, 30% are organic, 40% psychogenic, 25% both, and 5% other.

- Orgasmic disorders
  - Female orgasmic disorder
    - Key characteristic: persistent delay in or absence of orgasm during sexual intercourse
  - Male orgasmic disorder
    - Key characteristic: analogue of female orgasmic disorder
  - Premature ejaculation
    - Key characteristic: ejaculation with minimal sexual stimulation or before the man wishes it, accounting for social situation
- Sexual pain disorders
  - Dyspareunia
    - Key characteristic: recurrent genital pain associated with intercourse for either male or female
  - Vaginismus
    - Key characteristic: persistent, involuntary vaginal spasm that interferes with intercourse

- Go to **Panel 10.**

Panel 8: Characterizing Primary Disorders of Sexual *Direction* (Paraphilias)

Note: In querying for these disorders, be sure to assess for broader interpersonal difficulties, including personal or relationship problems or personality disorders (see *Module 15*).

- Exhibitionism
  - Key characteristic: exposing one's genitals to a stranger because of sexual arousal, or distress over such urges
- Fetishism
  - Key characteristic: recurrent sexual urges/fantasies/behaviors involving nonliving objects [except as part of dressing as the opposite sex ("cross-dressing"); see "transvestic fetishism" below]
- Frotteurism
  - Key characteristic: rubbing or touching one's genitals against a non-consenting partner, or distress over such urges
- Pedophilia
  - Key characteristic: sexual activity with a prepubescent child (typically ≤ 13 years old), or distress over such urges
- Sexual masochism
  - Key characteristic: recurrent sexual urges/fantasies/behaviors involving being humiliated or made to suffer
- Sexual sadism
  - Key characteristic: recurrent sexual urges/fantasies/behaviors involving making another suffer physically or psychologically
- Transvestic fetishism
  - Key characteristic: recurrent sexual urges/fantasies/behaviors involving dressing as the opposite sex
- Voyeurism
  - Key characteristic: recurrent sexual urges/fantasies/behaviors involving observation of an unsuspecting person who is naked, disrobing, or engaging in sexual activity

Note: Recall that disorders are not typically diagnosed unless they cause notable dysfunction or cause distress. Thus, if these behaviors do not cause distress or dysfunction, disorders are not typically diagnosed. Examples:

- Cross-dressing for sexual stimulation without a sense of distress
- Sadistic or masochistic sexual practices between consenting partners without a sense of distress or coercion.

- Go to **Panel 10.**

**Panel 9: Characterizing Primary Disorders
of Sexual *Match* (Gender Identity Disorder)**

Note: In querying for these disorders, be sure to assess for broader
interpersonal difficulties, including personal or relationship problems or
personality disorders (see *Module 15*).

Key characteristics:

- Persistent desire to be or belief one is in essence of the opposite sex
- Desire without any obvious cultural advantage or primary/secondary
  gain (see *Module 14* for discussion of primary/secondary gain)
- Persistent discomfort with current sex
- History of or current identification with the opposite sex, for example
  by:
  - Preference for cross-dressing
  - Current/childhood preference for cross-sex role in make-believe
    games/pastimes
  - Childhood strong preference for playmates of opposite sex

Note: According to the DSM system, a diagnosis of gender identity
disorder is not made in the context of gender reassignment procedures or
other "intersex condition." It is also open to question whether this disorder will continue at all in the next DSM version.

- For full criteria for gender identity disorder, see **Disorders Section**, page 228.
- Continue to **Panel 10.**

Panel 10: Treatment Planning for Sexual Problems in General

- The overall approach for this module, as for other modules, is to:
  - Identify and minimize causative factors, including:
    - Medical problems
    - Medications
    - Psychiatric problems
  - Treat symptoms that represent primary disorders
- Medical disorders: treatment focuses on:
  - Addressing underlying physiologic pathology
  - Minimizing fear, anxiety, fatigue, pain and other medical symptoms
- Medication side effects: treatment focuses on:
  - Substituting medications with fewer sexual side effects (e.g., serotonin reuptake inhibitor antidepressants may be replaced by tricyclic or monoamine oxidase inhibitor antidepressants or bupropion).
  - If this fails, and there are no contraindications, adding adjuvant medication to minimize sexual side effects. Examples with serotonin reuptake inhibitors:
    - Bupropion 75 to 200 mg every morning
    - Cyproheptadine 8 mg taken an hour prior to intercourse

Note: Neither drug is approved by the U.S. Food and Drug Administration for this indication. It is preferable to simply switch drugs and save the individual the additional cost, inconvenience, and exposure to side effects of adding a second drug. See *Treatment Section* for options.

- Psychiatric disorders: treatment focuses on:
  - Treating the underlying depressive, anxiety, or other disorder
  - Addressing the underlying personal/relationship problems due to adjustment disorders, neuroses, or personality disorders

- Continue to **Panel 11.**

Panel 11: Treatment Planning for Primary Sexual Disorders

- At least as arcane and foreboding as the classification of sexual problems is the area of "sex therapy."
  - As with other areas of psychiatry, there exist specialized treatments given by experts.
  - As with other areas of psychiatry, there are common-sense strategies that any trained clinician can implement that will help a large proportion of individuals.
- Among the primary sexual disorders above, consider treatment strategies as either:
  - **Facilitation strategies:** for the sexual dysfunctions and for the other sexual disorders where distress or dysfunction are caused by personal and noncriminal, nondamaging behaviors.
  - **Limitation strategies:** for those disorders where potentially criminal or damaging behaviors are involved.
    - Examples include nonconsenting sadism and pedophilia.
    - Treatment strategies must involve containment and may involve legal notifications (see *Module 6, Panel 13* in particular).
    - Specialist treatment is typically required and is not further discussed here.

- Continue to **Panel 12.**

Panel 12: Facilitation Strategies for Primary Sexual Disorders

- Most individuals requesting treatment for primary sexual disorders will have disorders of drive (i.e., sexual dysfunctions).
- It bears repeating that disorders of drive will commonly present as the tip of the iceberg for personal/relationship problems that need to be treated in their own right. However, for isolated primary disorders of drive, the ***ADEPT*** mnemonic can guide the clinician:
- **A**dd information, educate
- **D**ecrease performance pressure
- **E**xperimentation/strategies
- **P**ermission
- **T**oys/aids

- **Add information, educate**

Frequently, it can be helpful simply to provide information regarding sexual norms, expectations, and even specifics of physiologic function (e.g., the Kinsey Report indicates that typical sexual intercourse lasts 7 minutes and that it takes men between 30 seconds and 15 minutes to reach ejaculation). This can reduce anxiety, self-deprecation, or other emotions, and realign expectations. It is typically most helpful to work with a couple, not just the index individual.

- **Decrease performance pressure**

This should not be overlooked as a key precipitant to the vicious cycle of performance problems leading to increased pressure to perform leading to symptoms leading to more performance problems leading to . . . And so the cycle goes, until complete avoidance of physical intimacy results. With a supportive partner, frank discussion of feelings and expectations can often help to reduce this potent cause of dysfunction.

- **Experimentation/strategies**

Experimentation with different sexual techniques, positions, settings may help with desire, arousal, and orgasm or with specific problems. Techniques include, for example, varying the setting of intercourse, changing foreplay habits, and trying different positions for intercourse. Specific techniques may help for premature ejaculation (stop/start techniques as orgasm nears), vaginismus, or pain (e.g., lubricants).

- **Permission**

Permission—verbal assent from a supportive partner—can be an important therapeutic component of reducing performance pressure, experimenting, or (below) use of sexual aids. Do not overlook the importance of supportive communication between the partners—your primary intervention is support and modeling of acceptance and communication in the office, which hopefully will carry over to their bedroom.

- **Toys/aids**

Sexual aids ("toys") can help in stimulation, in changing routine, in giving and receiving permission, in stimulating healthy fantasies, and in sharing. In some situations such as vaginismus, aids can be very helpful (e.g., objects of graduated size from fingers to dilators). In addition, aids now include pharmacologic aids such as sildenafil (Viagra).

Note: Several of the strategies above may apply to individuals with disorders of direction (i.e., paraphilias), although by and large, treatment of paraphilias *without* a primary personal/relationship problem is left to specialists in sex therapy.

Panel 13: Specialized Treatments for Primary Sexual Disorders

Specialized therapies for specific primary sexual disorders are not covered here. These may include specific psychotherapies or specific pharmacotherapies (e.g., alprostadil or sildenafil for male erectile disorder or female gonadal steroids for pedophilia and related sexual disorders). Further information on these issues can be found in the sexual disorders section of the *Key References*.

Module 13

Chronic Pain and Its Management in "The House of Pain"

Orienting Notes

- Pain is a subjective experience.
- Pain can be acute or chronic; the former rarely comes to psychiatric attention, so our focus will be the latter.
  - The valid subjective experience of chronic pain does not correlate well with objective findings on computed tomography, magnetic resonance imaging, radiography, and so forth.
- Pain is routinely undertreated. This is especially true in vulnerable populations:
  - The elderly
  - Those with terminal diseases
- Pain is routinely overtreated with opiates and other addictive substances.
- A key pain treatment principle:
  - *Antiinflammatory agents* (e.g., NSAIDs, aspirin) are analgesic.
  - *Analgesics* (e.g., acetaminophen, opiates) are *not* antiinflammatory.
- And two more:
  - It's hard to relieve pain if you don't remove the cause.
  - Standing, rather than as-needed (p.r.n.) doses of pain medications are preferable for chronic pain.
- Treatable psychiatric disorders can exacerbate pain and warrant treatment.

Differential Diagnosis

Treatable Psychiatric Disorders that May Worsen Independent Pain

Depressive disorders (see *Module 1*)

Anxiety disorders (see *Module 3*)

Situational fear, including adjustment disorders (see *Disorders Section,* page 204)

Psychiatric Disorders that May Produce Pain as a Prominent Symptom

Somatoform and related disorders (see *Module 14*)

Sexual disorders (see *Module 12*)

Factitious disorders and malingering (see *Module 14*)

Panel 1: The Simple-Minded Clinician's Guide to Pain

- The pain pathway has three steps:

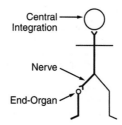

- Treatments can target any or all steps

- Continue to **Panel 2.**

Panel 2: Queries in Chronic Pain Assessment

- What sites?
- How severe?
  - Simple quantitative scales can help track response to treatment:
    - Visual analogue scale (put an "X" on a 100-mm line that runs from "no pain" to "worst pain I've ever felt.")
    - Likert scale (0–10, with same anchor points), either written or verbal.

No   Worst pain
pain   I've ever felt

  - Do no more frequently than each evening, summing over the past 24 hours (more frequent increases obsessiveness).
- How frequently?
- What makes worse?
- What makes better?
- What functional limitations do pain cause? Examples:
  - Sleeping
  - Walking
  - Carrying
  - Work roles
  - Family role disruption?
  - Hobby reduction?

- Continue to **Panel 3.**

Panel 3: Approach to Chronic Pain Treatment Planning

- Two major types of chronic pain:
  - Mechanical (due to ongoing end-organ dysfunction). Examples:
    - Degenerative disk disease
    - Osteoarthritis
  - Neuropathic (due to nerve signaling and/or central integration)
    - Phantom limb pain
    - Diabetic neuropathy
- Treatment options differ somewhat for mechanical versus neuropathic pain.
- Frequently, there are components of both.
- Treatment logic:
  - Remove/minimize the inciting/perpetuating factors.
  - Treat the residual pain.
- Treatments may be:
  - Nonpharmacologic
  - Pharmacologic

- The "**House of Pain**" provides a coherent approach to treating chronic pain.
- Continue to **Panel 4.**

Panel 4: The House of Pain: Overview

- The stable House of Pain includes a well built:
  - Foundation
  - Ground floor
  - Upper floor
  - Attic

INTACT HOUSE OF PAIN

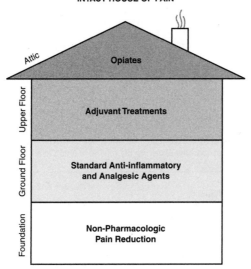

- However, many pain regimens start at the attic.
- Without a solid foundation and substructure, the plan will collapse:

CRUMBLED HOUSE OF PAIN

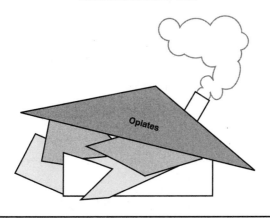

• Continue to **Panel 5** for construction plans for the stable House of Pain.

Panel 5: The House of Pain: Foundation

• The foundation consists of **nonpharmacologic methods to reduce the inciting factors.**
• This includes:
  • Removing cause of pain. Examples:
    • Ergonomic changes to reduce carpal tunnel
    • Work duty change to minimize back stress
    • Lifestyle/exercise change to reduce stress on degenerative knee
  • Reducing sequelae of pain. Examples:
    • Heat/cold
    • Immobilization and bracing
    • Physical therapy

Note: It is impressive how many pain regimens jump directly to pharmacologic treatment *without* reducing ongoing pain precipitants—for example, one will never "cure" carpal tunnel syndrome with antiinflammatory agents without changing the repetitive strain itself.

• Continue to **Panel 6.**

Panel 6: The House of Pain: Ground Floor

- The Ground Floor consists of *standing* **antiinflammatory or analgesic agents.**
- For chronic pain, standing dosing is preferable to p.r.n.[a] (as-needed) dosing:
  - Stop pain before it starts—otherwise you're always "playing catch-up."
  - Consider as-needed dosing the "stairway" from the basement to the ground floor.
- *For inflammatory processes, antiinflammatory agents are preferable to pure analgesics (acetaminophen/Tylenol).*
- Antiinflammatory agent classes include:
  - Aspirin—Don't neglect this: it works for pain!
  - Nonsteroidal antiinflammatory drugs (NSAIDs)
    - Nonselective prostaglandin cyclooxygenase (COX) inhibitors
      - Examples: ibuprofen (Motrin, Advil), naproxyn (Naprosyn), sulindac (Clinoril)
    - Highly selective COX-2 inhibitors
      - Examples: celecoxib (Celebrex), rofecoxib (Vioxx)
    - Relatively selective COX-2 inhibitors
      - Examples: etodolac (Lodine), nabumetone (Relafen)
  - All are efficacious. Costs and benefits differ:
    - Aspirin
      - Plus: low cost
      - Minus: gastrointestinal side effects, tinnitus (ringing in ears)
    - NSAIDs
      - Plus: low cost
      - Minus: gastrointestinal side effects, medication interactions (e.g., lithium)
    - Highly selective COX-2 inhibitors:
      - Plus: few gastrointestinal side effects
      - Minus: high cost, hepatic toxicity
    - Relatively selective COX-2 inhibitors:
      - Plus/minus: midway between (non)selectives in side effects and cost
  - Try multiple agents in a class before giving up.

[a] p.r.n.: "pro rerum natura," "according to the nature of things"

- Continue to **Panel 7.**

Panel 7: The House of Pain: Upper Floor

- If several days to weeks with a solid foundation and ground floor does not sufficiently reduce pain, additional **adjuvant treatments** may be necessary.
- Adjuvant treatments are aimed at:
  - End-organ mechanical processes
  - Neuropathic sources or contributions
- Adjuvant treatments are:
  - Nonpharmacologic
  - Pharmacologic
- To address end-organ mechanical processes:
  - Steroid injections
  - Oral steroids
  - Capsaicin cream
  - Muscle relaxants (only if prominent spasm)
    - Diazepam
    - Baclofen
    - Butalbital
    - Cyclobenzaprine
    - Carisoprodol (*Note:* Metabolized to meprobamate; may lead to barbiturate dependence)
- To address neuropathic sources or contributions:
  - Tricyclic antidepressants
    - Low doses may work, although full doses may be required.
    - Work in the absence of depressive symptoms.
    - Serotonin reuptake inhibitors don't work.
  - Selected anticonvulsants
    - Carbamazepine
    - Phenytoin
    - Perhaps:
      - Clonazepam
      - Gabapentin
      - Valproate
  - Nerve blocks
  - Acupuncture/acupressure
  - Transcutaneous electrical nerve stimulation (TENS)
- Other culturally specific nonallopathic interventions

Note: Depending on cultural setting and individual preference, certain upper floor interventions, particularly acupuncture, may be moved to the ground floor, that is, become primary interventions.

- Continue to **Panel 8.**

Panel 8: The House of Pain: Attic

- For chronic pain that has not responded despite a solid foundation, ground floor, and upper floor, **standing or as-needed opiates** comprise the attic.
  - Standing doses are often appropriate for chronic pain.
  - As with NSAIDs, use standing doses to stop pain before it starts
- Remember (see *Module 5*):
  - Tolerance and withdrawal (beyond recurrence of pain) are risks and are *physiologically* based.
  - Dependence is a *behavioral* disorder.
  - Standing doses may, paradoxically, be better for those with addictive tendencies (e.g., obsessive pain vigilance, less looking for the drug, waiting for effect, etc.).
- No role for barbiturates/benzodiazepines (except as specifically noted above).

Note: For details regarding selection of opiates, go to *Appendix 9, Guide to Oral Opiate Selection for Chronic Pain.*

- Continue to **Pain Management Summary, Panel 9.**

Panel 9: The Stable House of Pain

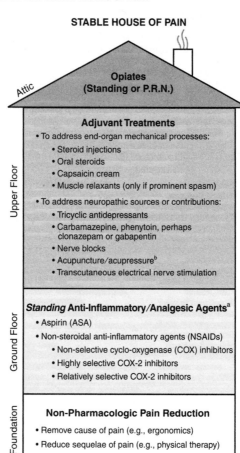

STABLE HOUSE OF PAIN

Attic

**Opiates
(Standing or P.R.N.)**

Adjuvant Treatments
- To address end-organ mechanical processes:
  - Steroid injections
  - Oral steroids
  - Capsaicin cream
  - Muscle relaxants (only if prominent spasm)
- To address neuropathic sources or contributions:
  - Tricyclic antidepressants
  - Carbamazepine, phenytoin, perhaps clonazepam or gabapentin
  - Nerve blocks
  - Acupuncture/acupressure[b]
  - Transcutaneous electrical nerve stimulation

Upper Floor

***Standing* Anti-Inflammatory/Analgesic Agents[a]**
- Aspirin (ASA)
- Non-steroidal anti-inflammatory agents (NSAIDs)
  - Non-selective cyclo-oxygenase (COX) inhibitors
  - Highly selective COX-2 inhibitors
  - Relatively selective COX-2 inhibitors

Ground Floor

Non-Pharmacologic Pain Reduction
- Remove cause of pain (e.g., ergonomics)
- Reduce sequelae of pain (e.g., physical therapy)

Foundation

[a] For *pure* neuropathic pain, when anti-inflammatory agents may not be required, consider the House of Pain a raised ranch!

[b] As per Panel 7, cultural or individual preference factors may move some non-pharmacologic interventions to the Ground Floor.

Note: For *pure* neuropathic pain, when antiinflammatory agents may not be required, consider the House of Pain a raised ranch!

- For additional information on comprehensive pain assessment and management, see *Key References.*
  - Borsook et al.
  - McCaffery and Pasero

Module 14

Multiple Unexplained Physical Complaints

Orienting Notes

- Individuals with difficult-to-explain physical symptoms are frequently encountered in mental health, primary care, and medical/surgical in-patient settings.
- Their presentation is often confusing.
- Not surprisingly, the DSM classification system is also confusing.
- The overall assessment strategy is:
  - First, rule out nonsomatoform disorders.
  - Then assess, categorize, and treat the somatoform disorder(s).
- Somatization disorders are *not* diagnoses of exclusion. A psychologic component contributing to the presentation *must* be identified.
  - This module discusses clinical presentations that closely dovetail with those in several other modules (see *Differential Diagnosis*).
- Take particular care in assessing pain: The subjective perception of pain does not correlate well with "objective" physical findings; pain "disorders" are diagnosed *only* if psychologic symptoms can be demonstrated to have a key role in producing the pain.

Differential Diagnosis

Disorders not Primarily Somatoform
- Depressive disorders (see *Module 1,* page 17)
- Anxiety disorders (see *Module 3,* page 28)
  - Panic disorder (see *Disorders Section* page 174)
  - GAD (see *Disorders Section,* page 180)
- Psychosis (see *Module 4,* page 36)
- Medical syndromes
- Pain inadequately treated (see *Module 13*)

Somatoform Disorders and Related Disorders
- Somatization disorder (see *Disorders Section,* page 210)
- Hypochondriasis (see *Disorders Section,* page 214)
- Pain disorder (see *Disorders Section,* page 212)
- Factitious disorder (see *Disorders Section,* page 217)
- Malingering (not officially a DSM system disorder)
- Anorexia nervosa (see *Disorders Section,* page 220)
- Bulimia (see *Disorders Section,* page 221)
- Body dysmorphic disorder (see *Disorders Section*, page 218)

Panel 1: Organizing Queries about Physical Complaints

A number of nonsomatoform psychiatric disorders can present primarily with physical complaints. Classic examples include:

- Major depressive disorder
- Panic disorder
- Medical disorders must be ruled out with appropriate evaluation and consultation.

- If psychiatric disorders are suspected, go to appropriate **Module.**
- If medical syndromes and psychiatric disorders have been ruled out, continue to **Panel 2.**

Panel 2: Sorting through Disorders that Present Primarily with Physical Complaints

- If the complaints are primarily related to weight or a specific aspect of appearance, go to *Module 10.*
- To be considered a somatoform disorder, there must be a positive identification of a psychologic component that produces, maintains, or exacerbates the symptom.
  - Somatoform disorders are *not* diagnoses of exclusion.
  - Some symptoms are, simply, unexplained for a time.
  - Leaving them unexplained is preferable to labeling them "psychosomatic," which tends to end critical diagnostic consideration.

- Do the findings appear to be produced *de novo* by the individual out of nothing, that is, "made up" or "faked"?
- Or do they appear to be a secondary elaboration, concern, or focus of an existing, plausible complaint?
- In the case of unexplained *signs* (findings observed by the clinician), the clinician is directed toward the former. Examples include:
  - Seizures
  - Weakness
  - Numbness
  - Fainting
  - Unexplained bleeding
  - Unexplained diarrhea
- In the case of unexplained *symptoms* (the individual's report of subjective sensations to the clinician), either is possible. Examples include:
  - Abdominal pain
  - Bloating
  - Headaches
  - Joint pain
  - Reports of the above signs

- If the findings appear by clinical judgment to be produced *de novo* by the individual, go to **Panel 3.**
- If the findings appear by clinical judgment to be exacerbations or overinterpretations of existing physical symptoms, go to **Panel 5.**

Panel 3: Findings that Appear to be Produced *de novo* by the Individual

- Is the individual judged to produce the findings *unconsciously* (i.e., without clear choice or intent)?
  - If so, the diagnosis is most likely conversion disorder.

Note: Conversion disorder may coexist with other similar, physiologically based disorders; for example, pseudo-seizures most commonly are found in individuals with a documented seizure disorder.

- Is the individual judged to produce the findings voluntarily, consciously?
- If so, what does the individual seek to gain?
  - Continuation of the patient or sick role?
    - This is considered *primary gain.*
    - If so, the diagnosis is most likely factitious disorder. Go to *Disorders Section,* page 217.
  - Some other type of end; e.g., compensation, sick time, avoidance of duty or responsibility?
    - This is considered *secondary gain.*
    - If so, the diagnosis is most likely malingering. Go to *Disorders Section,* page 217.

- If the likely diagnosis is conversion disorder, go to **Disorders Section,** page 215.
- Otherwise, continue to **Panel 4.**

Panel 4: Notes on Factitious Disorder and Malingering

- Factitious disorder is diagnosed when an individual manufactures symptoms or findings in order to continue in the sick role, without prominent role of secondary gain.
  - "Münchausen's syndrome" is another name for factitious disorder, named after the 18th century German soldier, traveler, and teller of fantastic tails.
  - Findings can be complex or simple, evanescent or tenaciously consistent.
  - Individuals can go to great lengths to produce clinical findings. For example:
    - Laxatives to produce diarrhea
    - Injection of pyrogens to produce fever
    - Ingestion of blood to mimic gastrointestinal bleeding
    - Fabrication of medical records
  - Individuals sometimes have studied the disorder they take on and can produce accurate emulation of complex, multisystem disorders.
  - Psychiatric syndromes also can be feigned in factitious disorder.
  - Note that factitious disorder also can be by proxy (also called "Münchausen's by proxy"), particularly if the individual being presented for treatment is a child or elderly person.
    - The criterion here is whether the individual fabricates the findings, so that he or she can remain involved with the medical system (vs. for secondary gain, such as compensation).
    - Legal issues may arise and state law may require the clinician to report findings to the relevant social service agency (e.g., departments of elderly affairs, youth/family services).
- Malingering is not classified "officially" as a disorder in the DSM system.
  - However, both malingering and factitious disorder have as their core finding the manufacture of symptoms.
  - The differentiation is in the end that is desired:
    - Primary gain: factitious disorder
    - Secondary gain: malingering

- If factitious disorder, go to **Disorders Section,** page 217.
- If malingering, go to **Disorders Section,** page 217.

127

Panel 5: Findings that Appear to be Exaggerations or Overinterpretations

- Does the individual's concern focus on a specific symptom or cluster of symptoms?
  - If the focus is primarily pain, the diagnosis is likely pain disorder (if pain is the focus).
  - If other symptoms or findings are the focus, the diagnosis is likely hypochondriasis.
- Does the individual have a history of *many* complaints across *multiple* systems? Did the complaints begin before age 30?
  - If so, the diagnosis is likely somatization disorder.

- If likely hypochondriasis or somatization disorder, continue to **Panel 6.**
- If likely pain disorder, go to **Panel 7.**

Panel 6: Notes on Hypochondriasis and Somatization Disorder

- The terms *hypochondriasis* and *somatization* are often used imprecisely, even colloquially.
- However, the disorders differ substantially in presentation and course.
  - Hypochondriasis: The individual has a specific symptom and misinterprets it.
    - Examples:
      - Rectal bleeding due to hemorrhoids produces fear of colon cancer.
      - Headaches produce fear of brain tumor.
    - Onset any age; may or may not be chronic.
  - Somatization: Many symptoms over multiple organ systems.
    - Onset in early adulthood or earlier; typically chronically symptomatic.
    - Fear/worry may or may not be a part of the presentation.

  Note: Each of these diagnoses assumes:

- Appropriate medical evaluation has been done.
- Medical evaluation does not substantiate the preoccupation.
- Reasonable reassurance has not diminished symptoms.

- If hypochondriasis, go to **Disorders Section,** page 214.
- If somatization disorder, go to **Disorders Section,** page 210.

Panel 7: Evaluating Pain

- Recall that the subjective experience of pain does not correlate well with objective findings (e.g., lower back pain does not correlate well with imaging findings of degenerative disk or other disease).
- Recall that pain is routinely undertreated.
- Recall that a diagnosis of somatoform disorder requires a positive identification of a psychologic component that initiates, maintains, and exacerbates the pain.
- Therefore, a diagnosis of pain disorder is made *only* if a psychologic component can be demonstrated.
- Pain disorder usually exists in the context of pain due to valid physiologic cause.

- For management of pain, go to **Module 13.**
- Some suggestions for managing psychologic components of pain are found in the **Disorders Section** under the entry for hypochondriasis, page 214.

Module 15

Relationship and Personal Problems

Orienting Notes

- Personal problems (e.g., "I don't like myself," "I am having trouble coping with stress") and relationship problems ("My wife and I aren't getting along," "I'm not coping well at work") are common reasons for presentation in mental health and primary care settings.
- These presenting complaints can represent a wide range of disorders, or no disorder at all (see *Differential Diagnosis*).
- Picking one's way through the assessment of such complaints can be time-consuming and frustrating.
- An efficient and accurate assessment strategy will include consideration of whether the complaints are:
  - Acute or chronic
  - Focal or general
  - Secondary to an underlying psychiatric disorder or not

Differential Diagnosis

- Adjustment disorder (see *Disorders Section,* page 204)
- Depressive disorders (see *Module 1*)
- Manic-depressive disorders (see *Module 2*)
- GAD (Generalized Anxiety Disorder) (see *Disorders Section,* page 180)
- Psychosis (see *Module 4*)
- Substance use disorders (see *Module 5*)
- Personality disorder (see *Disorders Section,* page 236)
- "Neurosis" (see *Panels 5–6*).

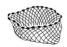

Panel 1: Approach to Assessing Relationship and Personal Problems

- Are the problems chronic, or time-limited with a defined onset?
- Are the problems focal and related only to a specific relationship or issue, or wide-ranging or pervasive?
- Examples:
  - Work is fine. Marriage has been a problem for the past 6 months (focal, time-limited).
  - Work and marriage have been problems for the past year (wide-ranging, time-limited).
  - Work and marriage have always been problems, so has child rearing, so have friendships (pervasive, chronic).

- If time-limited and focal, consider adjustment disorder. Go to **Disorders Section,** page 204.
- If time-limited and wide-ranging, strongly consider underlying psychiatric disorders. Continue to **Panel 2.**
- If chronic, go to **Panel 3.**

Panel 2: Psychiatric Disorders Presenting as Personal/Relationship Problems

- Personal and relationship problems are often the presenting "tip of the iceberg" of more extensive, treatable psychiatric illnesses:
  - Individuals often don't think in "syndromes" like clinicians do; for example, they may not even know the words *depression* or *anxiety*.
  - These are frequently the issue that is most evident, or most troubling, to the individual.
- Screening for psychiatric disorder is of great importance:
  - Useful treatments exist.
  - Presenting complaints are often not resolvable without treatment of the underlying disorder.
- If an underlying psychiatric disorder is responsible, the relationship and personal problems are typically not chronic and lifelong, but have their onset coincident with the disorder.

Note: Particularly during a major depressive episode or dysthymia, relationship and personal problems can be presented as chronic and pervasive—even if they are not. This is due to recall bias because of cognitive distortions ("I am a bad person . . . I've always been a bad person . . . I ruin all my relationships . . . and always have"). Remarkably, such an apparently "neurotic" approach to one's life and relationships may be fully reversible with appropriate treatment for depression.

- Screen for relevant psychiatric disorders in the **Differential Diagnosis** using the relevant **Modules.**
- If no underlying psychiatric disorders are identified, continue to **Panel 3.**

Panel 3: "Official" Categorization of Primary Relationship/Personal Problems

The DSM system does not handle personal and relationship problems particularly well.

- The system accommodates such focal and time-limited problems that fall under the rubric of adjustment disorders.
- The system accommodates chronic and pervasive problems that fall under the rubric of personality disorders.
- However, other findings on the spectrum of personal and relationship problems are not well accommodated.
- "Neurosis" no longer officially exists in the DSM system, but it remains a useful construct (see *Panel 5*).

- Continue to **Panel 4.**

Panel 4: Personality Disorders

- The hallmarks of a personality disorder are relationship and/or personal problems presenting as beliefs and patterns of behaviors that are:
  - *Pervasive:* involving multiple relationships or domains in life
  - *Inflexible:* not easily changeable, despite failure or negative feedback
  - *Lifelong:* with onset in young adulthood or before
- A virtue of the DSM system is that it specifies explicit criteria by which a *positive* diagnosis is made.
  - The diagnosis of a personality disorder is categorical (either the individual has it or does not).
  - However, "personality *traits*" can be identified for subsyndromal but characteristic variants.

Note: This "dimensional" approach will likely turn out to be more accurate than the currently official "categorical" approach.

- Personality Disorders:
  - Are *not* diagnoses of exclusion.
  - Are *not* diagnosed based on the clinician's feelings toward the individual ("countertransference").
  - Do *not* have acute onset later in life (e.g., with debilitating medical illness or psychiatric disorder).
  - Personality disorders are grouped into three classes based on their characteristics:
    - Cluster A: the "odd"
    - Cluster B: the "dramatic"
    - Cluster C: the "anxious"

Note: Once a personality disorder diagnosis appears on a medical chart, it seldom comes off—be careful in using this persisting and often stigmatizing term!

- To assess criteria for individual personality disorders, go to **Disorders Section,** page 236.
- Otherwise, continue to **Panel 5.**

Panel 5: Neurosis and Its Continuing Utility

- For primary personal/relationship problems, there is much not covered between the focal, time-limited presentation of adjustment disorders and the chronic, pervasive presentation of personality disorders. The concept of neurosis remains helpful.
- *Neurosis* is a psychoanalytically derived term that designates patterns of symptoms or maladaptive behaviors that are:
  - produced by intrapsychic (internal) conflicts that
  - are due to conflicts that arise during development
  - are not in the individual's awareness (i.e., are "unconscious").
- The diagnosis implies that the *syndrome* (pattern of symptoms or maladaptive behaviors) is driven by a *mechanism* (unconscious conflicts laid down in childhood).
- The utility of the concept is that it encompasses relationship/personal findings that:
  - Are chronic
  - May be wide-ranging but are less pervasive than those of personality disorders
  - Cause suffering
  - May be amenable to certain types of psychotherapy, although not to medications.

- Continue to **Panel 6.**

**Panel 6: A Historical Note on Neuroses
and the DSM System**

- Neuroses were gradually expurgated from the DSM system as it moved away from explicit mention of "mechanisms" for disorders and toward its current "*atheoretic*" basis.
- Through DSM-III and DSM-IIIR (third edition and third revised edition), several disorders retained dual titles as "neuroses":
  - Anxiety or phobic neuroses (anxiety disorders)
  - Obsessive-compulsive neuroses (OCD)
  - Depressive neurosis (dysthymic disorder)
  - Hysterical neurosis (conversion disorder)
  - Hypochondriacal neurosis (hypochondriasis)
  - Depersonalization neurosis (depersonalization disorder)
- However, their designation as neuroses is no longer accurate either because:
  - Non-neurotic mechanisms have subsequently been identified as likely predominant for these disorders, and/or
  - Their criteria have evolved in the DSM-IV categorization scheme to designate a different syndrome.

- Although categorization, diagnosis, and psychotherapeutic management of neuroses are beyond the scope of this book, several modern, time-limited, manual-based, psychoanalytically derived psychotherapies are geared toward assessing and treating neurotic aspects of personal and relationship problems. Several can be found in the **Key References,** including those by:
  - Luborsky
  - Davanloo
  - Sifneos

135

Module 16

Competency

Orienting Notes

- "Competency" (or "competence," "capacity") is the ability to carry out a specific task. In the medical context, it refers to one's ability to make medical and self-care decisions.
- Competency is assessed with regard to a specific, individual decision, not globally.
- Competency is *not* determined by diagnosis, or even by score on cognitive tests such as the MMSE.
- Competency has legal and clinical components.
  - The role of the clinician, usually a physician and typically a psychiatrist, is to make a clinical assessment.
  - The final decision of how to proceed in an individual situation is based on legal precedent, which varies among jurisdictions.
- Four basic abilities must be established in order to establish competency:
  - To understand the relevant facts
  - To appreciate their relevance to one's own personal situation
  - To rationally manipulate the information to arrive at a choice
  - To communicate that choice
- Disagreements in decision making between an individual and clinician can often be resolved by utilizing a few basic strategies (see *Panel 9*).

Differential Diagnosis

- Unlike other modules, no specific diagnoses are listed here because:
  - Having a specific disorder does not mean that an individual is incompetent.
  - Even if symptoms of a disorder render an individual incompetent for a specific decision, they may be competent for other decisions.
  - Competency assessments may be required for individuals with any, or no, evident psychiatric diagnosis.
- Nonetheless, certain psychiatric symptoms may compromise competence around specific decisions. These include:
  - Delirium
  - Cognitive disorders, including mental retardation
  - Psychosis
  - Severe depression
  - Severe mania
  - Severe personality disorders
  - Substance use

Panel 1: Competency Decisions—Who Does What?

- Clinicians are frequently nervous about competency assessments because they believe that their decision will dictate treatment. *This is not correct!*
- Competency decisions have two components:
  - Clinical—determines decision-making *capacity*
  - Legal—exercises decision-making *authority*
- Legal procedures determine what will be done, based on:
  - Clinical competency assessment
  - Other societal and legal parameters that are independent of the clinician's assessment.
- The clinical component:
  - The clinician evaluating competency is usually a physician, and most typically a psychiatrist.
  - He or she *does not* decide what to do.
  - He or she *does* assess the individual clinically to determine whether the individual has the abilities necessary to make and communicate a rational decision about his or her own well-being.
- The legal component:
  - Using this clinical information, the legal system–based on its statutes and prior rulings–then determines whether decision making resides with the individual or passes to another agency (e.g., family, next of kin, health-care institution or representative).
  - This is based on legal precedent.
  - This varies from jurisdiction to jurisdiction.
  - The legal deliberations balance two sets of principles:
    - *Autonomy:* the individual's wishes are foremost (rights-driven).
    - *Beneficence:* the individual's well-being is foremost (treatment-driven)

- Continue to **Panel 2.**

Panel 2: Common Occasions for Competency Assessment

- Clinical competency assessment is frequently requested in the case of:
  - Refusal of medical/surgical treatment
  - Refusal of psychiatric treatment (see also *Module 6*)
  - Refusal of higher level of living support (e.g., nursing home)
  - Establishment of guardian of person (ongoing health-care and housing decision making)
  - Establishment of financial guardian
- The basic clinical competency assessment is the same.
- The subsequent legal procedures may differ (e.g., psychiatric treatment refusal may be handled in district court while finances/housing may be handled in probate).
- Disagreements between the individual and clinician can often be negotiated without recourse to legal means (see *Panel 9*).

Note: In many states, the physician is allowed to turn to surrogate decision makers (e.g., family) without consulting the courts in situations of medical urgency involving an individual who cannot make competent decisions.

- Continue to **Panel 3.**

Panel 3: The Basics of Clinical Competency Assessment

Note: This approach to clinical competency assessment draws heavily on that of Slavney and of Grisso and Appelbaum (see *Key References*).

- Establishment of competency requires **FIRM Communication:**
  - Understanding **F**acts
  - Appreciating personal **I**mplications
  - **R**ationally **M**anipulating the information
  - **Communication** of the decision in a coherent manner.

Note: What is critical is the *process* that an individual uses, not the *content* of the decision or the individual's values.

- Continue to **Panel 4.**

Panel 4: The Basic Abilities: Understanding Facts

An individual must be able to understand basic information about the illness in question and its treatment. For instance:

- Diabetes is a problem in controlling blood sugar.
- If it is untreated, nerves can be damaged, infections can occur easily, and amputations may be necessary.
- Diabetes can be treated with insulin injections.
- Proper use of insulin can make it less likely that complications of diabetes will occur.

- Continue to **Panel 5.**

Panel 5: The Basic Abilities: Appreciating Personal Implications

- An individual must understand and accept that the relevant generic information pertains to *his or her own specific situation.* For instance:
  - Yes, I have diabetes.
  - Yes, the doctors recommend that I use insulin.
  - Yes, I may have the following complications if I do not use insulin.
  - Yes, the doctors recommend that I have my right big toe removed.
- It is not uncommon for individuals to understand the facts in a rational manner but then deny their applicability to their own situation.
  - In its most obvious form, such *denial* can be seen in psychosis or dementia.
  - However, appreciation of personal implication of information is a graded ability rather than either/or and may be seen in other situations of limited insight (e.g., depression, severe personality disorders, mental retardation, or even adjustment disorders due to illness).

- Continue to **Panel 6.**

Panel 6: The Basic Abilities: Rationally Manipulating Information

- An individual must have a coherent and logical method for weighing the options, based on the information relevant to their specific case. The issue for clinical competency assessment is:
  - How they use the information at their disposal, that is:
  - *Not* the decision he or she comes to, but rather *how* he or she makes the decision.
- Typically, this involves an explicit weighing of the relative *risks* and *benefits* of available options, based on personal *values.* For instance:
  - I would rather avoid suffering the side effects of chemotherapy even though I know my life will be shorter.
  - I would rather live out my days in my apartment with some sense of autonomy than go to a nursing home, even though I know I may die much sooner without the support a nursing home would give me.
- The basis of an individual's decision making may not appear "rational" or "logical" in an intellectual sense, but if it has an internal rationale ("*ratio*" = order), then this ability is considered present. For instance:
  - I do not want my children immunized because my faith prohibits it.

Note: In some legal jurisdictions, weighted more toward *beneficence* than *autonomy,* legal factors may override an individual's wishes more readily than in others. This is *not* relevant to the *clinical* competency assessment: the clinical assessment seeks to determine whether the decision making has a logical basis.

- Even with understanding and appreciation, rational manipulation may fail. For instance:
  - Individuals may understand and appreciate their need for psychiatric hospitalization to remain safe, and they may *typically* place a high priority staying safe, yet may refuse to stay because of the need to pay bills that day, or because the food is poison, or because the staff are CIA operatives. Individuals may understand and appreciate their need for a nursing home for their well-being, and they may *typically* place a high priority on preserving their well-being, yet may want to go home to be with their cat.

- Continue to **Panel 7.**

Panel 7: The Basic Abilities: Communication of the Decision

- It goes (almost) without saying that the individual must be able to communicate his or her understanding and explicit choice.
- This is frequently not the case in delirium, and sometimes not the case in severe dementia or psychosis.

- Continue to **Panel 8.**

Panel 8: A Rubric to Elicit Competence Information

Grisso and Appelbaum (see *Key References*) provide a useful rubric by which to elicit information relevant to the abilities necessary to establish competence:

- *Disclose* information if necessary.
- *Inquire* about specifics to determine if they understand the facts and personal implications.
- *Probe* if the individual is not initially forthcoming with the needed information.
- Continue the cycle of *disclose/inquire/probe* until it is clear that the individual does or does not possess the competence ability in question.

- Continue to **Panel 9.**

Panel 9: Disagreements in Medical/Psychiatric Decision Making

- The psychiatrist is often called to "assess competence for medical decision making."
  - However, the agenda also often includes a request by the medical/surgical staff to "work with" or "talk to" the individual to solve the conflict.
  - This latter agenda on the part of the medical/surgical staff may be explicit or unspoken.
- Any skilled and empathic clinician is able to assess and negotiate around conflicts in decision making. "Talking with" an individual is not the special province of the psychiatrist.
- With a few simple considerations, a consultant "outsider" may not be necessary.

Note: This issue also comes up frequently in psychiatric treatment decision making (e.g., involuntary commitment, medication choice).

- Continue to **Panel 10.**

Panel 10: Getting to Yes: A Few Basics to Consider

- The individual owns the disease, not the clinician.
- A *collaborative* approach to joint decision making typically goes further than a paternalistic approach (see Collaborative Practice Model in *Section IV, Psychotherapy* and in *Key References*):
  - Establish *joint* treatment priorities based on:
  - *The individual's* values and needs, and
  - *The clinician's* technical expertise
- Make sure the individual understands what is going on.
  - An incredible amount of information bombards the individual during treatment, much of which we clinicians take as self-evident.
  - The individual is usually not in tip-top shape for information processing because of pain, fear, anxiety, and fatigue.
- Explain half as fast, and be twice as redundant, as you think you need to be.
- Explain half as fast, and be twice as redundant, as you think you need to be.
- Write down information; give education handouts regarding the condition and treatment.
- Involve the family or significant friends. They will often:
  - Provide additional clinical information
  - Provide essential values information
  - Be constructive in helping the individual make rational choices

---

Module 17

Assessment and Management of Psychotropic-Induced Movement Disorders

Orienting Notes

- Major psychotropic-induced movement disorders can be categorized as:
  - Neuroleptic-associated
    - Acute onset
      - Acute dystonia ("dystonic reaction")
      - Akathisia
      - Parkinsonism
    - Late onset (tardive)
      - Tardive dyskinesia
      - Tardive dystonia
  - Tremor associated with other psychotropics
- The term *extrapyramidal symptoms* (EPS) is typically used to encompass the three neuroleptic-associated acute-onset syndromes (acute EPS), and occasionally the tardive syndromes as well.
- Treatments of varying efficacy exist for each of these.
- The best strategy is prevention through minimization of exposure to the inciting drug.

Differential Diagnosis

Neuroleptic-Associated, Acute Onset

- Acute Dystonia
  - Catatonia (see *Module 7*)
  - Myoclonus
  - NMS (see *Module 7*)
  - OCD with compulsions (see *Module 3*)
  - Other movement disorders (e.g., Huntington disease)
  - Tic disorders
- Akathisia
  - Attention-deficit hyperactivity disorder (see *Module 9*)
  - Intoxication with alcohol or use/intoxication with stimulants (see *Module 5*)
  - Manic-depressive (bipolar) disorder with mania or hypomania (see *Disorder Section*, page 169)
  - Psychosis (see *Module 4*)
  - Withdrawal from alcohol or sedatives (see *Module 5*)
- Parkinsonism
  - Catatonia with hypokinesia (see *Module 7*).
  - Dementia with hypokinesia (see *Module 8*)
  - Major depressive episode with hypokinesia (see *Module 1*)
  - Idiopathic parkinsonism
  - Side effects or toxicity due to:
    - Carbon monoxide poisoning
    - Methyldopa
    - Manganese poisoning
    - MPTP (methylphenyltetrahydropyridine) (an Ecstasy-like "designer" drug)
    - Serotonin reuptake-inhibiting antidepressants
  - Tremor due to other psychotropics or medications
  - Schizophrenia with negative (hypokinetic) symptoms (see *Disorders Section*, page 197)

Neuroleptic-Associated Tardive Dyskinesia/Dystonia

- Catatonia (see *Module 7*)
- Myoclonus
- NMS (see *Module 7*)
- OCD with compulsions (see *Disorders Section*, page 182)
- Other movement disorders (e.g., Huntington disease)
- Tic disorders

Tremor Due to Other Psychotropics

- Alcohol/sedative withdrawal (see *Module 5*)
- Essential/familial tremor
- Generalized anxiety disorder (see *Disorders Section*, page 180)
- Hepatic cirrhosis with asterixis (see *Panel 1*)
- Panic disorder (see *Disorders Section*, page 174).
- Parkinsonism
- Stimulant use:
  - Beta-agonists (oral/inhaled)
  - Caffeine
  - Decongestants
  - Drugs of abuse (see *Module 5*)
  - Theophylline
- Tic disorders

Panel 1: Some Definitions

- *Akathisia:* Motor restlessness or subjective need to move described in *Panel 8.*
- *Akinesia:* Cessation of spontaneous motor movements.
- *Apical/axial:* Terms useful in describing the location of abnormal movements:
    - *Apical* movements are those that affect the upper or lower extremities.
    - *Axial* movements are those that affect the trunk and neck.
- *Asterixis:* Intermittent loss of muscle tone due to interruption of neuro-muscular transmission; characteristic of hepatic cirrhosis, where demonstrated by loss of muscle contraction during dorsiflexion of the wrist. May be related to more generalized *cataplexy* (see *Module 11, Panel 1*).
- *Athetosis:* Writhing, smooth, typically slow movements of the extremities, or less typically the trunk.
- *Chorea:* Jerky, nonrhythmic movements of the extremities, or less typically the trunk. Contrast with rhythmic *tremor* below.
- *Cogwheeling or cogwheel rigidity:* Ratcheting or "catching" during apical movements best detected on examination with thumb lightly pressed on biceps brachialis tendon. Characteristic of (but not specific for) parkinsonism.
- *Dyskinesia:* General term denoting "abnormal movements."
- *Dystonia/dystonic reaction:* Acute, sustained muscle spasm described in *Panel 6.*
- *Extrapyramidal symptoms:* A general term denoting movements due to abnormalities of central pathways not under voluntary control. Typically, the term is applied specifically to the three neuroleptic-associated movement disorders (acute EPS, described in *Panels 6, 8, and 10*) and sometimes to the tardive syndromes (described in *Panel 12*).
- *Hypokinesia:* Reduction in spontaneous or elicited motor movements.
- *Myoclonus:* Irregular jerking of individual apical muscles or muscle groups. May occur during waking hours, sleep, or the transition between (see also *Module 11*).
- *Parkinsonism:* Constellation of signs described in *Panel 10.* May be idiopathic (Parkinson *disease*), neuroleptic associated, or due to other causes.
- *Pill-rolling tremor:* Rotary tremor of the upper extremities characteristic of (but not specific for) parkinsonism.
- *Pseudoparkinsonism:* Term sometimes used to differentiate psychotropic-induced parkinsonism from Parkinson disease.
- *Rabbit syndrome:* Perioral "sniffing" tremor characteristic of (but not specific for) parkinsonism.
- *Tardive:* Late-occurring (tardy).
- *Tardive dyskinesia/dystonia:* Neuroleptic-associated late-occurring movement disorders described in *Panel 12* below.
- *Tic disorders:* Disorders characterized by stereotypic movements that may range from simple nonrhythmic choreic jerks to complex movements including guttural vocalizations or short phrases.
- *Tremor:* Rhythmic movements of the extremities, or less typically the trunk. Contrast with nonrhythmic *chorea* above. Movements may be fine, high amplitude or coarse, low amplitude. See also *pill-rolling* above.

- Continue to **Panel 2.**

Panel 2: Categorizing Psychotropic-Associated Movement Disorders

- Psychotropic-associated movement disorders are by definition associated with, and likely caused by, specific psychotropic medications.
- The two major groups of psychotropic-associated movement disorders are:
  - **EPS** associated with neuroleptics
  - **Tremors** associated with other psychotropic medications

Note: For rates for a specific neuroleptic agent (also called *antipsychotics* or in earlier days *major tranquilizers*), go to *Treatment Section,* page 300.

- If movements are primarily associated with a non-neuroleptic psychotropic, continue to **Panel 3.**
- If movements are primarily associated with a neuroleptic, go to **Panel 4.**
- If unclear, or movements are associated with both, continue to **Panel 3.**

Panel 3: Assessment of Tremors Associated with Psychotropic Medications

- As described in *Panel 1, Tremors* are *rhythmic* movements of extremities, or less typically the trunk.
- Useful descriptive terms:
  - Axial or apical
  - Unilateral or bilateral
  - Movements may be:
    - Fine, low amplitude
    - Coarse, high amplitude (sometimes called "gross" tremors)
    - Pill-rolling [characteristic of (but not diagnostic of) parkinsonism]
- Examination for tremors (in order of increasing sensitivity to detect tremors):
  - At rest, unobserved, from a distance
  - At rest during examination
  - With outstretched arms, hands palm down
  - Finger-to-nose with stationary examiner's finger
  - Finger-to-nose with examiner's finger moving

Note: Tremors are usually worse on intention with nondominant hand, although solely unilateral tremors suggest a focal lesion rather than diffuse medication effects.

Note: Analogous examination can be done with lower extremities, using heel-to-shin maneuver (individual places heel on knee and slides it down along shin to ankle).

- Tremors are fairly nonspecific and may occur in a variety of clinical situations. See *Differential Diagnosis* above.
- Most frequent culprits among psychotropics are:
  - Lithium
  - Valproate
  - Stimulating antidepressants (e.g., bupropion, venlafaxine, fluoxetine)
  - Stimulants

- Continue to **Panel 4.**

Panel 4: Management of Psychotropic-Associated Tremor

- Reduce/remove other inciting agents (e.g., caffeine).
- Reduce dose if possible.
- For lithium or valproate: single daily dosing at bedtime with non-sustained release preparation.
- Switch to other medication
- Beta-blockers, e.g.:
  - Atenolol 25 to 50 mg orally twice daily (b.i.d.)
  - Propranolol 20 to 60 mg orally b.i.d. or sustained-release preparation 80 mg every morning

- Continue to **Panel 5,** if applicable.

Panel 5: Characteristics of Neuroleptic-Associated Disorders

- Classification of **neuroleptic-associated movement disorders** is based on:
  - Time of onset
    - *Acute:* Onset within hours to weeks of starting neuroleptic agent; cessation of symptoms with reduction or cessation of neuroleptic agent.
    - *Tardive:* Onset after weeks to years of starting neuroleptic agent; symptoms continue after cessation of neuroleptic agent.
  - Description of specific movements
- If **acute:**
  - Movements may be primarily spasms (**acute dystonia**).
  - Movements may reflect primarily urge to move or walk; secondary anxiety or irritability may be presenting finding (**akathisia**).
  - Movements may be primarily akinetic or tremulous (**parkinsonism**).

Note: Acute dystonia may be the most uncomfortable symptom that an individual in mental health treatment will encounter, and akathisia may well be the second most uncomfortable. Thus, each may *profoundly reduce compliance and may compromise treatment alliance.* Avoidance or prompt resolution is critical.

- If **tardive,** movements may be one or the other or both of:
  - Choreiform or athetotic (**tardive dyskinesia**)
  - Dystonic (**tardive dystonia**)
- For each of the above syndromes, refer to *Differential Diagnosis* above to rule out other causes. The following assumes movement disorder is due to treatment with neuroleptics.

- If likely acute dystonia, continue to **Panel 6.**
- If likely akathisia, go to **Panel 8.**
- If likely parkinsonism, continue to **Panel 10.**
- If likely tardive dyskinesia or dystonia, continue to **Panel 12.**

Panel 6: Assessment of Acute Dystonia

- Acute dystonia is characterized by:
  - Apical or axial protracted muscle spasms, especially:
    - Neck (*torticollis, retrocollis*)
    - Extraocular muscles (*oculogyric crisis*)
    - Jaw (*trismus*)
    - Spine (*opisthotonus*)
  - Dysarthria, tongue spasms, or vague complaints of "stiff tongue"
  - Waxing/waning sense of stiffness in apical/axial musculature
- Severe complications:
  - Laryngeospasm and respiratory arrest
  - Discoordination of swallowing muscles and aspiration pneumonia
  - Diaphragmatic spasm and difficulty breathing
  - Cessation of cooperation in treatment
- Prevalence and incidence:
  - 3% to 15% of individuals treated with neuroleptics
  - May occur within minutes to hours of first dose; onset typically by first 2 weeks
- Risk factors (as with akathisia):
  - Younger
  - Male
  - High-potency typical neuroleptics (e.g., haloperidol, fluphenazine); may be as high as 50% with high doses of high-potency neuroleptics
  - Not associated with future development of tardive dyskinesia
- Mechanism: All three types of acute EPS are typically ascribed to deficiency of dopamine at D2 receptors in the nigrostriatal pathway; however, actual data support this mechanism primarily for parkinsonism.

- Continue to **Panel 7.**

Panel 7: Management of Acute Dystonia

- Prophylaxis with agents below may or may not be warranted:
  - Benefits of prophylaxis: prevention
  - Costs of prophylaxis: chronic treatment with a second drug that has its own side effects
- Preferable to prevent by using:
  - Atypical neuroleptics
  - Lower potency typical neuroleptics (which have their own built-in anticholinergic effects)
  - Lowest possible doses of high-potency neuroleptics
- Continue for duration of neuroleptic treatment plus at least several days if acute symptoms have occurred:
  - Anticholinergics
    - Benztropine 0.5 to 2 mg intramuscularly (i.m.) or orally twice daily
    - Triphenhexidyl 2 to 5 mg orally b.i.d.
    - Side effects: dry mouth, blurry vision, constipation, urinary retention, tachycardia, acute worsening of narrow-angle glaucoma, confusion in the elderly
  - Antihistamines
    - Diphenhydramine 25 to 50 mg orally or i.m. b.i.d.
    - Side effects: sedation, dry mouth, constipation
  - Dopamine agonists
    - Amantadine 100 mg orally two to three times daily
    - Side effects: mania, worsening of psychosis, insomnia

Note: Acute dystonic reactions require immediate treatment, typically intramuscularly. Benztropine 1 mg or diphenhydramine 25 mg is a reasonable dose for most, with repeat treatment if no relief in 15 minutes. Then begin oral dosing. Adjunctive benzodiazepines are typically not needed. Debriefing with the patient usually is.

Panel 8: Assessment of Akathisia

- Akathisia is characterized by:
  - Excessive physical movement, especially walking.
  - Not stereotypic or delirious; individuals typically relate: "I don't know why, I just have to keep moving."
  - May be limited to subjective urge or need to move.
  - Is not necessarily associated with a subjective sense of anxiety— may be a completely somatic (from the neck down) sensation.
- Severe complications:
  - Agitation
  - Extreme irritability, particularly in less verbal patients
  - Cessation of cooperation in treatment
- Prevalence and incidence:
  - 10% to 50% of individuals treated with neuroleptics
  - May occur within hours of first dose; onset typically by first several weeks
- Risk factors (as with acute dystonia):
  - Younger
  - Male
  - High-potency typical neuroleptics (e.g., haloperidol, fluphenazine); may be as high as 75% with high doses of high-potency neuroleptics
  - May be associated with future development of tardive dyskinesia
- Mechanism: All three types of acute EPS are typically ascribed to deficiency of dopamine at D2 receptors in the nigrostriatal pathway; however, data support this mechanism primarily for parkinsonism.

- Continue to **Panel 9.**

Panel 9: Management of Akathisia

- Prophylaxis with agents below may or may not be warranted:
  - Benefits of prophylaxis: prevention
  - Costs of prophylaxis: chronic treatment with a second drug that has its own side effects
- Preferable to prevent by using:
  - Atypical neuroleptics
  - Lower potency typical neuroleptics (have their own built-in anti-cholinergic effects)
  - Lowest possible doses of high-potency neuroleptics
- Agents for acute and continuation treatment differ from those for acute dystonia and parkinsonism
- Continue for duration of neuroleptic treatment plus at least 1 week if acute symptoms have occurred, and longer if necessary.
  - Benzodiazepines (any), for example:
    - Diazepam 2 to 10 mg orally b.i.d.
    - Lorazepam 0.5 to 1 mg orally b.i.d.
  - Lipophilic beta-blocker antihypertensives, for example:
    - Propranolol 20 to 40 mg orally three times daily (t.i.d.)
  - Second-line agents:
    - Clonidine (α_2 agonist antihypertensive) 0.1 to 0.2 mg orally t.i.d.
    - Anticholinergics or diphenhydramine (see *Panel 7*)

Note: Treatment of akathisia usually requires prompt but not emergent treatment; oral medications are usually sufficient, although i.m. benzodiazepines may be helpful to begin treatment of acute discomfort. As with acute dystonia, debriefing with the individual usually mitigates sequelae of this acutely uncomfortable syndrome.

Panel 10: Assessment of Neuroleptic-Associated Parkinsonism

- Neuroleptic-associated parkinsonism is characterized by the same symptoms as idiopathic Parkinson disease:
  - Akinesia or hypokinesia including:
    - Slow ambulation
    - Decreased arm movements when walking
    - Overall decrease in nonessential task movements
    - Masklike facial expression
  - Cogwheel rigidity (see *Panel 1*)
  - Coarse tremor
  - Pill-rolling tremor (see *Panel 1*)
  - Rabbit syndrome (see *Panel 1*)
- Severe complications:
  - Misdiagnosis as depression, dementia, catatonia
  - Cessation of cooperation in treatment
- Prevalence and incidence:
  - 10% to 15% of individuals treated with neuroleptics
  - May occur within hours of first dose; onset typically by first 3 months
  - May persist for several months after cessation of neuroleptic agent
- Risk factors:
  - Older
  - Female
  - High-potency typical neuroleptics (e.g., haloperidol, fluphenazine)
  - May be associated with future development of tardive dyskinesia
- Mechanism: deficiency of dopamine at D2 receptors in the nigrostriatal pathway

- Continue to **Panel 11.**

Panel 11: Management of Parkinsonism

- Prophylaxis with agents below may or may not be warranted:
  - Benefits of prophylaxis: prevention
  - Costs of prophylaxis: chronic treatment with a second drug that has its own side effects
- Preferable to prevent by using:
  - Atypical neuroleptics
  - Lower potency typical neuroleptics (have their own built-in anticholinergic effects)
  - Lowest possible doses of high-potency neuroleptics
- Acute and continuation treatment is similar to that for acute dystonia.
- Continue for duration of neuroleptic treatment plus at least 1 week if acute symptoms have occurred, and longer if necessary.
  - Anticholinergics
    - Benztropine 0.5 to 2 mg orally b.i.d.
    - Triphenhexidyl 2 to 5 mg orally b.i.d.
    - Side effects: dry mouth, blurry vision, constipation, urinary retention, tachycardia, acute worsening of narrow-angle glaucoma, confusion and falls in the elderly
  - Antihistamines
    - Diphenhydramine 25 to 50 mg orally b.i.d.
    - Side effects: sedation, dry mouth, constipation, confusion and falls in the elderly
  - Dopamine agonists
    - Amantadine 100 mg orally b.i.d. to t.i.d.
    - Side effects: mania, worsening of psychosis, insomnia

Note: Unlike for acute dystonia, treatment is typically by the oral route and not emergent.

Panel 12: Assessment of Tardive Dyskinesia and Tardive Dystonia

- Tardive syndromes include:
  - Tardive dyskinesia, characterized by:
    - Apical or axial athetotic or choreiform movements.
    - Most common are perioral movements including lip pouting, sniffing movements, tongue writhing, and chewing as if chewing gum.
    - Movements can sometimes be voluntarily suppressed, may worsen with stress or anxiety, and disappear during sleep.
    - Muscles of swallowing and respiration may be affected.
  - Tardive dystonia, characterized by chronic symptoms identical to those of acute dystonia (see *Panel 6*).
  - The standardized Abnormal Involuntary Movement Scale (AIMS) categorizes and rates symptoms of tardive dyskinesia/dystonia (see *Appendix 8*).
  - A rarer *tardive akathisia* also has been described.
- Severe complications:
  - Dysphagia with aspiration pneumonia or weight loss
  - Respiratory compromise
  - Disfiguration and social stigmatization
  - Painful, chronic spasms in tardive dystonia
- Prevalence and incidence:
  - 10% to 20% of individuals treated with neuroleptics.
  - 2% to 4% per year over first 7 years of exposure.
  - Persists indefinitely after cessation of neuroleptic.
  - Some dyskinesias remit several months after cessation of neuroleptic.
  - Resumption or increase of neuroleptic will temporarily suppress dyskinesias.
- Clear risk factors:
  - Older
  - Female
  - Duration of treatment with neuroleptics
  - Mood disorder (vs. schizophrenia)
    - Possibly due to genetic factors or medication interactions
    - Possibly due to on/off pattern of neuroleptic use
  - Use of typical (as opposed to atypical) neuroleptics
  - Anticholinergics may exacerbate choreoathetotic movements
- Possible risk factors:
  - Cumulative exposure to neuroleptics (years × dosage)
  - Prior neuroleptic-induced akathisia or parkinsonism
  - Neurologic disease or brain damage
  - Ethnicity (African Americans > Caucasians > Asians)
  - Diabetes
- Mechanism: hypothesized supersensitivity of dopamine at D2 receptors in the nigrostriatal pathway

Note: Minimization of tardive dyskinesia/dystonia has been made possible by the development of the newer atypical neuroleptics. However, it should be recalled that:

- Atypical neuroleptics are *relatively* not *absolutely* unlikely to cause tardive dyskinesia/dystonia.
- Several atypical neuroleptics are likely to cause severe health problems, including type 2 diabetes and obesity, which can itself also be:
  - Disfiguring
  - Socially stigmatizing

- Tardive dyskinesia often occurs without tardive dystonia. However, tardive dystonia rarely occurs without tardive dyskinesia. Therefore, continue to **Panel 13.**
- See **Appendix 8** for AIMS.

Panel 13: Management of Tardive Dyskinesia

- There are no prophylactic agents for tardive dyskinesia/dystonia.
- *Prevention* is key:
  - Avoid neuroleptic use whenever possible.
  - Lowest possible doses of any neuroleptic.
  - Atypical rather than typical neuroleptics.

Note: Recall that administration or increased dosing of neuroleptics may temporarily suppress symptoms of tardive dyskinesia. Do not be fooled: symptoms will reemerge later.

- There are no clearly effective *treatments* for tardive dyskinesia/dystonia.
- Comprehensive evidence-based reviews to date by the Cochrane Collaboration (see *Key References*) indicate that:
  - No agents studied in randomized controlled trials have consistently been shown to reduce tardive dyskinesia/dystonia.
  - However, treatment with vitamin E may reduce the *progression* of tardive dyskinesia.
- Although tardive dyskinesia and dystonia have no regularly effective treatments, they are chronic and disabling. Use of agents with only anecdotal evidence may be justified. Agents with some evidence for efficacy include:
  - Clozapine, the one neuroleptic that may reduce dyskinesia long-term. See entry in *Treatment Section.*
  - Vitamin E 400 IU orally t.i.d. to 800 IU orally b.i.d.
  - Reserpine 0.1 to 0.5 mg orally b.i.d.
  - High-dose buspirone: 45 to 90 mg orally b.i.d.
  - Clonidine 0.1 to 0.2 mg orally b.i.d.
  - Propranolol 20 to 40 mg orally t.i.d.
  - Valproate in standard neurologic doses
  - Additional agents of with inconsistent data for efficacy (see *Key References* for details):
    - Anticholinergics
    - Baclofen and other gabaergic drugs
    - Benzodiazepines
    - Calcium channel blockers
    - Cholinomimetics
    - Insulin in low doses
    - Alphamethyldopa
    - L-dopa

- If symptoms of tardive dystonia are present, continue to **Panel 14.**

Panel 14: Management of Tardive Dystonia

- The presence of the painful muscle spasms of dystonia, in addition to tardive dyskinesia, may require more focal treatment with muscle relaxants.
- Although no treatments have clear efficacy, antispasmodic treatments may provide some relief, including:
  - Baclofen 5 to 10 mg orally t.i.d.
  - Diazepam 2 to 10 mg orally t.i.d.
  - Anticholinergics as dosed for acute dystonia (see *Panel 7*)

Module 18

When the Black Dog Comes Back: Thinking Through Recurrence

Orienting Notes

- Winston Churchill, despite his incredible political leadership through-out much of the twentieth century, was dogged by recurrent major depressive episodes. These crippling episodes came on, pinned him down, and then left of their own accord. Churchill anticipated these periods and called them his "Black Dog."
- Unlike the other modules, this module does not address a specific symptom constellation.
- Rather, it provides the clinician with a cognitive drill to go through when psychiatric symptoms of any type recur in previously stable individuals.

Note: In the study of mood disorders, the terms *recurrence, relapse,* and the like have specific technical meanings. In this module, we use the term *recurrence* in its less technical sense—as Churchill would have used it when he saw his Black Dog come back.

Differential Diagnosis

- Compliance?
  - If not compliant, why not—*specifically:*
    - Side effects?
    - Expense or change in financial situation?
    - Perception of no effect?
    - Hopelessness, demoralization?
    - Frustration with/anger at provider?
    - Switch to alternative/complementary treatment?
    - Loss of transportation?
    - Pharmacy problem?
    - Other glitch?
    - My mistake?
  - What changes need to be made to get the individual back on medications?
- Medical illness
  - Example: Carcinoma leading to weight loss, fatigue, feeling of being "not right" in an individual with remitted depression
  - Urinary tract infection leading to cognitive decline or delirium in an individual with previously stable dementia
- Medication side effects
  - Example: Hypothyroidism leading to depressive symptoms in an individual with manic-depressive disorder previously stabilized with lithium
  - Example: Steroids for rheumatoid arthritis leading to psychotic symptoms in an individual with previously stable schizophrenia
- Medication interactions
  - Example: Addition of carbamazepine for neuropathic pain in an individual with previously stable schizoaffective disorder leading to increased metabolism of haloperidol and subsequent recurrence of psychosis.
  - Note that nicotine increases metabolism—and reduces levels—of many psychotropic drugs, including:
    - Antidepressants: imipramine, clomipramine, fluvoxamine, trazodone (but not buproprion).
    - Neuroleptics: chlorpromazine, clozapine, fluphenazine, olanzapine
    - Benzodiazepines: alprazolam, diazepam, lorazepam, oxazepam
    - See also *Appendix 12*
- Concurrent substance use, including:
  - Intoxication
  - Withdrawal
  - Don't forget changes in use of nicotine, which
    - is psychoactive
    - interacts with psychotropic drugs as above
- Psychosocial stressors
  - Anniversaries or exposure to triggers leading to exacerbation of symptoms in an individual with previously stable PTSD.
  - Increased job stress in an individual with previously stable anxiety disorder leading to increased symptoms (e.g., panic, generalized anxiety, or social phobia symptoms).
  - Stress that is "good" may also lead to recurrence of symptoms (e.g., job promotion, marriage, new love interest).
- Physical stress
  - Example: Seasonal—spring and fall (times of highest rate of change of day length) are times of greatest risk for mania/depression in manic-depressive disorder.
  - Example: Environmental change leading to cognitive deterioration in an individual with previously stable dementia (e.g., change in room, roommate, or staff in nursing home).
  - Example: New baby leading to sleep deprivation and subsequently to manic symptoms in father with previously stable manic-depressive disorder.
- Spontaneous/breakthrough
  - This is an attribution of exclusion.
  - Rule-out above causes first.

SECTION III

Disorders

INTRODUCTION

This section supports the third of the four core tasks of psychiatric assessment and treatment planning (**Section I, Panel 1**):

1. Characterize symptoms and signs.
2. Build symptoms and signs into syndromes.
3. Build syndromes into disorders.
4. Treat the disorders.

In particular, this reflects attention to the fourth of the **Five Principles of Assessment and Treatment Planning (Section I, Panels 2 and 3)**:

• Diagnosis drives treatment.

Although it should go without saying, it is necessary to emphasize this point more than ever because we now have more and more broad-spectrum treatments that reduce the symptoms of multiple disorders—and correspondingly we have greater temptation to "shot-gun" symptoms.

There are two major reasons to be meticulous with diagnosis. First, treatment can further muddy the clinical picture. If one does not have a good grasp of the diagnosis at the beginning, it will be even more difficult to figure out later. Second, comorbidity among psychiatric disorders is the rule rather than the exception in many clinical settings. To miss a comorbid disorder is to hamper treatment planning as well as diagnosis. Unfortunately, we have all had the experience of being well into treatment when a comorbid diagnosis is discovered and treatment must be changed—for example, a history of bipolar disorder revealed when mania develops during serotonin reuptake inhibitor treatment for panic disorder, a substance use disorder revealed when benzodiazepines are overused for primary insomnia, or pathologic gambling revealed during treatment for alcohol dependence.

The clinician has typically arrived at the present section on disorders through **Section II, Symptom-Driven Assessment.** He or she has arrived at a specific disorder diagnosis or is considering several. The entries in this section assist the clinician by providing specific diagnostic criteria, providing data regarding clinical features, and reviewing overall management and specific treatment strategies.

Each entry in **Section III** represents a distinct disorder based on the *American Psychiatric Association's Diagnostic and Statistical Manual* (DSM) system, fourth revision (DSM-IV-TR; see **Key References**). The majority of DSM diagnoses that affect adults are included here, either as individual entries [e.g., manic-depressive (bipolar) disorder] or within a group (e.g., personality disorders). Although the DSM system is not accepted worldwide, and is not typically used for billing purposes, it is the *lingua franca* for most scientific communications worldwide and for clinical discussions at least in the United States. Moreover, it is closely coordinated with the disorder categories in the broader International Classification of Diseases (ICD) system.

There are a number of important strengths to the DSM system. For instance, its diagnostic categories are based on explicit criteria and not intuition or imputation by the clinician. The reliability and reproducibility of most of its categories have been well established in many studies over many years. It attempts to be devoid of theoretic or partisan grounding.

However, there are also some weaknesses. It is important to note, for instance, that the DSM (as well as the ICD) system is a *categorical* system: either one has a disorder, or one does not. This may or may not represent reality in all cases. For instance, it may be that the DSM categories of major depressive episode, dysthymia, and normalcy represent the major, and distinct, states in which one can find one's self with regard to depressive symptoms. Alternatively, however, depression may be a continuously distributed population trait—that is, a *dimensional* (spectrum of severity) rather than a *categorical* (yes/no) characteristic, and what we call dysthymia or a major depressive episode simply represents the most severe end of the spectrum. The same may be true, for example, for personality disorders.

There are also a number of gaps in the DSM system that render it unable to easily conceptualize certain problems that commonly underlie individuals' requests for help. For instance, as pointed out in **Module 15, Relationship and Personal Problems,** by doing away with the theoretically based concept of "neurosis" the DSM system makes it difficult to conceptualize patterns of untoward feeling, thought, and behavior that are more widespread than an adjustment disorder but less severe, pernicious, and inflexible than a personality disorder.

Nonetheless, it is imperative that clinicians learn and think along the categorical DSM/ICD lines as the basis for their diagnoses and treatment planning. Consider learning the categories like learning to play a musical instrument: once the basics are mastered, the experienced clinician can then perform variations on these well-known themes. But not to recognize the basic categories and their distinct boundaries is to leave one's self mired in mushy diagnostic thinking.

Each diagnostic entry in **Section III** begins with the name of the disorder and relevant DSM-IV codes. Each entry then contains a series of key components that are listed below with specific explanatory notes. "N/A" means "not applicable" or "not available," depending on context.

ADAPTED DSM-IV CRITERIA

These criteria closely follow the DSM criteria. The language is purposely made less arcane than in the DSM, and some of the diagnostic considerations that are related primarily to research or specialty clinic tasks are glossed over, although without loss of diagnostic precision for general clinical practice. Those seeking the research or specialty level of diagnostic sophistication are urged to consult the DSM materials and the general and specific texts listed among the **Key References.**

Note also that three key DSM diagnostic characteristics that apply to *all* disorders are not listed repetitiously in each entry, but are given here:

- To be considered a disorder, the individual must experience *distress* or *dysfunction*. Thus, lack of gender identity clarity or atypical sexual practices are not disorders unless they cause distress or dysfunction to the individual.
- Culturally sanctioned beliefs or behaviors—for instance, hearing voices, or seeing visions, or religious beliefs shared by the community—are not considered pathologic.
- Each diagnostic entity in the DSM includes a criterion that says something to the effect of "Not due to medications, medical conditions, or other psychiatric diagnoses including . . ." **Section II, Symptom-Based Interviewing.** guides the clinician through these differential diagnosis complexities.

CLINICAL HIGHLIGHTS

This section includes several characteristics of each disorder that will help the clinician to understand the core features of presentation. This will help the clinician not only to get a better "feel" for the nuances of the disorder but will also help them diagnostically by revising their evidence-based predictive values (see **Section I, Panel 10**) based on relevant diagnostic information.

- **Features.** This section describes key clinical features not covered in the DSM criteria. These include, for instance, suicide rates for several disorders, notes on additional clinical diagnostic systems (such as the Bleulerian "4 As" and Schneiderian "first rank" symptoms for schizophrenia), and various diagnostic subtleties not addressed in the modules of **Section II.**
- **Gender Issues.** Differences in occurrence or pattern of presentation across genders are noted here.
- **Cultural Issues.** Cultural issues relevant to differential diagnosis are noted here.
- **Adult Life Cycle Issues.** Differences in occurrence, pattern of presentation, or course across various ages of adulthood are noted here.

PREVALENCE

This section assists the clinician with regard to the very important issue of the underlying probability that a specific disorder is present in the individual you are interviewing. All of our interview questions simply revise that underlying probability or predictive value (**Section I, Biopsychosocial Assessment, Panel 10**). To use an absurd example: If a man has monthly bouts of depressive and irritable symptoms that last about a week, it's not likely to be premenstrual dysphoric disorder (PMDD) since its prevalence in men is zero. A less absurd example is provided in **Section I, Panel 16.** The diagnostic old saw alluded to in that panel—"When you hear hoofbeats in Wyoming, think horses, not zebras"—captures the importance of this perspective succinctly.

The underlying principle is that common things are common. What is not necessarily appreciated is that the populations seen in different settings are not always the same. What is common in the general population is not necessarily common in primary care practice is not necessarily common in outpatient mental health settings is not necessarily common in inpatient settings.

An example is the prevalence of comorbid substance use disorders in manic-depressive disorder. The rates of current substance use disorders among those with manic-depressive disorder in outpatient mental health treatment facilities are typically below 10%. However, rates of current substance use disorders among those with manic-depressive disorder in inpatient mental health settings are on the order of 30% to 40%. Thus, when one sits interviewing an individual with manic-depressive disorder who has been admitted to an inpatient unit, one is well advised to pay particular attention to the review of systems for substance use disorders.

The importance of specific prevalence figures to you as a clinician is determined by where you happen to be sitting at that particular time. Thus, we have attempted to gather prevalence data for each disorder, or group of disorders across the various settings in which this Field Guide might be used.

As might be expected, prevalence data outside the community setting are scarce. We attempted to locate as many sources as possible for prevalence rates in various clinical treatment settings and were successful to varying degrees. The user of this guide is therefore urged to consider that these rates may not be as stable as those for the community. "N/A" denotes data not available. Sources for available data are:

- **Community.** These data come primarily from the Epidemiologic Catchment Area and National Comorbidity Studies, as well as several other specialized investigations reported in peer-reviewed journals.
- **Primary Care Practice.** These data come from various studies in peer-reviewed journals.
- **Outpatient Mental Health Practice.** We were able to locate only two studies delineating rates of various psychiatric disorders in outpatient mental health practice settings. Each is listed among the **Key References.** The Zimmerman study took place in a clinic located within a nonprofit academically affiliated medical center in an urban area in New England. Data from the Segal study are taken from a group of publicly funded community mental health centers across six counties in the San Francisco Bay area. Both studies collected data in the 1990s.
- **Among Mental Health Admissions.** We were unable to find published studies that delineated rates of various psychiatric disorders among unselected admissions in inpatient mental health settings. We therefore obtained annual discharge diagnosis data from two New England hospitals and averaged the rates to provide prevalence rates for groups of diagnoses in this sector.

COURSE

This information is provided to help with treatment planning and with the education of the individuals and families affected by the disorder.

COMMON COMORBIDITIES

This information supports the important task of identifying comorbidities that impact on diagnosis, course, and treatment planning (see also **Section I, Panel 14**).

TREATMENT CONSIDERATIONS

This section contains several types of information that will help in treatment planning, and will specifically assist the clinician to move to the appropriate treatment modality found in **Section IV, Treatment.**

- **Criteria for Urgent Intervention.** This section reminds the clinician of situations in which particularly aggressive intervention or monitoring is required.
- **Medication Options.** This section outlines the overall classes of medication options, with classes cross-referenced to **Section IV.** Further considerations in choosing among these options are outlined in the section below.
- **Psychotherapeutic Options.** This section briefly highlights considerations in using psychotherapeutic interventions for the given disorder. It is important to note that the **Psychotherapy** section in **Section IV** is divided into two components:
  - **Supportive Psychotherapy (Panels 1–4)** provides an overview of important points in treating any disorder with any treatment, psychotherapeutic or pharmacologic.

- **Formal, Structured Psychotherapies (Panels 5–21)** help the clinician to identify those specific, specialized, and usually manual-based psychotherapies that have been shown to be effective in controlled trials for a given disorder.
- **Considerations in Choosing Among Treatments.** This section provides a series of suggestions regarding choice among various treatments. These suggestions are based on a combination of empirical data and accumulated clinical experience, with an emphasis on the latter for the many clinical situations for which evidence-based trials have not been brought to bear.

MOOD DISORDERS

Disorder: Major Depressive Disorder
DSM-IV Codes: 296.2x (Single Episode)
                    296.3x (Recurrent)

Adapted DSM Criteria
For Major Depressive Disorder

Single Episode: One major depressive episode lifetime
Recurrent: Two or more major depressive episodes

For Major Depressive Episode

A.   Five (or more) of the following symptoms for at least 2 weeks
B.   Including either or both of:
     (1)   Depressed mood most of the day, nearly every day, as indicated by either subjective report or observation (can be irritability in children and adolescents), or
     (2)   Markedly diminished interest and pleasure in all, or almost all, activities most of the day, nearly every day (as indicated by either subjective account or observation made by others).
C.   Plus:
     (3)   Decrease or increase in appetite nearly every day or weight change of at least ±5%
     (4)   Insomnia or hypersomnia nearly every day
     (5)   Psychomotor agitation or retardation nearly every day observable by others
     (6)   Fatigue or loss of energy nearly every day
     (7)   Feelings of worthlessness or excessive guilt or inappropriate guilt (not merely self-approach or guilt about being sick)
     (8)   Decreased concentration or indecisiveness
     (9)   Recurrent thoughts of death or suicidal ideation or plan

Clinical Highlights
Features

- The *disorder* diagnosis is built from *episode* diagnoses as above:
  - One major depressive *episode* = major depressive *disorder, single episode.*
  - More than one *episode* = major depressive *disorder, recurrent.*
  - A major depressive episode is characterized by a down or depressed mood occurring most of the day, more days than not. It can also be characterized by a lack of interest and pleasure in activities most of the day, more days than not.

- It typically represents a change from baseline function, although some patients have long-term chronic mild or even severe depressive symptoms.
- See **Module 1** for episode and disorder subtypes.
- Up to 35% of individuals presenting for treatment of a major depressive episode have manic-depressive disorder.

Gender Issues

- Women have at least a twofold higher incidence of depression than men. This may be due to biologic and/or social factors.
- Some studies show worse outcome in women than men.
- The first four postpartum weeks is the time of highest risk for depression. Psychotic symptoms may be present during postpartum episodes of depression. Risk of recurrence with subsequent parturition is increased, and careful monitoring is warranted. Hormonal, circadian, and psychosocial stressors may all contribute.

Cultural Issues

- In some cultures, depression may present with primarily physical complaints with little or no report of mood symptoms.
- There are large variations in depression cross-nationally, but the reasons are not clear.

Adult Life Cycle Issues

- The incidence increases significantly at puberty.
- The incidence of depressive symptoms increases with increasing age, although the prevalence of DSM-defined major depressive disorder declines.

Prevalence
Community

- Males:
  - Lifetime 10% to 15%
  - 12-month 5% to 8%
- Females:
  - Lifetime 15% to 20%
  - 12-month 10% to 15%
- Total (males and females)
  - Lifetime 15% to 20%
  - 12-month 10% to 15%
  - Community point-prevalence of 16.5% for at least one depressive symptom
  - Community point-prevalence of 0.4% for major depressive episode with psychotic features

In Primary Care Practice

- Lifetime risk is 5% to 10% for both men and women.

In Outpatient Mental Health Practice

- 37% in a private university-affiliated hospital-based clinic
- 10% as secondary diagnosis in a private university-affiliated hospital-based clinic
- 68% in a community mental health center

Among Mental Health Admissions

- Depressive disorders comprise approximately 30% of inpatient mental health admissions.

165

Course

- 20% to 30% of episodes persist for months without treatment.
- 5% to 10% of episodes last more than 2 years.
- 60% with one episode will have a second, 70% with a second episode will have a third.

Common Comorbidities

- Substance use disorders
- Anxiety disorders

Treatment Considerations
Criteria for Urgent Intervention

- Suicidal ideation, plan, or attempt
- Psychosis
- Maladaptive substance use
- Inability to care for self

Medication Options

- Tricyclic antidepressants
- Serotonin reuptake inhibitor antidepressants
- Other heterocyclic antidepressants
- Monoamine oxidase inhibitor antidepressants
- Alprazolam, perhaps unique among benzodiazepines, appears to have anti-depressant effects at moderate to high doses (1 mg t.i.d. or above).
- Adjuvant agents to add in case of nonresponse to antidepressant agent: lithium, triiodothyronine (T_3)

Psychotherapeutic Options

- Supportive care should focus on supporting medication management and role function. Where possible, it should include education of the patient and his or her family.
- For formal psychotherapy options, see Psychotherapy in **Section IV.**

Other

See Devices in **Section IV.**
- Electroconvulsive therapy (ECT)
- Bright light for seasonal pattern

Considerations in Choosing Among Treatments

- Formal, structured psychotherapy versus medication management based on:
  - Severity of depression (unclear benefit of psychotherapy in more severe depression)
  - Availability of formal, structured psychotherapy
  - Individual preference
- It is not clear whether combining medications and formal psychotherapy offers any benefit over either alone. However, general supportive measures (see **Psychotherapy** in **Section IV**) are always indicated.
- Medication choice is based on side effects that are to be avoided and those to be desired. For instance, for a patient sensitive to sexual side effects, it may be best to avoid the serotonin reuptake inhibitors. A patient with prominent

insomnia may do better, or not need additional hypnotics, with a sedating anti-depressant such as mirtazapine, imipramine, or trazodone.

- The widespread adoption of serotonin reuptake inhibitor antidepressants is based more on ease of provider use than on differences in efficacy versus older agents (if anything, tricyclics may be more effective) or side effects (each class has its own toxicity; serotonin reuptake inhibitors are, taken together, slightly better tolerated than the older tricyclics against what they are usually tested).
- No evidence of greater benefit with one type of psychotherapy than another.
- No evidence of greater benefit with one type of medication than another, except that monoamine oxidase inhibitors appear better for atypical depression.
- Consider ECT for psychotic or severely agitated depression or during pregnancy.
- ECT may be more effective than medication for individuals hospitalized with depression.
- Treat 6 to 9 months for first two episodes; lifetime prophylaxis after the third.

Disorder: Dysthymic Disorder
DSM-IV Codes: 300.40

Adapted DSM Criteria
A. Depressed mood for most of the day, for at least 2 years
B. Two or more of the following:
    (1) Poor appetite or overeating
    (2) Insomnia or hypersomnia
    (3) Low energy or fatigue
    (4) Low self-esteem
    (5) Poor concentration or difficulty making decisions
    (6) Feelings of hopelessness
C. No more than 2 months without symptoms in those 2 years
D. No major depressive episode in the first 2 years; that is, dysthymia is not a chronic or partially remitted major depressive disorder
E. No history of bipolar disorder or cyclothymia

Clinical Highlights
Features

- Criteria differ in minor aspects from those for major depressive disorder, but the core is the same.
- Symptoms are chronic and low grade.
- However, functional disability from dysthymic disorder equals or exceeds that from major depressive disorder.
- A chronic course of dysthymic disorder is frequently punctuated by major depressive episodes (so-called "double depression").

Gender Issues

- Women are two to three times more likely to develop this disorder.

Cultural Issues

- N/A

Adult Life Cycle Issues

- N/A

167

Prevalence
Community
- Males:
  - Lifetime 5%
  - 12-month 2%
- Females:
  - Lifetime 8%
  - 12-month 3%
- Total (males and females)
  - Lifetime 5% to 8%
  - 12-month 2% to 3%
  - Community point-prevalence of 16.5% for one or more depressive symptoms.

In Primary Care Practice
- N/A

Outpatient Mental Health Practice
- 1% in a private university-affiliated hospital-based clinic
- 6% as secondary diagnosis in a private university-affiliated hospital-based clinic

Among Mental Health Admissions
- Depressive disorders comprise approximately 30% of inpatient mental health admissions; dysthymia alone is uncommon among admissions.

Course
- Early onset, usually in childhood, adolescence, or early adulthood.
- This disorder is chronic by definition.

Common Comorbidities
- Major depressive disorder
- Personality disorders
- Anxiety disorders
- Substance use disorders

Treatment Considerations
Criteria for Urgent Intervention
- Suicide ideation, plan, or intent
- Maladaptive substance use

Medication Options
- Tricyclic antidepressants
- Serotonin reuptake inhibitor antidepressants
- Other heterocyclic antidepressants
- Monoamine oxidase inhibitor antidepressants

Psychotherapeutic Options
- Supportive care should focus on supporting medication management and role function. Where possible, it should include education of the patient and his or her family.
- For formal psychotherapy options, see Psychotherapy in **Section IV.**

168

Considerations in Choosing Among Treatments

- There is developing evidence that for this chronic disorder, the addition of cognitive-behavioral therapy to medication may provide greater benefit than medication alone.
- Otherwise, choice between formal psychotherapy and medication can be based on:
  - Availability of formal psychotherapy
  - Individual preference

Disorder:	Manic-Depressive (Bipolar) Disorder
DSM-IV Codes:	296.xx (Type I)
	296.89 (Type II)

Adapted DSM Criteria
Manic-Depressive Disorder

Type I

- Manic episode(s) alone (296.0x)
- Manic episode(s) + major depressive episode(s) (296.4x if manic, 296.5x if depressed)
- Mixed episode(s) + manic episode(s) or depressive episode(s) (296.6x)
  - Note: a single mixed episode alone qualifies only for a "bipolar, not otherwise specified" diagnosis because of questions of diagnostic stability.

Type II

- Hypomanic episode(s) + major depressive episode(s)
  - Note: a single hypomanic episode alone qualifies only for a "bipolar, not otherwise specified" diagnosis because of questions of diagnostic stability.

Major Depressive Episode

See page 164.

Hypomanic Episode

A. At least 4 days of abnormally and persistently elevated, expansive, or irritable mood
B. Three (or more) of the following symptoms have persisted (four if the mood is only irritable):
    (1) Inflated self-esteem or grandiosity
    (2) Decreased *need* for sleep (e.g., feels rested after only 3 hours of sleep)
    (3) More talkative than usual or pressure to keep talking
    (4) Flight of ideas or subjective experience that thoughts are racing
    (5) Distractibility
    (6) Increase in goal-directed activity (either socially, at work or school, or sexually) or physical agitation
    (7) Excessive involvement in risky activities (e.g., spending sprees, promiscuity, gambling, impulsive investments)

169

Manic Episode

Symptoms of hypomanic episode are met for at least 1 week plus at least one of the following:

(1) Psychosis
(2) Need for hospitalization (with any symptom duration)
(3) Severe impairment in role function or relationships (typically, this means total inability to follow important role, e.g., work or spousal or parenting. Another way to think about it is: "This person is so impaired that he or she *should* be hospitalized.")

Mixed Episode

The criteria are met both for a manic episode and for a major depressive episode diagnosis (simultaneously or rapidly alternating) during at least a 1-week period.

• Note: meeting criteria for a *hypo*manic episode and major depressive episode diagnoses does not meet DSM criteria for a mixed episode diagnosis because of questions of diagnostic stability but this syndrome is quite common.

Clinical Highlights
Features

• The terms "manic-depressive" and "bipolar" are interchangeable. The older term, manic-depressive, is more accurate because (a) manic episodes are not typically the euphoric, polar opposite of depressive episodes and (b) depressive episodes predominate during course and cause most dysfunction.
• *Disorder* diagnosis is built on *episode* diagnoses, as for major depressive disorder.
• Core symptom features of manic and hypomanic episodes are the same except for severity.
• Episodes are typically demarcated from normal mood and can be recognized by a gradual or abrupt change from normal. Chronic symptoms (e.g., irritability for years) are not likely to be due to manic-depressive disorder.
• The rapid cycling form of manic-depressive disorder has by definition four or more discrete full-length episodes of any type in any order in 12 months.
  • This occurs in about 15% of patients with manic-depressive disorder.
  • Episodes may occur back-to-back or may be scattered over the course of 12 months.
• Up to 35% of individuals presenting for treatment of a major depressive episode have manic-depressive disorder.

Gender Issues

• Equal in men and women.
• Rapid cycling is more common in women (60%–85% are women).

Cultural Issues

• No reports of prevalence differences based on race or ethnicity.
• However, compared with Caucasians, African Americans with psychosis appear to be overdiagnosed with schizophrenic spectrum disorders and underdiagnosed with manic-depressive disorder.

Adult Life Cycle Issues

• Episode intervals decrease as age increases.
• Mean age of onset is early twenties.

Prevalence
Community
- Type I lifetime 0.4% to 1.6%
- Type II lifetime 0.5%
- Gender distribution is equal

In Primary Care Practice
- N/A

In Outpatient Mental Health Practice
Type I
- 1.8% in a private university-affiliated hospital-based clinic
- 0.3% as secondary diagnosis in a private university-affiliated hospital-based clinic

Type II
- 3.3% in a private university-affiliated hospital-based clinic.
- 0.5% as secondary diagnosis in a private university-affiliated hospital-based clinic.
- Manic-depressive disorders represent 3% in a community mental health center.

Among Mental Health Admissions
- Manic-depressive disorders comprise approximately 16% of inpatient mental health admissions.

Course
- Depression predominates and is responsible for much of the functional compromise that is seen.
- Suicide attempt rate 1 in 50 each year.
- Average age of onset is early twenties for both men and women.
- Greater than 90% of individuals who have a single episode will have additional episodes.
- 60% to 70% of manic episodes occur before or after a major depressive episode.
- Delay in accurate diagnosis may be as long as 7 years.

Common Comorbidities
- Substance use disorders (current substance use disorders in up to 10% of outpatients and 30% of inpatients; lifetime substance use disorders in 60% to 70%)
- Posttraumatic stress disorder
- Panic disorder with or without agoraphobia
- Obsessive-compulsive disorder

Treatment Considerations
Criteria for Urgent Intervention
- Suicidal ideation, plan, or attempt
- Severe compromise in personal or family financial or social well-being due to manic excesses

171

- Psychosis
- Maladaptive substance use
- Inability to care for self

Medication Options

- For manic, hypomanic, or mixed episodes:
  - Lithium
  - Anticonvulsants (valproate, carbamazepine; possibly lamotrigine, oxcarbazepine, topiramate, verapamil)
  - Typical and atypical neuroleptics (especially if psychosis)
  - Alternative agents (e.g., verapamil, lorazepam, clonazapam)
  - ECT (especially if catatonic, medication intolerant, or first trimester pregnant)
  - Gabapentin add-on is no better than placebo
- For major depressive episodes:
  - Lithium alone or lamotrigine alone
  - Antidepressant added to lithium or other antimanic agent
  - ECT (especially if psychotic, catatonic, medication intolerant, or first trimester pregnant)
- For continuation/maintenance or prophylactic treatment:
  - The best data to date are for lithium, which appears to be prophylactic both for manic/hypomanic episodes and for depressive episodes.
  - Lamotrigine also has promise for prophylaxis of both types of episodes.
  - The acute antimanic agents above are probably useful in prophylaxis of manic episodes, but their efficacy in prophylaxis of depression is uncertain at best. Combination with antidepressants is usually necessary.
  - Until recently, most experts recommended brief treatment of depressive episodes with antidepressants (< 2 months). More recent data indicates standard treatment lengths (6 months) may be warranted.
  - For rapid cycling, agents with some evidence for efficacy include lamotrigine, valproate, and high-dose thyroxine (T_4).
  - For rapid cycling, minimize exposure to antidepressants.

Psychotherapeutic Options

- Supportive care should focus on supporting medication management and role function. Where possible, it should include education of the patient and his or her family.
- Several formal, structured psychotherapies *in addition to* medication management have been demonstrated to help in reducing depressive symptoms or improving course or improving function. See Psychotherapy in **Section IV.**

Considerations in Choosing Among Treatments

- The term *mood stabilizer* is inconsistently used [and not currently defined by the U.S. Food and Drug Administration (FDA)], so that many medications that have an indication for *any* aspect of manic-depressive disorder (usually for acute mania) are marketed as "mood stabilizers." However, more precise usage limits that term to agents efficacious in both acute treatment and prevention of both (hypo)manic and depressive episodes. Controlled trial data indicate that only lithium currently meets those criteria.
- For prophylaxis of individuals who do not respond to, or are intolerant of, lithium, an ongoing combination of antimanic and antidepressant agents may be necessary.

- Formal, structured psychotherapy is based on:
  - Availability of formal, structured psychotherapy
  - Patient preference
- As for major depressive disorder, agents should be chosen based on side effects to be avoided and those that are desired.
- No antidepressant agent has been shown to have greater efficacy than any other in bipolar depression.
- Monoamine oxidase inhibitor antidepressants may be more effective for depressive episodes with atypical features.
- Despite small studies and some but not all retrospective analyses, there is no clear evidence that one class of antidepressants is more or less likely than others to cause (hypo) mania.

Disorder: Cyclothymic Disorder
DSM-IV Codes: 301.13

Adapted DSM Criteria

A.   For at least 2 years, the presence of numerous periods with hypomanic symptoms and numerous periods with depressive symptoms that do not meet criteria for a major depressive episode

B.   No more than 2 months without symptoms in those 2 years

C.   No major depressive episode, manic episode, or mixed episode in the first 2 years

Clinical Highlights
Features

- Cyclothymic disorder is characterized by having a chronic, fluctuating mood that has numerous periods of hypomanic and depressive symptoms.
- Cyclothymic disorder may be a precursor to manic-depressive disorder.
- If a person already has an established diagnosis of manic-depressive disorder, a subsequent cyclothymic pattern does not merit a separate diagnosis of cyclothymic disorder. Rather, the mood instability is considered part of the manic-depressive disorder.

Gender Issues

- Equal in men and women

Cultural Issues

- N/A

Adult Life Cycle Issues

- N/A

Prevalence
Community

- Lifetime prevalence rate of cyclothymic disorder is 0.4% to 1%.

In Primary Care Practice

- N/A

173

In Outpatient Mental Health Practice
- N/A

Among Mental Health Admissions
- N/A

Course
- The disorder usually begins in adolescence or early adulthood.
- It is a chronic disorder.
- 15% to 50% risk that the individual will develop bipolar type I or II disorder.

Common Comorbidities
- N/A. May be similar to manic-depressive disorder.

Treatment Considerations
Criteria for Urgent Intervention
- Suicidal ideation, plan, or attempt
- Severe compromise in personal or family financial or social well-being due to manic excesses
- Maladaptive substance use

Medication Options
- Not well studied; likely the same as for manic-depressive disorder

Psychotherapeutic Options
- Not well studied

Considerations in Choosing Among Treatments
- Individuals with cyclothymic disorder frequently do not present for treatment until they develop a major mood episode or significant life stress.
- Mood stabilizers should be considered, and treatment can be expected to be chronic, given illness course.
- Antidepressants should be used with caution because of concern for worsening manic symptoms.
- Psychotherapy or supportive counseling should be used to help address functional problems or stress associated with depressive symptoms, manic symptoms, and the overall mood inconsistency of the disorder.

ANXIETY DISORDERS

Disorder: Panic Disorder
DSM-IV Codes: 300.01 (Without Agoraphobia)
                        300.21 (With Agoraphobia)

Adapted DSM Criteria
Panic Attack
Note: A panic attack is a symptom, not a disorder.

   A discrete period of intense fear or discomfort, with four or more of the following symptoms that come on abruptly and peak quickly (e.g., in 5–10 minutes):

(1) Palpitations, racing heart rate
(2) Sweating
(3) Trembling
(4) Shortness of breath
(5) Choking sensation
(6) Chest discomfort
(7) Nausea
(8) Feeling faint or dizzy
(9) Derealization or depersonalization (feelings of being outside of one's body watching the proceedings)
(10) Fear of losing control or going crazy
(11) Fear of dying
(12) Numbness or tingling sensations
(13) Chills or flushing

Panic Disorder

Both (1) and (2):

(1) Recurrent unexpected panic attacks
(2) Followed by at least 1 month of worry or behavior change because of the attacks

May or may not also have agoraphobia (see Phobias).

Clinical Highlights
Features

- Panic attacks often come out of the blue.
- They may wake an individual from sleep, but typically occur outside of rapid eye movement (REM) sleep.
- Individuals often say they are one of the most excruciating experiences of their lives.
- Fear of recurrence can dramatically change one's lifestyle, truncating activities and leading to avoidant "work-arounds" and disability.

Gender Issues

- Diagnosed two to three times more often in women than men.

Cultural Issues

- Panic attacks in some cultures are ascribed to intense fear of witchcraft or magic.
- Panic symptoms may occur in various cultures as part of syndromes that do not align well with the Western cultural notion of panic disorder.

Adult Life Cycle Issues

- May worsen over time if left untreated.
- Women have a greater increase in prevalence as they get older.

Prevalence
Community

- Males:
  - Lifetime 2%
  - 12-month 1% to 2%

- Females:
  - Lifetime 5%
  - 12-month 3% to 4%
- Total (males and females)
  - Lifetime 3% to 5%
  - 12-month 2% to 4%

In Primary Care Practice
- Of those with panic disorder, 46% are seen in primary care practices

In Outpatient Mental Health Practice
- *Anxiety disorders represent 9% in a community mental health center.*

Panic Disorder without Agoraphobia
- 0.8% in a private university-affiliated hospital-based clinic
- 3.8% as secondary diagnosis in a private university-affiliated hospital-based clinic

Panic Disorder with Agoraphobia
- 4.8% in a private university-affiliated hospital-based clinic
- 8.5% as secondary diagnosis in a private university-affiliated hospital-based clinic

Among Mental Health Admissions
- Anxiety disorders comprise approximately 4% of inpatient mental health admissions.

Course
- Onset is usually late adolescence through mid-thirties.
- Relapses are frequent.

Common Comorbidities
- Other anxiety disorders
- Major depressive disorder
- Manic-depressive disorder
- Personality disorders
- Substance use disorders

Treatment Considerations
Criteria for Urgent Intervention
- Suicidal ideation, plan, or intent
- Maladaptive substance use
- Truncation of normal activities or agoraphobia

Medication Options
- Tricyclic antidepressants
- Serotonin reuptake inhibitor antidepressants
- Monoamine oxidase inhibitor antidepressants
- Alprazolam and probably other benzodiazepines

176

Psychotherapeutic Options

- Supportive care should focus on supporting medication management and role function. Where possible, it should include education of the patient and his or her family.
- For formal psychotherapy options, see Psychotherapy in **Section IV.**

Considerations in Choosing Among Treatments

- Medication treatments appear to be equally efficacious; choose based on side effects desired or to be avoided.
- Use antidepressants as first-line treatment in individuals with comorbid major depressive disorder.
- Serotonin-reuptake inhibiting antidepressants may require higher doses than for major depressive disorder (e.g., up to 60 mg/day paroxetine or equivalent).
- Tricyclic monoamine oxidase inhibitor antidepressants are given at the same doses as for major depressive disorder.
- Formal psychotherapy versus medication based on:
  - Availability
  - Individual preference
- Development of agoraphobia demands early, aggressive intervention using supportive and behavioral techniques (see Psychotherapy in the **Treatment** section). Once an individual begins to truncate his or her activities due to panic attacks, it is difficult to reestablish those activities. Preventing of loss of function is key.
- Avoid benzodiazepines in active substance use disorders.

Disorder:	Phobias
DSM-IV Codes:	300.29 (Specific)
	300.23 (Social)
	300.22 (Agoraphobia)

Adapted DSM Criteria
Specific Phobia

A.   Persistent and excessive or unreasonable fear that is due to presence or anticipation of a specific object or situation (e.g., heights, needles, insects).
B.   Exposure almost invariably provokes an immediate anxiety response such as a panic attack.
C.   The person recognizes that the fear is excessive or unreasonable.
D.   The situation is avoided or endured only with intense distress.

Social Phobia

A.   Persistent fear of performance situations.
B.   Exposure to the situation almost invariably provokes anxiety or panic attacks.
C.   The person recognizes that the fear is excessive.
D.   The feared situations are avoided or endured only with intense distress.

Agoraphobia

A.   Fear of being in situations from which escape might be difficult or embarrassing, especially if fearful of panic attacks; and

177

B.   Avoidance of such situations.
C.   If only in social/performance situations, diagnosis is social phobia. If only with specific trigger, diagnosis is specific phobia.
D.   Can be a modifier of panic disorder.

Clinical Highlights
Features

- Phobias tend to be circumscribed with other areas of life minimally affected, except for agoraphobia.
- Development of agoraphobia can be crippling because it truncates a broad spectrum of important life functions.
- In clinical settings, those with social phobia typically fear more than one type of social situation.

Gender Issues

- Social, specific, and agoraphobia are more common in women than in men by as much as 2:1.

Cultural Issues

- Both specific and social phobias vary with culture and ethnicity.

Adult Life Cycle Issues

- Prevalence rates of phobias decline in the elderly.

Prevalence

Community:	Specific	Agoraphobia	Social
• Males:			
Lifetime	7%	4%	11%
12-month	4%	2%	7%
• Females:			
Lifetime	16%	7%	16%
12-month	13%	4%	9%
• Total (males and females)			
Lifetime	11%	5%	13%
12-month	9%	3%	8%

In Primary Care Practice

- N/A

In Outpatient Mental Health Practice

- Anxiety disorders represent 9% in a community mental health center.

Specific

- 0.5% in a private university-affiliated hospital-based clinic
- 9.5% as secondary diagnosis in a private university-affiliated hospital-based clinic

Social

- 1% in a private university-affiliated hospital-based clinic
- 27.8% as secondary diagnosis in a private university-affiliated hospital-based clinic

<u>Agoraphobia</u>
- 0% in a private university-affiliated hospital-based clinic
- 1.5% as secondary diagnosis in a private university-affiliated hospital-based clinic

Among Mental Health Admissions
- Anxiety disorders comprise approximately 4.1% of inpatient mental health admissions.
- Phobias are rarely the reason for admission to inpatient settings.

Course
Social
- Onset is usually mid-teens.
- Course is continuous.
- Duration is life-long, but may remit during adulthood.
- Severity of impairment can fluctuate with life stressors and demands.

Specific
- Onset occurs in childhood or early adolescence and may occur at a younger age for women than men.

Agoraphobia
- Little is known about the course.
- Typically persists for years and has considerable impairment.

Common Comorbidities
Social
- Anxiety disorders
- Major depressive disorder
- Manic-depressive disorders
- Dysthymia
- Substance use disorders
- Avoidant personality disorder

Specific
- Agoraphobia

Agoraphobia
- Panic disorder
- Specific phobia
- Major depressive disorder
- Manic-depressive disorders
- Dysthymia

Treatment Considerations
Criteria for Urgent Intervention
- Suicidal ideation, plan, or intent
- Maladaptive substance use
- Truncation of normal activities or agoraphobia

179

Medication Options

Specific

• As-needed benzodiazepines for unavoidable exposures

Social

• Selective serotonin-reuptake inhibitor (SSRI) antidepressants
• As needed benzodiazepines for particular social events
• Beta-blockers for individuals with prominent peripheral symptoms of anxiety (e.g., tremors)
• Monoamine oxidase inhibitor antidepressants

Agoraphobia

• Treat associated features (e.g., panic disorder) and comorbidities (e.g., major depressive disorder) as indicated.
• Occasionally, as-needed benzodiazepines for particular time-limited situations may help to minimize morbidity (e.g., to go to a relative's wedding, to attend a court date).

Psychotherapeutic Options

• Supportive care should focus on supporting medication management and role function. Where possible, it should include education of the patient and his or her family.
• For formal psychotherapy options, see Psychotherapy in **Section IV.**

Considerations in Choosing Among Treatments

• Medication recommendations above mention classes rather than specific agents. Typically, one or two agents in a class have been well studied, but most members of that class are in broad clinical usage (e.g., SSRIs).
• Benzodiazepines should be used with great caution, preferably less than daily, to prevent habitual use, tolerance, or dependence.

Disorder: Generalized Anxiety Disorder
DSM-IV Codes: 300.02

Adapted DSM Criteria

A.   Excessive anxiety and worry more days than not for at least 6 months about a number of life issues (such as work or school performance).
B.   The worry cannot easily be controlled.
C.   The anxiety and worry are associated with at least three of the following, with some present more days than not for the past 6 months:
    (1)   Restlessness or feeling keyed up or on edge
    (2)   Being easily fatigued
    (3)   Difficulty concentrating
    (4)   Irritability
    (5)   Muscle tension
    (6)   Difficulty falling or staying asleep or restless unsatisfying sleep

Clinical Highlights
Features

• Many people have real-world worries.

- However, generalized anxiety disorder should be considered when worry is chronic, uncontrollable, and causes dysfunction or marked distress.
- Other psychiatric or medical disorders may cause the psychological or physical symptoms of generalized anxiety disorder. (e.g., major depressive disorder, panic disorder). These should be ruled out before a diagnosis of generalized anxiety disorder is made.
- The physical symptoms of generalized anxiety disorder are general and chronic, while those for panic disorder, are time-limited or panic-related.

Gender Issues

- Diagnosed more often in females than in males (55%–60% female)

Cultural Issues

- Considerable variations among cultures. Some cultures express anxiety through somatic symptoms while others present symptoms through cognitive symptoms.

Adult Life Cycle Issues

- Onset in up to half of cases is in childhood and adolescence, but can occur after age 20.

Prevalence
Community

- Males:
  - Lifetime 4%
  - 12-month 2%
- Females:
  - Lifetime 7%
  - 12-month 4%
- Total (males and females)
  - Lifetime 5%
  - 12-month 3%

In Primary Care Practice

- Lifetime rate is 5%

In Outpatient Mental Health Practice

- 2% in a private university-affiliated hospital-based clinic
- 6% as secondary diagnosis in a private university-affiliated hospital-based clinic
- Anxiety disorders represent 9% in a community mental health center

Among Mental Health Admissions

- Anxiety disorders comprise approximately 4% of inpatient mental health admissions.

Course

- Chronic and may worsen during stressful times

Common Comorbidities

- Social phobia
- Panic disorder

- Major depressive disorder
- Dysthymia
- Substance use disorders

Treatment Considerations
Criteria for Urgent Intervention
- Suicidal ideation, plan, or intent
- Maladaptive substance use

Medication Options
- Buspirone
- Serotonin reuptake inhibitors
- Venlafaxine
- Benzodiazepines
- Some older studies indicate tricyclic antidepressants may have efficacy as well, but slower onset of action than benzodiazepines.

Psychotherapeutic Options
- Supportive care should focus on supporting medication management and role function. Where possible, it should include education of the patient and his or her family.
- For formal psychotherapy options, see Psychotherapy in **Section IV.**

Considerations in Choosing Among Treatments
- Onset of action for buspirone and antidepressants is days to several weeks.
- Onset of action of benzodiazepines is within a day to several days.
- Be careful of benzodiazepine use in individuals with potential for substance use disorders.

Disorder: Obsessive-Compulsive Disorder
DSM-IV Codes: 300.3

Adapted DSM Criteria
A.   Either obsessions:

(1)   Recurrent intrusive and subjectively inappropriate thoughts, impulses, or images that cause marked anxiety or distress, **and**

(2)   Are not simply excessive real-life worries, **and**

(3)   The person tries to ignore or suppress or neutralize them, **and**

(4)   Recognizes that they are a product of his or her own mind.

Or compulsions:

(1)   Repetitive behaviors (e.g., hand washing, ordering, checking) or mental acts (e.g., praying, counting, repeating words silently) that the person feels compelled to do because of an obsession or other rigid mental rules, **and**

(2)   The behaviors or mental acts are aimed at preventing or reducing distress but are unrealistic or excessive.

B.   The person recognizes that the obsessions or compulsions are excessive or unreasonable.

C.   The obsessions or compulsions cause marked distress or consume more than 1 hour a day or significantly interfere with a person's normal activities or relationships.

Clinical Highlights
Features

- May be associated with profound lack of insight, sometimes to psychotic proportions.
- Differs *substantially* from obsessive-compulsive personality disorder (see page 239–240).

Gender Issues

- Among adults, slightly more common in women
- More common in boys than girls when onset begins during childhood

Cultural Issues

- Should not be confused with culturally or religiously sanctioned rituals

Adult Life Cycle Issues

- Intensity does not decline with age.

Prevalence
Community

- Lifetime prevalence is 2.5%.
- One-year prevalence rates for adults is 0.5% to 2%.

In Primary Care Practice

- Outpatient rate is 1% to 2%

In Outpatient Mental Health Practice

- 2% in a private university-affiliated hospital-based clinic.
- 7% as secondary diagnosis in a private university-affiliated hospital-based clinic.
- Anxiety disorders represent 9% in a community mental health center.

Among Mental Health Admissions

- Anxiety disorders comprise approximately 4% of inpatient mental health admissions.

Course

- Onset is gradual.
- Obsessive-compulsive disorder usually begins in adolescence or early adulthood but could also begin in childhood.
- Mean age of onset is 21 to 35, earlier for males.
- 15% of people have marked deterioration in occupational and social functioning.

Common Comorbidities

- Major depressive disorder
- Other anxiety disorders
- Substance use disorders
- Eating disorders
- Avoidant personality disorder
- Dependent personality disorder

Treatment Considerations
Criteria for Urgent Intervention

- Suicidal ideation, plan, or intent
- Maladaptive substance use
- Truncation of normal activities or agoraphobia
- Marked loss of insight

Medication Options

- Clomipramine
- Fluvoxamine
- Other serotonin reuptake inhibitors, typically at higher doses than used to treat depression (e.g., sertraline 200 mg/day)

Psychotherapeutic Options

- Supportive care should focus on supporting medication management and role function. Where possible, it should include education of the patient and his or her family.
- For formal psychotherapy options, see Psychotherapy in **Section IV.**

Considerations in Choosing Among Treatments

- Meta-analyses have shown higher response rates with the tricyclic clomipramine (70%–80%), a bit higher than the 60% to 70% typically seen with the serotonin reuptake inhibitors.
- Neuroleptics in low doses (e.g., 1–5 mg/day haloperidol or risperidone) may be helpful with comorbid psychotic symptoms or marked loss of insight.
- Some specialty centers are exploring the utility of psychosurgery using gamma knife technology for severely incapacitated individuals refractory to medications plus psychotherapy.

Disorder: Posttraumatic Stress Disorder
DSM-IV Codes: 309.81

Adapted DSM Criteria

A. Traumatic event including both:

    (1)   Experience or witness of an event with actual or threatened death or serious injury or a threat to the physical integrity of self or others

    (2)   Response of fear, helplessness, or horror

    And at least one month of:

B. Event persistently reexperienced with at least one of:

    (1)   Intrusive distressing recollections, images, thoughts, or perceptions of the event

    (2)   Recurrent distressing dreams of the event

    (3)   Feeling as if event were recurring (e.g., sense of reliving the experience, illusions, hallucinations)

    (4)   Distress from internal or external cues of the traumatic event (real or symbolic)

    (5)   Physiologic reactivity on exposure to such cues

    And

C. Avoidance of cues and emotional numbing including at least three of:

    (1) Avoidance of thoughts, feelings, or conversations associated with the trauma

    (2) Avoidance of activities, places, or people associated with the trauma

    (3) Inability to recall an important aspect of the trauma

    (4) Diminished interest or participation in activities

    (5) Detachment or estrangement from others

    (6) Emotional numbing (e.g., unable to have loving feelings)

    (7) Sense of foreshortened future (e.g., does not expect to have a career, marriage, children, or a normal life span)

And

D. Persistent increased arousal including at least two of:

    (1) Difficulty falling or staying asleep

    (2) Irritability

    (3) Difficulty concentrating

    (4) Hypervigilance

    (5) Exaggerated startle response

Clinical Highlights
Features

- Common traumatic events include motor vehicle accidents, rape, other violent crime, combat, or childhood physical or sexual abuse.
- Among men, childhood physical and sexual abuse frequently are not reported unless asked for, and in some non-posttraumatic stress disorder clinical samples, rates may be as high as, respectively, 35% and 25%.
- Traumatic events may include serious threat of harm, as well as harm (e.g., near-miss motor vehicle accident, serious threat of physical injury).
- Traumatic events may include those witnessed, as well as those directly experienced.

Gender Issues

- More common in women than men except for combat-related posttraumatic stress disorder.

Cultural Issues

- Individuals from other cultures with considerable social unrest and civil conflict have higher rates of posttraumatic stress disorder.
- Rates of combat posttraumatic stress disorder may vary with organizational characteristics of the military (e.g., "well-run" vs. "poorly run" wars) and with the social context of the war.

Adult Life Cycle Issues

- Incidence tracks with incidence of trauma
- Does not "burn out" with age

Prevalence
Community

- Males:
  - Lifetime 5%
  - 12-month 2%

- Females:
  - Lifetime 10%
  - 12-month 5%
- Total (males and females)
  - Lifetime 8%
  - 12-month 4%

In Primary Care Practice
- N/A

Outpatient Mental Health Practice
- 5% in a private university-affiliated hospital-based clinic.
- 10% as secondary diagnosis in a private university-affiliated hospital-based clinic.
- Anxiety disorders represent 9% in a community mental health center.

Among Mental Health Admissions
- Anxiety disorders comprise approximately 4% of inpatient mental health admissions.

Course
- Can occur at any age.
- Chronic with people remaining symptomatic for years after initial event.
- Symptoms usually begin within the first 3 months after the trauma, but symptoms can be delayed for months or even years (e.g., with major life role changes, e.g., retirement).
- Duration for symptoms can vary. Recovery can occur anytime within 3 months up to longer than a year.
- Symptoms frequently worsen around anniversaries of trauma.
- May first become evident when buffering social structures are lost (e.g., retirement, loss of spouse).
- May first become evident when life patterns lead to more cue exposures (e.g., parenthood, job change).

Common Comorbidities
- Major depressive disorder
- Manic-depressive disorder
- Dysthymia
- Substance use disorders
- Panic disorder
- Agoraphobia
- Obsessive-compulsive disorder
- Generalized anxiety disorder
- Bipolar disorder

Treatment Considerations
Criteria for Urgent Intervention
- Suicidal ideation, plan, or attempt
- Psychosis
- Maladaptive substance use

186

- Inability to care for self
- Homicidality, assaultiveness, or severe or dangerous family role problems (e.g., excessive physical discipline of one's children or spouse abuse)

Medication Options

- Sertraline has received FDA approval for posttraumatic stress disorder, but with the caveat that it is no better than placebo in men.
- Serotonin reuptake inhibitors and nefazodone are widely used, especially in the presence of comorbid mood disorders.
- The α_1 antagonist prazosin has been reported to be useful in reducing nightmares and sleep disturbance.
- The α_2 agonist clonidine has also been reported to be useful in reducing hypervigilance and autonomic arousal.
- Buspirone is often used to reduce intrusive cognitions.
- Benzodiazepines or neuroleptics are often used to reduce anxiety.
- Neuroleptics and sometimes antimanics are often used to reduce impulsivity and aggression.

Psychotherapeutic Options

- Supportive care should focus on supporting medication management and role function. Where possible, it should include education of the patient and his or her family.
- For formal psychotherapy options, see Psychotherapy in **Section IV.**

Considerations in Choosing Among Treatments

- Treatment is typically symptomatic and multimodal.
- Aggressive treatment of comorbid disorders—especially substance and mood disorders—is essential.
- Particular attention must be directed to potential for violence toward self or others (see **Module 6**).

Disorder:	Acute Stress Disorder
DSM-IV Codes:	308.3

Adapted DSM Criteria

A.   Traumatic event including both:
  (1)   Experience or witness of an event with actual or threatened death or serious injury, or a threat to the physical integrity of self or others
  (2)   Response of fear, helplessness, or horror
B.   During or after the event, at least three of:
  (1)   Numbing, detachment, or absence of emotional responsiveness
  (2)   Reduced awareness of his or her surroundings (e.g., "being in a daze")
  (3)   Derealization (see **Module 4**)
  (4)   Depersonalization (see **Module 4**)
  (5)   Inability to recall an important aspect of the trauma
C.   The traumatic event is persistently reexperienced by recurrent images, thoughts, dreams, illusions, flashback episodes, or a sense of reliving the experience; or distress on exposure to reminders of the traumatic event.
D.   Marked avoidance of trauma cues.

187

E.   Anxiety or increased arousal (e.g., difficulty sleeping, irritability, poor concentration, hypervigilance, exaggerated startle response, motor restlessness).

F.   Disturbance lasts 2 days to 4 weeks and occurs within 4 weeks of the traumatic event.

Clinical Highlights
Features
• Little is known about this new DSM diagnosis.

Gender Issues
• N/A

Cultural Issues
• Different coping behaviors among cultures.
• Severity and pattern of response can be different among cultures.

Adult Life Cycle Issues
• N/A

Prevalence
Community
• 14% to 33% exposed to severe trauma

In Primary Care Practice
• N/A

In Outpatient Mental Health Practice
• N/A

Among Mental Health Admissions
• N/A

Course
• Occurs during or immediately after the trauma
• Typically may last 2 days to as long as 4 weeks

Common Comorbidities
• Posttraumatic stress disorder
• Substance use disorders

Treatment Considerations
Criteria for Urgent Intervention
• Suicidal ideation, plan, or attempt
• Maladaptive substance use
• Prominent or severe dissociative symptoms (e.g., criteria B.2, B.5)

Medication Options
• As-needed benzodiazepines or hypnotics may provide symptomatic relief for the short term.
• Benzodiazepine use should be short-term and preferably less than daily to prevent habitual use, tolerance, or dependence.

Psychotherapeutic Options
- Supportive care should focus on supporting medication management and role function. Where possible, it should include education of the patient and his or her family.
- Stress debriefing protocols may be helpful. Area Red Cross chapters or Veterans Affairs medical centers may be able to provide referral to competent clinicians.

Considerations in Choosing Among Treatments
- Single-session debriefing does more harm than good.
- Be careful using benzodiazepines in the context of suspected substance use.

SUBSTANCE USE DISORDERS AND PATHOLOGICAL GAMBLING

Disorder: Substance Use Disorders
DSM-IV Codes: See Chart

Adapted DSM Criteria for Substance Dependence
Maladaptive substance use manifested by three or more of the following in 12-months:

(1) Tolerance (needing increased amounts of the substance for intoxication or to stay out of withdrawal).
(2) Withdrawal when the substance is stopped.
(3) More substance used than was intended.
(4) Unsuccessful efforts to cut down or stop, or consistent desire to use.
(5) Great deal of time spent using or recovering.
(6) Important activities reduced because of use.
(7) Use continued despite awareness of physical or mental problems made worse by use.

Course specifiers:
Early full remission (at least 1 month but less than 12 months)
Sustained full remission (12 months or longer)
Early partial remission
Sustained partial remission
On agonist therapy
In a controlled environment

Adapted DSM Criteria for Substance Abuse
A. Maladaptive substance use manifested by one (or more) of the following in 12-months:
    (1) Failure to fulfill major role responsibilities such as work, school, and home
    (2) Use in physically hazardous situations (such as driving)
    (3) Recurrent legal problems
    (4) Continued use despite social or interpersonal problems
B. Never met criteria for substance dependence for that substance

Clinical Highlights
Features
- Dependence is a *behavioral* disorder.

189

- An individual need not have physiologic tolerance or withdrawal to have dependence.
- An individual may have physiologic tolerance or withdrawal and not be dependent.
- Dependence on multiple substances is common.
- Dependence and abuse have long-term, relapsing, and remitting courses.
- Suicidality, assaultiveness, and accidental danger to others are common.
- Functional deficits (family, work, leisure impairment) are the rule rather than the exception.
- Social/environmental factors (e.g., friends, family, work, stressors) may promote substance use.
- Substances can cause behavioral effects in up to three scenarios: intoxication, withdrawal, and long-term neuropsychologic effects:

Agent	Intoxication	Withdrawal Effects	Long-Term Neuropsychiatric Effects
Alcohol	X	X	X
Amphetamines	X	X	X
Caffeine	X	X	
Cannabis	X		
Cocaine	X	X	X
Hallucinogens	X	X	X
Inhalants	X	X	X
Nicotine		X	
Opioids	X	X	
Phencyclidine	X	X	X
Sedatives, hypnotics, or anxiolytics	X	X	

Gender Issues
- See Chart

Cultural Issues
- See Chart

Adult Life Cycle Issues
- See Chart

Prevalence

Community:	Alcohol Abuse	Alcohol Dependence	Drug Abuse	Drug Dependence
• Males:				
Lifetime	13%	20%	5%	9%
12-month	3%	11%	1%	4%
• Females:				
Lifetime	6%	8%	4%	6%
12-month	2%	4%	0.3%	2%
• Total (males and females)				
Lifetime	9%	14%	4%	8%
12-month	3%	7%	1%	3%

- Other prevalence statistics:
  - Alcohol: 90% in the United States have had a drink; 60% currently drink.
  - Amphetamines: Lifetime rate 1% to 2%; 6% ages 26 to 34; 2% ages 18 to 25
  - Cannabis: Lifetime rate up to 5% (abuse or dependence)
  - Cocaine: Lifetime rate up to 2% (abuse or dependence)
  - Hallucinogens: Lifetime risk 1% (abuse or dependence)
  - Opioids: Lifetime risk 1% (abuse or dependence)
  - Sedatives, hypnotics, or anxiolytics: 6% ages 26 to 34; lifetime rate less than 1% (abuse or dependence)

Prevalence for U.S. High School Seniors

	Lifetime	30 Days	Daily
Alcohol	80%	51%	3%
Cigarettes	65%	35%	23%
Marijuana	50%	23%	6%
Cocaine	10%	3%	0.2%
Heroin	2%	1%	0.1%
Steroids	3%	1%	0.2%

In Primary Care Practice

- Over 60 years of age, 15% of men and 12% of women exceed alcohol consumption recommendation set by the National Institute on Alcohol Abuse and Alcoholism.

In Outpatient Mental Health Practice

Alcohol Abuse or Dependence

- 1% in a private university-affiliated hospital-based clinic.
- 5% as secondary diagnosis in a private university-affiliated hospital-based clinic.
- Alcohol abuse represents 6% in a community mental health center.
- Alcohol dependence represents 14% in a community mental health center.

Drug Abuse or Dependence

- 1% in a private university-affiliated hospital-based clinic.
- 4% as secondary diagnosis in a private university-affiliated hospital-based clinic.
- Substance abuse represents 3% in a community mental health center.
- Substance dependence represents 50% in a community mental health center.

  Note: Substance use disorders are several-fold more frequent above as a secondary diagnosis than as a chief complaint. Thus, screening with a thorough Review of Systems is of great importance.

Among Mental Health Inpatient Admissions

- Substance use disorders represent 27% of acute mental health admissions, including 7% for drug disorders and 20% for alcohol disorders.

Course

- See chart.

Common Comorbidities
- Other substance use disorders
- Manic-depressive disorder
- Anxiety disorders
- Personality disorders
- Schizophrenia and other psychotic disorders

Treatment Choice Criteria for Urgent Intervention
- Suicidal ideation, plan, or intent
- Assaultiveness
- Criminal involvement
- Potential for accidental harm to others (e.g., operating a vehicle under the influence).
- Serious medical complications (see **Module 5**)
- Psychosis
- Blackouts
- Dependence or substances with potential for high morbidity withdrawal, for example, use of large amounts of:
  - Barbiturates (including carisoprodol and butalbital)
  - Alcohol
  - Benzodiazepines
- Pregnancy

Medication Options
- See **Appendices 2** through **6** for detoxification protocols.
- Alcohol maintenance treatment:
  - Alcohol craving may be reduced by naltrexone 25 to 50 mg every morning.
  - Alcohol aversive therapy may be implemented with disulfiram 250 to 500 mg daily. (*Note:* Typically requires 3–4 days alcohol free, educational materials, medic alert bracelet, and written informed consent.)
- Opiate maintenance treatment:
  - Methadone maintenance through federally licensed programs has been shown to reduce morbidity and mortality in heroin dependence. Typically dosed 50 to 100 mg/day.
  - LAAM (l-α-acetylmethodolacetate), a long-acting opiate agonist, like methadone, is also dosed in federally licensed programs. Dosage is typically 20 to 80 mg three times per week.
  - See **Module 13** for management of chronic pain while minimizing opiate use.
  - Buprenorphine, an opiate mixed agonist/antagonist, can be used both for detoxification and for maintenance. Providers must be certified in addictions or formally trained in buprenorphine use. Dosage typically 4 to 16 mg/day.
  - Naltrexone, an opiate antagonist, reduces effects of opiates and therefore discourages use. Dosage is typically 25 to 50 mg/day or 100 mg every other day since duration of action is 24 to 72 hours. Should not be initiated until at least 5 days heroin free or 7 days methadone free.
- Cocaine maintenance treatment:
  - Several agents have been shown in several studies to reduce cocaine craving, but data overall are equivocal:
    - Amantadine 100 mg three times daily
    - Desipramine 100 to 150 mg/day

Psychotherapeutic Options

- Psychosocial interventions as outlined below are the mainstay of substance treatment.
- Supportive care should focus on supporting medication management and role function. Where possible, it should include education of the patient and his or her family.
- For formal psychotherapy options, see Psychotherapy in **Section IV.**

Considerations in Choosing Among Treatments

- Detoxification (see **Appendices 2–6**) and maintenance/rehabilitation are sequential stages of treatment, though some rehabilitative work (e.g., education) begins immediately.
- Individuals are frequently cognitively compromised during intoxication and withdrawal, so that they may not be able to participate maximally in rehabilitation until detoxified.
- Detoxification for most substances can be conducted in structured outpatient settings.
- Inpatient treatment should be considered if:
  - Criteria for urgent intervention are met
  - Dependence on multiple substances
  - Severe anxiety or mood symptoms
  - Psychosis
- 12-step programs (e.g., Alcoholics Anonymous) are useful adjuncts.
- Rehabilitation programs may include varied levels of structure:
  - Inpatient
  - Partial hospitalization
  - Halfway house (therapeutic communities)
  - Outpatient
  - Sober house (minimal to no therapeutic programming)
- The American Society for Addiction Medicine has developed criteria for matching individuals to level of treatment intensity based on clinical findings (see **Key References**).
- Pharmacologic maintenance strategies are adjunct to, not replacements for, psychosocial interventions.
- Use of pharmacologic interventions is limited by the individual's insight, motivation, and ability to comply. This is especially true for antagonists (e.g., naltrexone for alcohol or opiates).
- In an individual with substance use disorders and prominent symptoms of another disorder (e.g., mood, anxiety, or psychotic symptoms), it is often difficult to distinguish true comorbid disorders from effects of substance that will resolve as substance use and withdrawal cease. Strategies:
  - Is there an extended substance-free period to assess (e.g., months or years)? If symptoms were present, a comorbid disorder is likely and treatment will likely be necessary.
  - If no extended substance-free period, or no symptoms during that period, a comorbid diagnosis cannot be made, nor can it be ruled out.
  - In the latter situation, there is little evidence to guide treatment.
  - Clinically, it makes sense to treat those symptoms that prevent meaningful participation in substance treatment (e.g., depressive, anxiety, psychotic symptoms) regardless of whether an independent comorbid disorder can be diagnosed.

	Dependence	Abuse	Intoxication	Withdrawal	Gender
Alcohol	303.90	305.00	303.00	291.81	More common in males
Amphetamines	304.40	305.70	292.89	292.0	3 or 4:1 male: female ratio for i.v.
Caffeine		305.90 Other	305.90	292.0 Other	Greater in males than females
Cannabis	304.30	305.20	292.89		More common in males
Cocaine/crack	304.20	305.60	292.89	292.0	More common in males, 1.5–2.0:1
Hallucinogens	304.50	305.30	292.89		More common in males 3:1
Inhalants	304.60	305.90	292.89		More common in males
Nicotine	305.1				More common in males
Opioids	304.00	305.50	292.89	292.0	More common in males
Phencyclidine	304.60	305.90	292.89		More common in males
Sedatives, hypnotics, or anxiolytics	304.10	305.40	292.89	292.0	More common in males
Ecstasy and related compounds	304.90 Other	305.90 Other	305.90 Other		N/A

Cultural	Adult Cycle	Course
Forbidden by some religions (Islam). Amounts differ in what is culturally acceptable. In Asians, flushing common with small amounts. Some European and American cultures accept large amounts.	1.5 million alcoholics in the United States are 65 or older. Over 50 years of age, alcohol dependence has been found in 3.5% of men and 2% of women, with less in Caucasian than minority individuals. 15%–25% of alcohol-dependent individuals first report dependence over 60 years of age.	Males: increases between ages 18 and 20, decreases in early 30s, and peaks again at 35–40. Females: increases at 21–30, levels off in late 30s to 40s
i.v. use is more common in lower socioeconomic groups	More common in ages 18–30	N/A
N/A	N/A	Begins mid-tens. Caffeine intake increases during the 20s and decreases after 65.
Worldwide use	N/A	N/A
In 1970s mainly among affluent, now shifted to lower socioeconomic groups	N/A	N/A
Used in some religious practices, e.g., Native Americans	Decreases with age.	Begins in adolescence.
N/A	Decreases with age.	Begins at 9–12 years of age.
Higher levels in African-American males, nonmetropolitan areas	N/A	Peeks in adolescence. Begins in early teens and persists daily at higher rates than other substances (see high school prevalence rates).
Higher levels in metropolitan areas	Decreases with age.	N/A
N/A	N/A	N/A
More common in males living in metropolitan areas. Commonly prescribed (and commonly sought) muscle relaxants include barbiturates caprisoprodol (Soma) and butalbital	N/A	Teenagers and in 20s.
Increasing use in the United States in past several years to enhance peak experiences at parties ("raves")	Mainly teens and young adults across socioeconomic spectrum.	N/A

Disorder:			Pathological Gambling
DSM-IV Codes:		312.31

Adapted DSM Criteria
A.	Gambling is considered pathologic according to the DSM system if there is social dysfunction or personal suffering. Pathologic gambling is diagnosed with five or more of:
1.	Preoccupied with gambling-related activities
2.	Increasing amounts to achieve desired thrill
3.	Unsuccessful attempts to cut down
4.	Restless/irritable when cutting down
5.	Gambling to escape problems or to relieve bad mood
6.	Frequent returns to gambling to recoup losses
7.	Lying about gambling
8.	Illegal acts to finance gambling
9.	Jeopardized/lost role function because of gambling

B.	Reliance on gambling to repay debts from gambling

Clinical Highlights
Features
- Occurrence may vary with proximity and ease of access to gambling.
- Gambling access may be at a specific geographic locale or remote (e.g., through the Internet).
- Some activities not typically considered gambling may serve the same purpose (e.g., day trading of investments).

Gender Issues
- One third of gamblers are female.
- Females are underrepresented in treatment programs and represent 2% to 4% of those who attend Gamblers Anonymous.

Cultural Issues
- Gender ratios can vary in different areas and cultures.

Adult Life Cycle Issues
- N/A

Prevalence
Community
- 0.4% to 3.4% for adults; some areas are as high as 7%.
- 2.8% to 8% in adolescents and college students.

In Primary Care Practice
- N/A

In Outpatient Mental Health Practice
- 0.3% in a private university-affiliated hospital-based clinic
- 0.6% as secondary diagnosis in a private university-affiliated hospital-based clinic

Among Mental Health Admissions
- Impulse control disorders represent approximately 1% of inpatient mental health admissions.

Course
- Can be habitual or episodic
- Tends to be chronic
- Occurs earlier in males than females (early adolescence for males, later for females)

Common Comorbidities
- Substance use disorders

Treatment Considerations
Criteria for Urgent Intervention
- Suicidal ideation, plan, or attempt
- Extreme family or financial stress
- Criminal involvement

Medication Options
- **N/A**

Psychotherapeutic Options
- Supportive care should focus on supporting medication management and role function. Where possible, it should include education of the patient and his or her family.

Considerations in Choosing Among Treatments
- Treatment is psychosocial.
- Increasing recognition of pathologic gambling has led to development of therapeutic communities and 12-step programs built on the substance abuse model. See **Appendix 10** for relevant information for pathologic gambling.

SCHIZOPHRENIA AND OTHER PSYCHOTIC DISORDERS

Disorder: Schizophrenia
DSM-IV Codes: 295.30 (Paranoid Type)
                       295.10 (Disorganized Type)
                       295.20 (Catatonic Type)
                       295.60 (Residual Type)
                       295.90 (Undifferentiated Type)

Adapted DSM Criteria
For Schizophrenia Disorder
A.   At least 1 month of at least two of:
    (1)   Delusions
    (2)   Hallucinations
    (3)   Disorganized speech

           (4)   Grossly disorganized or catatonic behavior
           (5)   Negative symptoms, i.e., affective flattening, alogia, or avolition
B.   Significant decline in work function, school function, interpersonal relations, or self-care
C.   Continuous signs of the disturbance for at least 6 months, including pro-
dromal or residual symptoms

Paranoid Type

A.   Preoccupation with one or more delusions or frequent auditory hallucinations.
B.   None of the following is prominent: disorganized speech, disorganized or
catatonic behavior, or flat or inappropriate affect.

Disorganized Type

A.   All of the following are prominent:
           (1)   Disorganized speech
           (2)   Disorganized behavior
           (3)   Flat or inappropriate affect
B.   The criteria are not met for catatonic type.

Catatonic Type

See **Module 7.**

Residual Type

A.   Absence of prominent delusions, hallucinations, disorganized speech, and
grossly disorganized or catatonic behavior.
B.   Negative symptoms or two or more symptoms listed in criterion A for
schizophrenia present in an attenuated form.

Undifferentiated Type

Criteria are not met for the paranoid, disorganized, or catatonic type.
Schizophreniform disorder (295.40)   Criteria A and B met, but for fewer
                                             than 6 months.

Clinical Highlights
Features

- Up to 50% with schizophrenia attempt suicide at some time in their lives.
- Positive symptoms are those listed in criterion A.
- Negative symptoms include:
  - Flat affect.
  - Alogia (minimal speech).
  - Avolition (minimal impetus to do anything).
  - Anhedonia (minimal enjoyment in activities), but not depressed mood.
  - *Simple schizophrenia* is an older term denoting a purely negative symptom
    or residual presentation.
  - *Paraphrenia* is a broad, obsolete term connoting either or both of paranoia
    and marked disorganization.
- Kraepelin coined the term *dementia praecox* (early dementia) to differentiate
  schizophrenia from manic-depressive disorder based on the progressive
  downhill course of the former.
- Historically, Bleuler and Schneider proposed core characteristics for schizo-
  phrenia:

198

- Bleulerian "4 A's":
  - Associations (loose)
  - Affect (flat)
  - Autism (negative symptoms)
  - Ambivalence (inability to recognize and/or react appropriately to the mutually incompatibility of thoughts, feeling, interpretations of events that they may have)
- Schneiderian "first rank" symptoms:
  - Audible thoughts
  - Voices in dialogue
  - Voices commenting on the person's behavior
  - Sense of being controlled
  - Thought withdrawal or insertion
  - Thought broadcasting
  - Hallucinations
- Note that Bleulerian and Schneiderian symptom chapters are not specific for schizophrenia, nor do they comprise high-sensitivity probes. See **Section I, Panels 10 and 11.**

Gender Issues
- Gender ratio 1:1.
- Some studies show better outcome in women.
- Onset for men is 18 to 25 and 25 to mid-thirties for women.

Cultural Issues
- Evidence for overdiagnosis in African Americans and Asian Americans.
- Catatonic behavior may be more common in developing than in developed countries.
- Better outcome in developing nations than in industrialized ones.

Adult Life Cycle Issues
- Chronic, throughout the lifespan.
- Onset after age 40 is rare.

Prevalence
Community
- 0.5% to 1.5%
- Annual rates 0.5 to 5.0 per 10,000
- Lifetime rate of delusions: 1.6%

In Primary Care Practice
- N/A

In Outpatient Mental Health Practice
- 0.5% in a private university-affiliated hospital-based clinic.
- Schizophrenia and schizoaffective disorder represent 14% in a community mental health center.

Among Mental Health Admissions
- Schizophrenia and related psychotic disorders comprise approximately 12% of inpatient mental health admissions.

Course
- Onset is late teens to mid-thirties.
- Late onset is less common in men.
- Positive symptoms may wax and wane. With appropriate treatment, some go years between symptom bouts; others are chronically psychotic.
- Relapse rates are 40% over 2 years on medications and 80% over 2 years without.
- The functional decline tends to remain or progress.

Common Comorbidities
- Substance use disorders
- Nicotine dependence 80% to 90%
- Obsessive-compulsive disorder
- Panic disorder

Treatment Considerations
Criteria for Urgent Intervention
- Suicidal ideation, plan, or attempt
- Psychosis
- Gross disorganization or potential for accidental harm to self or others
- Maladaptive substance use
- Inability to care for self

Medication Options
- Neuroleptics, or antipsychotics, are the cornerstone of treatment.
- Medications to treat or prevent neuroleptic-induced movement disorders are important adjuvants (see **Module 17**).

Psychotherapeutic Options
- Supportive care should focus on supporting medication management and role function. Where possible, it should include education of the patient and his or her family.
- For formal psychotherapy options, see Psychotherapy in **Section IV.**

Considerations in Choosing Among Treatments
- Medications are the cornerstone of treatment, and psychosocial interventions are important adjuvants.
- Newer atypical neuroleptics have become first-line treatment because of their apparently lower incidence rates of tardive dyskinesia.
- However, some atypical neuroleptics are associated with obesity and type II diabetes; obesity can be as disfiguring as tardive dyskinesia and carries a higher morbidity rate.
- More sedating neuroleptics may be useful for highly agitated individuals and may make unnecessary the use of nonspecific sedative agents.
- Prior history of acute extrapyramidal symptoms should lead to consideration of low-potency typical or atypical agents.
- Clozapine is to date the only agent to have demonstrated efficacy in refractory schizophrenia.
- ECT has been used in those intolerant of or refractory to medication or in the first trimester of pregnancy.

- There are some reports of successful adjuvant treatment with the anticonvulsants carbamazepine and valproate added to neuroleptics.
- Catatonia should be treated *without* neuroleptics and with high doses of lorazepam or ECT. Neuroleptics can be gradually reintroduced when catatonia abates (see **Module 7**).
- Atypical neuroleptics may be considered "doing and undoing" drugs:
  - Dopamine-2 (D-2) receptor blockade diminishes dopamine neurotransmission and reduces positive symptoms.
  - Serotonin-2A receptor blockade stimulates dopamine release, to a degree mitigating the effects of D-2 blockade.
  - This balance across relevant dopamine pathways in the brain is probably responsible for their effect on negative symptoms, less acute extrapyramidal symptoms, and reduced incidence of tardive dyskinesia.
  - In some cases augmentation of an atypical agent with a typical agent (which predominantly blocks D-2 receptors) may be required for adequate positive symptom control.

Disorder: Schizoaffective Disorder
DSM-IV Codes: 295.70

Adapted DSM Criteria
A.   Mood episode (major depressive episode, a manic episode, or a mixed episode) plus concurrent criterion A/schizophrenia symptoms; and
B.   Psychosis for at least 2 weeks in the absence of prominent mood symptoms; or
C.   If chronic criterion A/schizophrenia symptoms are met, then symptoms that meet criteria for a mood episode must be present for a substantial portion of the total duration of the active and residual periods of the illness.
Specify type:
Bipolar type: if mania/mixed episodes have occurred
Depressive type: if depressive episodes only

Clinical Highlights
Features
- A "wastebasket" term for those who have too much chronic mood pathology to be considered purely schizophrenic and too much psychosis to be considered purely mood disordered.
- Boundaries are not well established empirically.

Gender Issues
- Equal in women and men

Cultural Issues
- N/A

Adult Life Cycle Issues
- N/A

Prevalence
Community
- Less than 1%
- Lifetime rate of delusions: 1.6%

In Primary Care Practice

- N/A

In Outpatient Mental Health Practice

- 1% in a private university-affiliated hospital-based clinic.
- Schizophrenia and schizoaffective disorder represent 14% in a community mental health center.

Among Mental Health Admissions

- Schizophrenia and related psychotic disorders comprise approximately 12% of inpatient mental health admissions.

Course

- Outcome is midway between schizophrenia and manic-depressive disorder in terms of symptoms and function.
- Onset is typically early adulthood but can occur anywhere from adolescence to late in life.
- Bipolar type more common in young adults.
- Depressive type more common in older adults.

Common Comorbidities

- Substance use disorders

Treatment Considerations
Criteria for Urgent Intervention

- Suicidal ideation, plan, or attempt
- Psychosis
- Maladaptive substance use
- Inability to care for self

Medication Options

- Treatment of psychotic symptoms as for schizophrenia
- Treatment of mood symptoms as for manic-depressive or major depressive disorder

Psychotherapeutic Options

- By extension, consider formal psychotherapies for schizophrenia and manic-depressive disorder. See Psychotherapy in **Section IV.**

Considerations in Choosing Among Treatments

- Since schizophrenia phenomenologically shares features of both schizophrenia and manic-depressive disorder, consideration of treatment options in these two disorders are relevant to schizoaffective disorder.
- Some individuals appear to have a course virtually identical to that of manic-depressive disorder, with just a bit too much psychosis (see criterion B); they can be treated as for manic-depressive disorder, with neuroleptics as needed.
- Others have a much more schizophrenic picture and require chronic neuroleptics.

Disorder: Delusional Disorder
DSM-IV Codes: 297.1

Adapted DSM Criteria
A.   At least 1 month of delusions regarding situations that could occur in real life, such as being followed, poisoned, infected, or deceived.
B.   Never schizophrenia
C.   Functioning not otherwise markedly impaired and behavior not odd.

Clinical Highlights
Features
- Delusions tend to be systematized but circumscribed.
- Delusions may be quite believable.
- Function not compromised as in schizophrenia.
- Often, if you didn't stumble upon the "sore spot," you wouldn't know the individual was ill.

Gender Issues
- No gender difference except for jealous type, which occurs more often in men.

Cultural Issues
- Cultural and religious background needs to be taken into account. Some beliefs in one culture could be considered a delusion in another.

Adult Life Cycle Issues
- Occurs middle to late life

Prevalence
Community
- 0.03%
- Lifetime rate of delusions: 1.6%

In Primary Care Practice
- Uncommon in clinical settings

In Outpatient Mental Health Practice
- 0.3% as secondary diagnosis in a private university-affiliated hospital-based clinic

Among Mental Health Admissions
- Schizophrenia and related psychotic disorders comprise approximately 12% of inpatient mental health admissions, but delusional disorder represents a small percentage of these.

Course
- Can be chronic and lifelong.
- First admission is usually between the ages of 35 and 55.

Common Comorbidities
- Major Depressive Disorder
- Obsessive-compulsive disorder

203

- Paranoid personality disorder
- Schizoid personality disorder
- Avoidant personality disorder

Treatment Considerations
Criteria for Urgent Intervention
- Suicidal ideation, plan, or attempt
- Psychosis
- Maladaptive substance use
- Inability to care for self
- Danger to others or potential for this (e.g., delusions lead to perception of persecution and possible need to protect one's self or strike back).

Medication Options
- Neuroleptics are the cornerstone of treatment.
- Medications to treat or prevent neuroleptic-induced movement disorders are important adjuvants (see **Module 17**).

Psychotherapeutic Options
- No specific psychotherapy.
- See Supportive Psychotherapy outline.

Considerations in Choosing Among Treatments
- Basic approach is similar to that for schizophrenia.
- However, insight is often, paradoxically, worse because the delusions are credible, circumscribed, and do not profoundly impair function.
- Therefore, empathic alliance building followed by reframing of events and perceptions is a reasonable approach.
- It is important to get corroborating information to determine the degree to which concerns are actually warranted. The situation is often not black or white, true or false in nature. There is sometimes an element of truth in the situation, or it is at least understandable how the individual could have drawn the conclusions.

ADJUSTMENT DISORDERS

Disorder: Adjustment Disorders
DSM-IV Codes: 309.0 With Depressed Mood
                       309.24 With Anxiety
                       309.28 With Mixed Anxiety and Depressed Mood
                       309.3 With Disturbance of Conduct
                       309.4 With Mixed Disturbance of Emotions and Conduct
                       309.9 Unspecified

Adapted DSM Criteria
A.   Symptoms in response to a stressor that begin within 3 months of the stressor.
B.   Not due to another axis I or axis II disorder or bereavement.
C.   Once the stressor (or its consequences) is over, symptoms remit within 6 months.

Clinical Highlights
Features
- Other diagnoses must be excluded (e.g., major depressive disorder with a identified stressor).
- Individuals usually make the connection between the stressor and the symptoms.
- If an individual meets criteria for another disorder (e.g., major depressive disorder), then that diagnosis is given, not adjustment disorder.

Gender Issues
- Women are given the diagnosis twice as often as men.

Cultural Issues
- N/A

Adult Life Cycle Issues
- Likely varies with stressor.
- Life transitions are times of high risk. For example:
  - High school to work or college
  - Marital status change
  - New child
  - Job change or relocation
  - Retirement
  - Physical illness

Prevalence
Community
- Adjustment disorders have been diagnosed in up to 12% of general hospital inpatients who are referred for a mental health consultation.

In Primary Care Practice
- N/A

In Outpatient Mental Health Practice
- 5% in a private university-affiliated hospital-based clinic
- 1% as secondary diagnosis in a private university-affiliated hospital-based clinic

Among Mental Health Admissions
- Adjustment disorders comprise approximately 4% of inpatient mental health admissions.

Course
- Time-limited by definition

Common Comorbidities
- Substance abuse

Treatment Considerations
Criteria for Urgent Intervention
- Suicidal ideation, plan, or attempt
- Maladaptive substance use

Medication Options
* Symptomatic treatment as below if necessary

Psychotherapeutic Options
* Supportive psychotherapy is indicated (see Psychotherapy entry in **Section IV**).

Considerations in Choosing Among Treatments
* Short-term as-needed medications for anxiety (benzodiazepines) or insomnia (hypnotics) may be useful.
* Benzodiazepine and hypnotic use should be short-term and preferably less than daily to prevent habitual use, tolerance, a or dependence.
* Chronic treatment (e.g., with antidepressants) is not necessary; if it appears so, reevaluate the diagnosis.

COGNITIVE DISORDERS

Disorder:	Dementia
DSM-IV Codes:	294.1x Alzheimer Type
	290.4x Vascular Type

Adapted DSM Criteria
Alzheimer Type

A. Multiple cognitive deficits including:

    (1) Memory impairment (impaired ability to learn new information or to recall previously learned information)

    (2) One (or more) of the following cognitive disturbances:

        (a) Aphasia (language disturbance)

        (b) Apraxia (impaired ability to carry out motor activities despite intact motor function)

        (c) Agnosia (failure to recognize or identify objects despite intact sensory function)

        (d) Disturbance in executive functioning (i.e., planning, organizing, sequencing, abstracting)

B. Gradual onset and continuing cognitive decline.

C. The cognitive deficits in criteria A1 and A2 are not due to other specific causes.

Vascular Dementia

A. Multiple cognitive deficits as for Alzheimer's dementia

B. Focal neurologic signs and symptoms or imaging evidence of cerebrovascular disease judged to be etiologically related to the disturbance.

C. The deficits do not occur exclusively during the course of a delirium.

Clinical Highlights
Features
* See **Module 8.**

Gender Issues
* For Alzheimer's dementia, there appears to be a predominance of women, although rates vary widely, from 1.2–3:1.

- For vascular dementia, men are affected more frequently than women, up to 2:1.

Cultural Issues
- Prevalence can vary among cultures, with some studies indicating lower prevalence or less severe course in developing nations compared with industrialized nations.

Adult Life Cycle Issues
- Primarily a disorder of the elderly
- Down syndrome associated with high prevalence and early onset of Alzheimer disease

Prevalence
Community
- 0.6% ages 65 to 69
- 1% ages 70 to 74
- 2% ages 75 to 79
- 3.3% ages 80 to 84
- 8.4% ages 85 and older

In Primary Care Practice
- N/A

In Outpatient Mental Health Practice
- 1% of outpatients

Among Mental Health Admissions
- Dementia and cognitive disorders comprise 4% of inpatient mental health admissions.

Course
- Chronic and typically progressive

Common Comorbidities
- Delirium (see **Module 7**)
- Major depressive disorder
- Substance use disorder
- Associated symptoms that are common and require treatment:
  - Anxiety
  - Psychosis

Treatment Considerations
Criteria for Urgent Intervention
- Suicidal ideation, plan, or attempt
- Psychosis
- Maladaptive substance use
- Inability to care for self

Medication Options
- Cognitive enhancers lessen progression and perhaps lead to some improvement.

- Some trials of vitamin E 800 to 1,600 IU/day have shown promising results.
- Treatment of associated symptoms and comorbid disorders as indicated.

Psychotherapeutic Options
- Supportive work with the individual and families is always indicated (see Psychotherapy in **Section IV**).
- No psychotherapy has been shown to be effective for core cognitive symptoms, and participation in psychotherapy for comorbid conditions may be limited by cognitive abilities.
- Cognitive retraining has not been clearly shown to be beneficial.

Considerations in Choosing Among Treatments
- As the disease progresses, the focus of treatment moves more from the individual to him or her plus family or living institution.
- Treatment of associated conditions—including physical and occupational therapy for neurologic deficits—is always indicated.
- Attention to caregiver burden, fatigue, and abuse (either direction) is necessary and accommodations are essential.
- Cognitive enhancer medications are well tolerated, and much dementia is mixed (Alzheimer type plus vascular type). Therefore although cognitive enhancers have shown efficacy only in Alzheimer type, one should err on the side of using them in uncertain or mixed cases.

Disorder: Attention-Deficit/Hyperactivity Disorder
DSM-IV Codes: 314.00 (Inattentive Type)
                    314.01 (Combined Type)
                    314.01 (Hyperactive-Impulsive Type)
                    314.9 [Not Otherwise Specified (NOS)]

Adapted DSM Criteria
A.   Six or more months of either (1) or (2):
   (1)   Six or more inattention symptoms of:
      (a)   Poor attention to details or careless mistakes in schoolwork, work, or other activities
      (b)   Difficulty sustaining attention in tasks
      (c)   Does not seem to listen when spoken to directly
      (d)   Does not follow through on instructions and fails to finish tasks
      (e)   Difficulty organizing tasks and activities
      (f)   Reluctant to engage in tasks that require sustained mental effort (such as schoolwork or homework)
      (g)   Often loses things necessary for tasks
      (h)   Easily distracted by extraneous stimuli
      (i)   Forgetful in daily activities
   (2)   Six or more hyperactivity-impulsivity symptoms of:
      (a)   Fidgets or squirms
      (b)   Often leaves seat in situations in which remaining seated is expected

(c)   Often has subjective feelings of restlessness
(d)   Difficulty engaging in leisure activities quietly
(e)   Often "on the go" or often acts as if "driven by a motor"
(f)   Talks excessively
(g)   Blurts out answers before questions have been completed
(h)   Has difficulty awaiting turn
(i)   Interrupts or intrudes on others

B.   Some hyperactive-impulsive or inattentive symptoms that caused impairment were present before age 7 years.

C.   Impairment from symptoms is in two or more settings (e.g., school, work, home).

Clinical Highlights
Features

- Commonly recognized in children, less so in adults.
- To diagnose in adults, symptoms must have been present in childhood.
- Expression of symptoms may be different in adults than children because environmental demands are different.
- Many adults with this disorder live their lives around their symptoms and avoid environments that lead to problems.

Gender Issues

- 2:1 to 9:1, males to females

Cultural Issues

- N/A

Adult Life Cycle Issues

- Chronic from childhood, by definition
- Characteristics in elderly ill defined

Prevalence
Community

- N/A

In Primary Care Practice

- N/A

In Outpatient Mental Health Practice

- 3% in a private university-affiliated hospital-based clinic
- 1% as secondary diagnosis in a private university-affiliated hospital-based clinic

Among Mental Health Admissions

- N/A

Course

- Chronic
- Differentiated from manic-depressive disorder with hypomania and cyclothymia by its chronic, rather than episodic, course

209

Common Comorbidities
- Major depressive disorder
- Manic-depressive disorder
- Anxiety disorders

Treatment Considerations
Criteria for Urgent Intervention
- Suicidal ideation, plan, or attempt
- Impending serious occupational compromise

Medication Options
- Methylphenidate
- Pemoline
- Amphetamine or dextroamphetamine 5 to 30 mg twice daily given in the morning and no later than early afternoon; several brand-name combination preparations have recently become available.
- Desipramine in antidepressant doses
- Bupropion in antidepressant doses

Psychotherapeutic Options
- Although medication treatment is typically beneficial, life structuring, problem solving, and family support are required to minimize morbidity.
- No structured, formal psychotherapies for adults are available.

Considerations in Choosing Among Treatments
- Among medications, stimulants are first-line treatment, with desipramine and bupropion typically reserved for situations where stimulants cannot be used or have failed.
- Nonresponse to one stimulant does not mean nonresponse to all.
- Use stimulants with care in situations of potential substance misuse (including in family members).

SOMATOFORM AND RELATED DISORDERS

Disorder: Somatization Disorder
DSM-IV Codes: 300.81

Adapted DSM Criteria
A. Several years of many physical complaints beginning before age 30 years, including treatment-seeking or significant functional impairment.
B. Each of the following at any time during the disturbance:
  (1) *Four pain symptoms:* a history of pain related to at least four different sites or functions
  (2) *Two gastrointestinal symptoms:* other than pain
  (3) *One sexual symptom:* other than pain
  (4) *One neurologic symptom*
C. Either (1) or (2):
  (1) Criterion B cannot be fully explained by a known general medical condition.
  (2) When there is a related general medical condition, complaints or impairment are in excess of what would be expected from the findings.

D. The symptoms are not intentionally produced or feigned (as in factitious disorder or malingering).

Clinical Highlights
Features
- Recurrent physical complaints
- Most pervasive somatoform disorder

Gender Issues
- More common in women

Cultural Issues
- Individuals from non-Western, developed, and some non-Anglo, cultures may present with prominent physical complaints. These may be:
  - Within cultural norms and nonpathologic if they do not cause distress
  - Part of culture-bound syndromes that do cause distress but are not well represented in the Western/Anglo psychiatric nomenclature
  - Somatically weighted presentations of DSM-defined mood, anxiety, or psychotic disorders

Adult Life Cycle Issues
- By definition, begins in young adulthood or earlier

Prevalence
Community
- 0.2% to 2% in women
- Less than 0.2% in men

In Primary Care Practice
- N/A

In Outpatient Mental Health Practice
- 0.5% as secondary diagnosis in a private university-affiliated hospital-based clinic

Among Mental Health Admissions
- Somatoform disorders comprise approximately 0.2% of inpatient mental health admissions.

Course
- Chronic and fluctuates, but rarely remits completely.
- Symptoms often start in adolescence, but criteria is usually met before age 25.

Common Comorbidities
- Because criteria overlap with other somatoform disorders, individuals may meet criteria for more than one. However, careful differential diagnosis is required to differentiate among them (see **Module 14**).
- Major depressive disorders
- Dysthymia
- Generalized anxiety disorder
- Substance use disorders

Treatment Considerations
Criteria for Urgent Intervention

- Suicidal ideation, plan, or attempt
- Maladaptive substance use
- Frequent or potentially high-morbidity but unnecessary medical interventions

Medication Options

- Treatment of comorbid conditions as indicated

Psychotherapeutic Options

- Supportive care should focus on supporting medication management and role function. Where possible, it should include education of the patient and his or her family.
- For formal psychotherapy options, see Psychotherapy in **Section IV.**

Considerations in Choosing Among Treatments

- The approach is primarily supportive psychotherapeutic, from a medical perspective.
  - Ensure there are no medical grounds for complaints.
  - Listen empathically rather than confront.
  - Take the approach of the individual's needing to "live with symptoms" but that careful follow-up will be arranged to monitor changes.
  - Minimize unnecessary tests and interventions.
  - Monitor for mood and anxiety comorbidities.
- Ensure that same message is delivered both by medical and by mental health providers.
- 20 minutes spent on the above will save 2 hours' time down the road.

Disorder: Pain Disorder
DSM-IV Codes: 307.80 (with psychologic factors only)
                       307.89 (psychologic factors and general medical condition)

Adapted DSM Criteria

A. Pain involving treatment seeking and significant dysfunction.
B. Psychologic factors are judged to have an important role in the onset, severity, exacerbation, or maintenance of the pain.
C. The symptom or deficit is not intentionally produced or feigned (as in factitious disorder or malingering).

Clinical Highlights
Features

- Most commonly occurs in the setting of pain due to a clear physical cause (i.e., "real pain")
- Symptoms of pain are exacerbated or maintained by psychologic factors
- If there is not clear physical cause for pain, carefully consider other somatoform disorders (e.g., somatization disorder, conversion disorder).

Gender Issues

- Occurs more often in females

Cultural Issues
- Cultures differ in acceptability of expressing pain; however, the core of the diagnosis of pain disorder is identifying a clear psychologic component.

Adult Life Cycle Issues
- Can occur at any age

Prevalence
Community
- N/A

In Primary Care Practice
- N/A

In Outpatient Mental Health Practice
- 0.3% in a private university-affiliated hospital-based clinic
- 0.8% as secondary diagnosis in a private university-affiliated hospital-based clinic

Among Mental Health Admissions
- Somatoform disorders comprise approximately 0.2% of inpatient mental health admissions.

Course
- Resolves in short periods if outside stressor is identified and resolved
- May become chronic

Common Comorbidities
- Substance use disorders
- Major depressive disorder

Treatment Considerations
Criteria for Urgent Intervention
- Suicidal ideation, plan, or attempt
- Maladaptive substance use
- Frequent or potentially high morbidity, but unnecessary, medical interventions
- Initiation of unnecessary opiates

Medication Options
- Ensure that physical pain is adequately managed in "The House of Pain" (**Module 13**).
- Treat comorbid disorders.

Psychotherapeutic Options
- Supportive care should focus on supporting medication management and role function. Where possible, it should include education of the patient and his or her family.
- No formal psychotherapeutic interventions have been identified.

Considerations in Choosing Among Treatments
- Overall approach is similar to that for somatization disorder.

Disorder: Hypochondriasis
DSM-IV Codes: 300.7

Adapted DSM Criteria

A.   At least 6 months of preoccupation with having a serious disease, based on misinterpretation of bodily symptoms.

B.   Preoccupation persists despite appropriate medical evaluation and reassurance.

C.   Not delusional (see **Module 4**) or due to body dysmorphic disorder.

Clinical Highlights

Features

- The core feature is misinterpreting actual symptoms and fearing that one may have a serious disease.
- Symptoms or deficits are not generated *de novo*—that is conversion disorder.
- Symptoms are not feigned—that is factitious disorder or malingering.

Gender Issues

- Equally common in men and women

Cultural Issues

- Cultures differ in acceptability of expressing physical symptoms; however, the core of the diagnosis of hypochondriasis is identifying a clear psychologic component that generates excessive concern.

Adult Life Cycle Issues

- Most common age of onset is early adulthood.

Prevalence

Community

- 1% to 5% among general population

In Primary Care Practice

- 2% to 7% among primary care outpatients

In Outpatient Mental Health Practice

- 0.5% in a private university-affiliated hospital-based clinic
- 0.8% as secondary diagnosis in a private university-affiliated hospital-based clinic

Among Mental Health Admissions

- Somatoform disorders represent approximately 0.2% of inpatient mental health admissions.

Course

- Chronic, but complete recovery can occur.
- 25% patients do poorly, 65% chronic but fluctuating course, and 10% recover after a specific episode.

Common Comorbidities

- Major depressive disorder
- Substance use disorder
- Dysthymia
- Anxiety disorders

Treatment Considerations
Criteria for Urgent Intervention

- Suicidal ideation, plan, or attempt
- Maladaptive substance use
- Frequent or potentially high morbidity but unnecessary medical interventions

Medication Options

- Treatment of comorbid disorder

Psychotherapeutic Options

- Supportive care should focus on supporting medication management and role function. Where possible, it should include education of the patient and his or her family.
- No specific formal psychotherapy has been shown to be effective.

Considerations in Choosing Among Treatments

- Overall approach is similar to that for somatization disorder.

Disorder:	Conversion Disorder
DSM-IV Codes:	300.11

Adapted DSM Criteria

A.   Voluntary motor or sensory symptoms or deficits that suggest a neurologic or other general medical condition (excluding pain or sexual dysfunction).

B.   Initiation or exacerbation of the symptom or deficit is preceded by conflicts or other stressors.

C.   The symptom or deficit is not intentionally produced or feigned (as in factitious disorder or malingering).

D.   The symptom or deficit cannot, after appropriate investigation, be fully explained by illness, substance, or culture.

Clinical Highlights
Features

- The core of this disorder is psychologically produced *signs or symptoms.*
- Solely *worry* about existing symptoms or signs is more consistent with hypochondriasis.
- Signs and symptoms are *unconsciously* produced.
- Purposely produced symptoms comprise factitious disorder (to take on or extend the patient role) or malingering (for financial or other secondary gain).
- Amobarbital interviewing or hypnosis may temporarily or permanently resolve findings.
- Some dramatic early psychoanalytic case reports describe treatment of conversion disorder, earlier called "hysteria" or "hysterical neurosis."

Gender Issues

- More common in women—2:1 to 10:1 ratios

215

Cultural Issues
- More common in rural populations and lower socioeconomic status.
- Conversion symptoms may accompany physiologically based symptoms (e.g., pseudo-seizures in epilepsy).

Adult Life Cycle Issues
- Onset in late childhood to early adulthood
- Rarely starts after age 35

Prevalence
Community
- 0.1% to 0.5% among the general population.
- In general medical/surgical inpatients, conversion symptoms range between 1% and 14%.

In Primary Care Practice
- N/A

In Outpatient Mental Health Practice
- 1% to 3% among outpatient psychiatric referrals

Among Mental Health Admissions
- Somatoform disorders comprise approximately 0.2% of inpatient mental health admissions.
- 5% to 24% among psychiatric outpatients.
- 5% to 14% among general hospital patients.

Course
- Acute, short duration.
- Recurrence is common, 20% to 25% within 1 year.

Common Comorbidities
- N/A

Treatment Considerations
Criteria for Urgent Intervention
- Suicidal ideation, plan, or attempt
- Maladaptive substance use
- Accidental self-injury from deficits
- Unnecessary but potentially high morbidity medical tests or treatments

Medication Options
- Amytal interviewing may lead to temporary or sometimes permanent resolution of symptoms.

Psychotherapeutic Options
- As noted above, successful experience has accumulated with psychoanalytic treatment and with hypnosis, but without controlled trial data.

Considerations in Choosing Among Treatments
- General approach is similar to that for somatization disorder.

Disorder:	Factitious Disorder and Malingering Disorder
DSM-IV Codes:	300.16 Factitious Disorder
	V65.2 Malingering

Adapted DSM Criteria

A. Feigning physical or psychological signs or symptoms, and

B. To assume the sick role (factitious disorder), **or**

C. For external incentives (e.g., economic gain, avoiding legal responsibility) (malingering)

Clinical Highlights

Features

- These syndromes are discussed together because their findings are the same (feigned findings) but their purpose is different:
  - Factitious disorder: to take on or maintain the patient role (*primary gain*)
  - Malingering: to achieve other ends such as financial gain, disability status, or work avoidance (*secondary gain*)
- Unconsciously produced signs or symptoms comprise conversion disorder, not factitious disorder or malingering.
- Factitious findings may be accompanied by comorbid disorders.
- Findings may be faked (e.g., heating a thermometer to stimulate fever) or may involve self-induced damage or danger (e.g., warfarin ingestion to induce anti-coagulation or a pyrogen injection to produce fever).
- Inducing findings in a dependent child or elder also has been reported ("by proxy").
- Another, more colorful name for factitious disorder is *Munchausen syndrome,* so-called after the nineteenth century nobleman, adventurer, and teller of tall tales.

Gender Issues

- More common in females (factitious)
- Most chronic and severe appears to be in males (factitious)

Cultural Issues

- Some cultures are characterized by expression of emotions through prominent somatic symptoms or somatically weighted culture-bound syndromes. However, neither is considered *feigning* symptoms.

Adult Life Cycle Issues

- N/A

Prevalence

Community

- Within large general hospitals, factitious disorder is diagnosed 1%, with higher rates in specialized treatment settings.
- 0.8% of all psychiatric consultations are for factitious disorder or malingering.

In Primary Care Practice

- N/A

217

In Outpatient Mental Health Practice
- N/A

Among Mental Health Admissions
- N/A

Course
- Intermittent episodes (factitious).
- Onset is usually early adulthood (factitious).

Common Comorbidities
- Substance abuse (factitious)
- Borderline personality disorder (factitious)

Treatment Considerations
Criteria for Urgent Intervention

- Unnecessary but potentially high morbidity medical tests or interventions
- Self-injury to produce findings

Medication Options
- N/A

Psychotherapeutic Options
- Explicit identification of goal of symptom/sign fabrication
- Limit setting, refocusing, and more appropriate problem solving

Considerations in Choosing Among Treatments
- Approach is similar to that for somatization disorder.
- If a dependent (child, elderly) is proxy, reporting to child welfare or elderly affairs services may be indicated or required by law.

Disorder: Body Dysmorphic Disorder
DSM-IV Codes: 300.7

Adapted DSM Criterion
- Preoccupation with an imagined or slight defect in appearance

Clinical Highlights
Features

- Preoccupation with one's appearance, especially a particular defect that may be imagined or exaggerated.
- There may, in fact, be a physical deformity, but its characteristics and impact are exaggerated.
- It is not typically considered psychotic, although there is a clear lack of insight and perspective.
- Severe cases may include psychotic symptoms.

Gender Issues
- Equally common in females and males in outpatient mental health settings

Cultural Issues
- Cultural concerns about appearance may influence an imagined deformity.

Adult Life Cycle Issues
- Begins typically in adolescence or young adulthood.

Prevalence
Community
- N/A

In Primary Care Practice
- 6% to 15% in cosmetic and dermatology settings

In Outpatient Mental Health Practice
- 1% in a private university-affiliated hospital-based clinic
- 2% as secondary diagnosis in a private university-affiliated hospital-based clinic
- 3% of outpatient referrals to mental health clinics

Among Mental Health Admissions
- N/A

Course
- Usually peaks in adolescence and early adulthood, but can begin in childhood.
- Onset can be gradual or abrupt.
- Chronic and continuous course.

Common Comorbidities
- Major depressive disorder
- Obsessive-compulsive disorder
- Social phobia

Treatment Considerations
Criteria for Urgent Intervention
- Suicidal ideation, plan, or attempt
- Psychosis
- Maladaptive substance use
- Frequent or potentially high morbidity medical-surgical interventions

Medication Options
- Clomipramine in doses for obsessive-compulsive disorder.
- Fluoxetine (60–80 mg/day).
- Possibly other serotonin reuptake inhibitors.
- Some studies indicate benefit from tricyclic, monoamine oxidase inhibitors, and other antidepressant medications.
- Some studies indicate benefit from neuroleptics.

Psychotherapeutic Options
- Supportive care should focus on supporting medication management and role function. Where possible, it should include education of the patient and his or her family.
- Some studies suggest benefit from cognitive-behavioral techniques.

219

Considerations in Choosing Among Treatments

- Serotonin reuptake inhibitors and clomipramine appear to have effects even in the absence of comorbid mood or anxiety disorders.

EATING DISORDERS

Disorder: Anorexia Nervosa
DSM-IV Codes: 307.1

Adapted DSM Criteria

A.   Refusal to maintain body weight at or above a minimally normal weight for age and height (e.g., weight reduction less than 85% of expected or failure to gain weight during growth to less than 85% of expected).
B.   Unrealistic fear of gaining weight or becoming fat.
C.   Unrealistic appraisal of body weight or shape or denial of seriousness of current low body weight.
D.   In postmenarcheal females, amenorrhea (i.e., the absence of at least three consecutive menstrual cycles).
   Note: May be restricting type or binge-eating/purging type.

Clinical Highlights
Features

- Anorexia nervosa is characterized by a clear misperception of body shape or size and a willful behavioral response based on their own perception.
- It is not considered a psychotic disorder, but there is a clear lack of insight and perspective.
- Nutritional, electrolyte, cardiac, and other significant medical problems may develop (see **Module 10**).
- Anorexia nervosa shares many features of body dysmorphic disorder.

Gender Issues

- At least 90% of individuals with this disorder are female.

Cultural Issues

- More prevalent in developed societies

Adult Life Cycle Issues

- Up 20% of individuals admitted to a hospital for anorexia nervosa will die within 20 to 30 years.

Prevalence
Community

- Lifetime prevalence for females is 0.5%, 0.05% for men

In Primary Care Practice

- N/A

In Outpatient Mental Health Practice
- Eating disorders comprise 0.3% in a nonspecialized private university-affiliated hospital-based clinic.

Among Mental Health Admissions
- Eating disorders comprise approximately 0.1% of nonspecialized inpatient mental health admissions.

Course
- The disorder typically begins in mid to late adolescence (age 14–18 years).
- Rarely occurs in women over 40 years old.
- Can recover fully after a single episode.

Common Comorbidities
- Obsessive-compulsive disorder
- Personality disorders
- Social phobia
- Body dysmorphic disorder
- Substance use disorders
- Medical complications (see **Module 10**)

Treatment Considerations
Criteria for Urgent Intervention
- Suicidal ideation, plan, or intent
- Maladaptive substance use
- Medical complications (see **Module 10**)
- Failure to achieve significant physical or psychosocial developmental milestones

Medication Options
- N/A

Psychotherapeutic Options
- Supportive care should focus on supporting medication management and role function. Where possible, it should include education of the patient and his or her family.
- For formal psychotherapy options, see Psychotherapy in **Section IV.**

Considerations in Choosing Among Treatments
- Treatment must include medical monitoring for complications of caloric restriction and purging (see **Module 10**).
- Family involvement, where applicable, is critical.
- Treat comorbid disorders (e.g., major depressive disorder) as indicated.

Disorder: Bulimia Nervosa
DSM-IV Codes: 307.51

Adapted DSM Criteria
A.   Recurrent episodes of binge eating:

(1) Eating, in a discrete period of time (e.g., in 2 hours), an amount of food that is definitely larger than most people would eat during a similar period of time and under similar circumstances

(2) A sense of lack of control during the episode

B. Inappropriate behavior to compensate (e.g., self-induced vomiting, laxatives, diuretics, fasting).

C. Eating and compensation at least twice a week for 3 months.

D. Self-evaluation is unduly influenced by body shape and weight.

E. Not due to anorexia nervosa.

May be **purging type** (e.g., induces vomiting or using laxatives) or **nonpurging type.**

Clinical Highlights
Features
- Individuals with bulimia may be of normal or low body weight.
- The latter should be differentiated from anorexia nervosa.

Gender Issues
- At least 90% of individuals with this disorder are female

Cultural Issues
- Similar across Western/developed countries.
- Only a few studies have been in other cultures, and appears to be more prevalent in developed countries.

Adult Life Cycle Issues
- Typically begins in adolescence or young adulthood
- Unclear if "burns out" with age

Prevalence
Community
- Lifetime prevalence rates among women are 1% to 3%. Rate among men is one tenth that of women.

In Primary Care Practice
- N/A

In Outpatient Mental Health Practice
- Eating disorders comprise 0.3% in a nonspecialized private university-affiliated hospital-based clinic.
- Bulimia nervosa comprise 0.5% as secondary diagnosis in a private university-affiliated hospital-based clinic.

Among Mental Health Admissions
- Eating disorders comprise approximately 0.1% of nonspecialized inpatient mental health admissions.

Course
- Begins in late adolescents or early adulthood
- Usually begins after the individual was dieting
- Persists for several years
- Can be chronic or intermittent with periods of remission alternating with binging

Common Comorbidities
- Major depressive disorder
- Dysthymic disorder
- Social phobia
- Anxiety disorders
- Substance use disorders
- Medical complications (see **Module 10**)

Treatment Considerations
Criteria for Urgent Intervention

- Suicidal ideation, plan, or intent
- Maladaptive substance use
- Medical disorders (see **Module 10**)

Medication Options

- Controlled trials indicate utility for certain antidepressant drugs, in contrast to the situation with anorexia nervosa. Not all studies have been positive, but the aggregated data indicate overall beneficial effects of antidepressant medications:
  - Desipramine
  - Imipramine
  - Phenelzine
  - Isocarboxazid
  - Fluoxetine (FDA-approved)
  - Possibly other serotonin reuptake inhibitors

Psychotherapeutic Options

- Supportive care should focus on supporting medication management and role function. Where possible, it should include education of the patient and his or her family.
- For formal psychotherapy options, see Psychotherapy in **Section IV.**

Considerations in Choosing Among Treatments

- Treatment must include medical monitoring for complications of purging (see **Module 10**).
- Psychosocial intervention is the cornerstone of treatment. Medications should be given in this context.
- Antidepressants have effects even in individuals who do not have comorbid mood disorders.
- Although there are some data indicating beneficial effects for bupropion, this drug is not first line due to reported increased incidence of seizures in individuals with bulimia (FDA "black box warning").

SLEEP DISORDERS

Disorder: Sleep Disorders
DSM-IV Codes: **Dyssomnias (Disorders of Sleep Pattern)**
     307.42 Primary Insomnia
     307.44 Primary Hypersomnia
     347 Narcolepsy
     780.59 Breathing-Related Sleep Disorder

307.45 Circadian Rhythm Sleep Disorder
307.47 Dyssomnia NOS
Parasomnias (Disorders of Sleep Events)
307.47 Nightmare Disorder
307.46 Sleep Terror Disorder
307.46 Sleepwalking Disorder
307.47 Parasomnia NOS

Adapted DSM Criteria for Dyssomnias (Disorders of Sleep Pattern)

Primary Insomnia: At least 1 month of difficulty initiating or maintaining sleep, or nonrestful sleep, and not due to other medical, sleep, or psychiatric disorders.

Primary Hypersomnia: At least 1 month of excessive sleepiness including either prolonged sleep episodes or daytime sleep episodes that occur almost daily, and not due to other medical, sleep, or psychiatric disorders

Narcolepsy

A.   At least 3 months of irresistible attacks of refreshing sleep that occur daily plus either of:

(1)   Cataplexy (i.e., brief episodes of sudden bilateral loss of muscle tone, most often in association with intense emotion)

(2)   REM sleep in the transition between sleep and wakefulness, with hypnopompic or hypnagogic hallucinations or sleep paralysis at the beginning or end of sleep (see **Panel 1, Module 11**)

* *Breathing-Related Sleep Disorder:* Sleep disruption, leading to excessive sleepiness or insomnia, due to obstructive or central sleep apnea or central alveolar hypoventilation (see **Panel 7, Module 11**).

* *Circadian Rhythm Sleep Disorder:* Sleep disruption with excessive sleepiness or insomnia due to a mismatch between the sleep-wake schedule required by a person's environment and his or her circadian sleep-wake pattern.

  * In delayed sleep-phase type, the individual's sleep-wake cycle is phase-delayed compared to most environmental and societal zeitgebers (see **Panel 1, Module 11**).

  * In shift-work type, the individual's sleep-wake cycle cannot re-synchronize sufficiently to the occupationally imposed demands of shifted or shifting work schedule.

Adapted DSM Criteria for Parasomnias (Disorders of Sleep Events)

Nightmare Disorder: Repeated awakenings due to nightmares, usually well remembered and usually during the second half of the sleep period. On awakening, the person rapidly becomes oriented and alert.

Sleep Terror Disorder: Recurrent episodes of abrupt awakening, usually occurring during the first third of the major sleep episode, beginning with a panicky scream, and with intense fear and autonomic arousal. There is relative unresponsiveness to efforts of others to comfort the person during the episode and no detailed dream is recalled.

Sleepwalking Disorder: Repeated episodes of walking about during sleep, usually occurring during the first third of the major sleep episode, always unresponsive to the efforts of others to communicate with him or her. On awakening, the person has amnesia for the episode and rapidly becomes alert.

Clinical Highlights
Features
- See **Module 11.**

Gender Issues
- Narcolepsy: Equally common in males and females.
- Breathing-related sleep disorder: Male-to-female ratio of obstructive sleep apnea is 2:1 to 4:1. Central apnea is more common in males.
- Nightmare disorder: Females report more nightmares than men (2:1 to 4:1).
- Sleep terror disorder: Equally common in males and females.
- Sleepwalking disorder
  - Violent activity during sleepwalking occurs more often in men.
  - Eating when sleepwalking occurs more often in women.
  - Sleepwalking occurs more often in females during childhood and more often in men during adulthood.

Cultural Issues
- Nightmare disorder: May vary with cultural background. Some cultures will relate nightmares to spiritual or supernatural phenomena while others see them as mental or physical disturbances.
- Sleep terror disorder: Significance and course of sleep terror episodes differ between cultures.

Adult Life Cycle Issues
- Circadian rhythm sleep disorder: increases with age

Prevalence
Community
- Primary insomnia: 1% to 10% in adult population and up to 25% in the elderly.
- Primary hypersomnia: Lifetime rate is 16%; 5% to 10% of individuals with complaints of daytime sleepiness are diagnosed with hypersomnia.
- Narcolepsy: 0.02% to 0.16% in adult population.
- Breathing-related sleep disorder: 1% to 10%, may be higher in the elderly.
- Circadian rhythm sleep disorder: Delayed sleep phase occurs in 0.1% to 4%; 60% of night shift workers may have shift-work type.
- Nightmare disorder: 50% report occasional nightmares. 3% of young adults report having frequent nightmares.
- Sleep terror disorder: Less than 1% in adults.
- Sleepwalking disorder: 1% to 7% in adults.

In Primary Care Practice
- N/A

In Outpatient Mental Health Practice
- N/A

Among Mental Health Admissions
- N/A

Course
Primary Insomnia
- Begins in young adulthood or middle age. Rare in childhood or adolescence.

- In clinics specializing in sleep disorders, only 15% to 25% of people with chronic insomnia are diagnosed with primary insomnia.
- Variable course, may be limited to several months or may be chronic.

Primary Hypersomnia
- Begins between ages 15 and 30.
- Gradual progression over weeks to months.
- Chronic and stable course.
- Usually resolves during middle age.

Narcolepsy
- Daytime sleepiness is the first symptom.
- Could be present as early as preschool and early school ages but becomes significant during adolescence.
- Onset after age 40 is unusual.
- Chronic course.

Breathing-Related Sleep Disorder
- Can occur at any age, but usually appears between ages 40 and 60.
- Females are more likely to develop obstructive sleep apnea after menopause.
- Insidious onset, gradual progression, and chronic course.
- Usually present for years before diagnosis.

Circadian Rhythm Sleep Disorder
- Delayed sleep phase begins between late childhood and early adulthood. Can last for years or even decades, though may correct itself with age.
- Shift work type will last for as long as the person has that schedule. It usually reverses within 2 weeks of normal sleep.

Nightmare Disorder
- Begins between ages 3 and 6

Sleep Terror Disorder
- Onsets during childhood between the ages of 4 and 12 and resolves spontaneously during adolescence. In adults, onset between the ages of 20 and 30.
- Chronic course.
- Episodes can occur for days or weeks.

Sleepwalking Disorder
- Can occur any time after a child learns to walk.
- Usually begins between the ages of 4 and 8. Peak age of onset is 12 years old.
- Rarely occurs for the first time in adults.

Common Comorbidities
- Substance use disorders (with chronic dyssomnics)

Treatment Considerations
Criteria for Urgent Intervention
- Maladaptive substance use
- Endangerment of self or others due to attentional or psychomotor compromise (e.g., driving, child care, operating equipment)

Medication Options

- Treat underlying medical or psychiatric disorders (see **Panels 4 and 5, Module 11**).
- Discontinue problematic medications (see **Panel 6, Module 11**).

Primary Insomnia

- Hypnotics
  - Benzodiazepine
  - Nonbenzodiazepine (zaleplon, zolpidem)
- Sedating antihistamines
  - Diphenhydramine 25 to 75 mg
  - Hydroxeyzine 10 to 25 mg
- Trazodone 25 to 200 mg

Narcolepsy

- Modafinil 200 to 400 mg divided between morning and noon
- Stimulants including:
  - Methylphenidate
  - Pemoline
  - Dextroamphetamine 5 to 60 mg/day divided up to four times in the morning and afternoon

Obstructive Sleep Apnea

- Some studies indicate benefit from the tricyclic protriptyline 20 to 30 mg divided t.i.d.; it is not clear whether other tricyclics share their effect.

Periodic Limb Movement of Sleep (Restless Legs Syndrome)

- Clonazepam 0.25 to 2 mg at bedtime; unclear if similar efficacy with other benzodiazepines

Psychotherapeutic Options

- See **Appendix 7** for Biopsychosocial Management of Sleep Complaints.

Considerations in Choosing Among Treatments

- The cornerstone of treating most sleep disorders is behavioral (see **Appendix 7**).
- Hypnotics are approved by the FDA for short-term use only, and have not been studied for more than 2 weeks.
- Melatonin, 2 to 20 mg/night is a popular alternative therapy
- Tachyphylaxis and tolerance are typical for hypnotics
- If chronic hypnotic use is necessary, limit to 4 to 5 nights per week to reduce likelihood of tachyphylaxis and tolerance.
- Benzodiazepines hypnotics act as GABA receptors that mediate both sleep and anxiety, whereas the nonbenzodiazepine hypnotic zaleplon and zolpidem are more selective for those GABA receptors that mediate sleep.
- However, *both groups* have been shown to have:
  - Addictive potential
  - Tachyphylaxis and tolerance
- For obstructive sleep apnea:
  - Avoid alcohol, sedatives
  - Weight reduction
  - Avoid prone sleeping position and elevate head of bed
  - Oral prosthesis

- Nighttime positive airway pressure delivered via mask or nasal cannula (CPAP/BIPAP)
- Protriptyline as above
- Surgery
  - Uvulopalato pharyngoplasty
  - Tracheostomy
  - Surgical treatment for morbid obesity

SEXUAL AND GENDER IDENTITY DISORDERS

Disorder: Sexual and Gender Identity Disorders
DSM-IV Codes:

Sexual Dysfunctions
(Disorders of Sexual Drive)
302.71 Hypoactive Sexual Desire Disorder
302.79 Sexual Aversion Disorder
302.72 Female Sexual Arousal Disorder
302.72 Male Erectile Disorder
302.73 Female Orgasmic Disorder
302.74 Male Orgasmic Disorder
302.75 Premature Ejaculation

Paraphilias
(Disorders of Sexual Object)
302.4 Exhibitionism
302.81 Fetishism
302.89 Frotteurism
302.2 Pedophilia
302.83 Sexual Masochism
302.84 Sexual Sadism
302.3 Transvestic Fetishism
302.82 Voyeurism

302.85 **Gender Identity Disorder**

Adapted DSM Criteria for Sexual Dysfunctions (Disorders of Sexual Drive; see also Panel 7, Module 12)
Hypoactive Sexual Desire Disorder: Lack of sexual fantasies or desire for sexual activity, taking into account factors that affect sexual functioning such as age and the context of the person's life.
Sexual Aversion Disorder: Extreme aversion to, or avoidance of, all (or almost all) contact with a sexual partner.
Female Sexual Arousal Disorder: Inability to attain, or maintain adequate lubrication/swelling response of sexual excitement.
Male Erectile Disorder: Inability to attain, or maintain adequate erection.
Female Orgasmic Disorder: Delay or absence of orgasm following a normal sexual excitement phase.
Male Orgasmic Disorder: Delay or absence of, orgasm following a normal sexual excitement phase.
Premature Ejaculation: Ejaculation with minimal sexual stimulation before, on, or shortly after penetration and before the person wishes it.

Sexual Pain Disorders
- Dyspareunia: Recurrent genital pain associated with intercourse in men or women.
- Vaginismus: Persistent, involuntary vaginal spasm interfering with intercourse.

Adapted DSM Criteria for Paraphilias (Disorders of Sexual Object) (see also Panel 8, Module 12)
Paraphilias (overall)
- Chronic, lifelong

228

- Begin in childhood or early adolescence, but is more elaborate in adolescence and early adulthood

Exhibitionism: At least 6 months of recurrent, intense sexually arousing fantasies, sexual urges, or behaviors involving the exposure of one's genitals to an unsuspecting stranger, and the person has acted on or is distressed by these sexual urges.

Fetishism: At least 6 months of recurrent, intense sexually arousing fantasies, sexual urges, or behaviors involving the use of nonliving objects (e.g., items of clothing).

Frotteurism: At least 6 months of recurrent, intense fantasies or sexual urges involving touching and rubbing against a nonconsenting person.

Pedophilia: At least 6 months of recurrent, intense fantasies or sexual urges involving sexual activity with a prepubescent child or children (generally age 13 years or younger).

Sexual Masochism: At least 6 months of recurrent, intense fantasies or sexual urges, involving the act (real, not simulated) of being humiliated, beaten, bound, or otherwise made to suffer, and the fantasies, sexual urges, or behaviors cause clinically significant distress or impairment.

Sexual Sadism: At least 6 months of recurrent, intense fantasies or sexual urges involving acts in which the real psychologic or physical suffering of the victim is sexually exciting to the person, and the person has acted on these urges with a nonconsenting person or been distressed by such fantasies.

Transvestic Fetishism: At least 6 months in a heterosexual male of recurrent, intense sexually arousing fantasies, sexual urges, or behaviors involving cross-dressing.

Voyeurism: At least 6 months of recurrent, intense fantasies or sexual urges, involving the act of observing an unsuspecting person who is naked, disrobing, or engaging in sexual activity.

Adapted DSM Criteria for Gender Identity Disorder (see also Panel 9, Module 12)

A.   A strong and persistent cross-gender identification causing intense distress or dysfunction. In adolescents and adults, the disturbance is manifested by symptoms such as a stated desire to be the other sex, frequent passing as the other sex, desire to live or be treated as the other sex, or the conviction that he or she has the typical feelings and reactions of the other sex.

B.   Persistent discomfort with his or her sex or sense of inappropriateness in the gender role of that sex. In adolescents and adults, the disturbance is manifested by symptoms such as preoccupation with getting rid of primary and secondary sex characteristics (e.g., request for hormones, surgery, or other procedures to physically alter sexual characteristics to simulate the other sex) or belief that he or she was born the wrong sex.

Clinical Highlights
Features

- See **Module 12.**
- Recall that the DSM requires that a *disorder* be associated with distress or dysfunction. Sexual *behaviors* that are not typical of the dominant culture are

therefore not necessarily considered pathological and need not necessarily be a focus of treatment.

Gender Issues
- See **Module 12.**

Cultural Issues
- Different cultures can have different norms for sexual behaviors, desires, expectations, and attitudes.

Adult Life Cycle Issues
- See **Module 12.**

Prevalence
Community
- Dyspareunia: Males 3%, females 15%
- Orgasm problems: Males 10%, females 25%
- Hypoactive sexual desire: 33%
- Premature ejaculation: 27%
- Female arousal problems: 20%
- Male erectile difficulties: 10%

In Primary Care Practice
- N/A

In Outpatient Mental Health Practice
- N/A

Among Mental Health Admissions
- N/A

Course
Hypoactive Sexual Desire Disorder
- Onset is puberty.
- The disorder develops in adulthood after a person experiences sexual interest, psychologic distress, stressful events, or interpersonal difficulties.
- Course can be continuous or episodic.

Male Erectile Disorder
- Onset varies.
- Can be chronic and lifelong.
- 15% to 30% of the time, it can remit spontaneously.

Female Orgasmic Disorder
- More prevalent in younger women
- Lifelong

Premature Ejaculation
- Particularly in younger men

Exhibitionism
- Usually onsets before age 18, but can occur later in life. Less severe after age 40.

Fetishism
- Begins by adolescence, but can occur in childhood
- Chronic course

Frotteurism
- Usually occurs between the ages of 15 and 25; will decline in frequency thereafter

Pedophilia
- Chronic

Sexual Masochism
- Age of onset varies; common by early adulthood.
- Chronic.
- Person tends to repeat the same acts.

Sexual Sadism
- Onset varies, usually present in childhood, but is common by early adulthood
- Chronic

Transvestic Fetishism
- Onset is usually before the age of 15.
- Chronic course.

Gender Identity Disorder
- Onset may be as early as 4 years old, but does not meet criteria until adolescence or adulthood.
- By late adolescence or adulthood, 75% of boys with a history of gender identity disorder as a child will have homosexual or bisexual orientation.
- 1 per 30,000 males and 1 per 100,000 females have sex-reassignment surgery.

Common Comorbidities
- Mood disorders
- Obsessive-compulsive disorder
- Panic with agoraphobia
- Specific phobia
- Other Sexual/Gender Identity Disorders

Treatment Considerations
Criteria for Urgent Intervention
- Maladaptive substance use
- Suicidality
- Danger to others
- Inadvertent danger to self/others

Medication Options, Psychotherapeutic Options, and Considerations in Choosing Treatment
- See **Module 12.**

231

PREMENSTRUAL DYSPHORIC DISORDER

Disorder: Premenstrual Dysphoric Disorder
DSM-IV Code: None (in DSM Appendix)

Adapted DSM Criteria
A.   Symptoms:
- During most menses
  - Over the past year
  - Onset in luteal phase
  - Offset with menses
- At least five of:
    (1) Depressed mood, hopelessness, self-depreciation
    (2) Anxiety, tension, feeling on edge
    (3) Affective lability or rejection sensitivity
    (4) Easy irritability or interpersonal conflicts
    (5) Decreased interest in usual activities
    (6) Difficulty concentrating
    (7) Easy fatigue
    (8) Marked change in appetite
    (9) Hypersomnia or insomnia
    (10) Sense of being overwhelmed or out of control
    (11) Other physical symptoms, such as breast tenderness or swelling, headaches, joint or muscle pain, subjective bloating, weight gain
- At least one symptom must be (1), (2), (3), or (4)
B.   Not merely worsening of another disorder

Clinical Highlights
Features
- Characterized by depressed mood, anxiety, marked affective lability, and decreased interest in activities during the last week of the luteal phase in menstrual cycles.
- Symptoms remit within a few days of onset.
- Overlapping syndromes, some with more exclusively physical symptoms, have also been described [e.g., premenstrual syndrome (PMS)].
- The older DSM name is "Late Luteal Phase Dysphoric Disorder."
- The syndrome is listed in the appendix of DSM-IV as "needing further study."

Gender Issues
- Occurs only in females with menstrual cycle

Cultural Issues
- N/A

Adult Life Cycle Issues
- Limited to years of active menstrual cycle

Prevalence
Community
- 3% to 5%.
- 5% to 9% of childbearing-age women meet criteria.

In Primary Care Practice
- N/A

In Outpatient Mental Health Practice
- N/A

Among Mental Health Admissions
- N/A

Course
- As per definition, regular pattern with menstrual cycle

Common Comorbidities
- Major depressive disorder
- Dysthymia
- Anxiety disorders

Treatment Considerations
Criteria for Urgent Intervention
- Suicidal ideation, plan, or attempt
- Maladaptive substance use

Medication Options
- Serotonin reuptake inhibitors in low to standard antidepressant doses (e.g., fluoxetine 10 to 20 mg/day).
- May be given only on premenstrual days or chronically.
- Lilly's Serafem is simply the repackaging of fluoxetine for PMDD and is FDA approved for PMDD.
- Other SSRIs are likely to be efficacious.

Psychotherapeutic Options
- As below

Considerations in Choosing Among Treatments
- Symptom management with psychosocial interventions may be a useful adjunct to medications. For example:
  - Education.
  - Work and social planning.
  - Couples intervention.
  - Cognitive techniques to assist in reframing depressive or anxious cognitions.
  - Behavioral techniques including sleep hygiene (see **Appendix 7**) and regular exercise.
  - Some sources also emphasize cessation of smoking, alcohol.
  - In evaluating the treatment literature for PMS or other closely related variants, be aware that not all syndrome criteria are the same. For instance, some PMS trials evaluate participants who have a much stronger weighting toward somatic symptoms (e.g., bloating) than psychiatric (e.g., dysphoria).
  - A number of other treatments have been used in PMS, none with efficacy evidence as strong as that for SSRIs in PMDD:
    - Vitamin B_6 to 100 mg/day
    - Vitamin E to 600 IU/day

233

- Calcium carbonate 1,200 to 1,600 mg/day
- Magnesium to 500 mg/day
- Spironolactone 100 mg/day
- Bromocriptine 2.5 mg three times daily
- Progesterone 200 to 400 mg/day
- Oral contraceptives (estrogen/progesterone)
- Gonadotropin-releasing hormone agonists
- Danazol 100 mg/day

DISSOCIATIVE DISORDERS

Disorder: Dissociative Disorders
DSM-IV Codes: 300.12 Dissociative Amnesia
300.13 Dissociative Fugue
300.14 Dissociative Identity Disorder
300.6 Depersonalization Disorder

Adapted DSM Criteria
Dissociative Amnesia Disorder

A.   Inability to recall important personal information, usually of a traumatic or stressful nature, beyond ordinary forgetfulness
B.   Not part of other dissociative or stress disorders

Dissociative Fugue

A.   Sudden, unexpected travel away from home or one's customary place of work, with inability to recall one's past
B.   Confusion about personal identity or assumption of a new identity
C.   Not due to dissociative identity disorder

Dissociative Identity Disorder

A.   Two or more distinct identities or personality states with their own pattern of perceiving, relating to, and thinking about the environment and self.
B.   At least two of these identities recurrently control behavior.
C.   Inability to recall important personal information beyond ordinary forgetfulness.

Depersonalization Disorder

A.   Persistent or recurrent experiences of feeling detached from, and as if one is an outside observer of, one's mental processes or body (e.g., feeling like one is in a dream).
B.   No delirium, dissociation, or psychosis.
C.   Not part of another disorder.

Clinical Highlights
Features

- The core feature of each of these is a disruption of consciousness, memory, identity, or perception.

Gender Issues

- Each is more common in women.

Cultural Issues
- N/A

Adult Life Cycle Issues
- Dissociative identity disorder becomes less manifest in individuals by the late forties, but can reemerge during times of stress, trauma, or substance abuse.

Prevalence
Community
- N/A

In Primary Care Practice
- N/A

In Outpatient Mental Health Practice
- N/A

Among Mental Health Admissions
- N/A

Course
Fugue
- Usually related to traumatic, stressful, and overwhelming events
- Usually in adults
- Episodes can last for hours to months
- Recovery is rapid, but amnesia may persist

Amnesia
- Can occur in young children to adults
- Can be minutes to years

Identity
- Chronic and fluctuating course that is recurrent
- Average time from first symptom to diagnosis is 6 to 7 years

Depersonalization
- Mean age of onset is 16
- Chronic, but also can be episodic

Common Comorbidities
- Posttraumatic stress disorder
- Major depressive disorder
- Cluster B personality disorders
- Anxiety disorders

Treatment Considerations
Criteria for Urgent Intervention
- Suicidal ideation, plan, or attempt
- Inadvertent harm to self or others

- Inability to care for self
- Maladaptive substance use

Medication Options
- Treatment of comorbid disorders or related features (e.g., anxiolytics for anxiety) is indicated.

Psychotherapeutic Options
- Supportive care should focus on supporting medication management and role function. Where possible, it should include education of the patient and his or her family.
- Historically, there is substantial experience using psychodynamically oriented therapies with dissociative disorders, but few formal outcome data.

Considerations in Choosing Among Treatments
- Treatment is typically empirically based, from a biopsychosocial perspective.
- Some techniques that are used in the management of personality disorders and posttraumatic stress disorder also may be useful in dissociative disorders if similar features are present. (See Psychotherapies in **Treatment Section**).

PERSONALITY DISORDERS

Disorder: Personality Disorders
DSM-IV Codes: **Cluster A**
                   301.0 Paranoid Personality Disorder
                   301.20 Schizoid Personality Disorder
                   301.22 Schizotypal Personality Disorder
                   Cluster B
                   301.7 Antisocial Personality Disorder
                   301.83 Borderline Personality Disorder
                   301.50 Histrionic Personality Disorder
                   301.81 Narcissistic Personality Disorder
                   Cluster C
                   301.82 Avoidant Personality Disorder
                   301.6 Dependent Personality Disorder
                   301.4 Obsessive-Compulsive Personality Disorder
                   301.9 Personality Disorder NOS

Adapted DSM Criteria
A.   An enduring pattern of inner experience and behavior that is:
- *pervasive:* across many relationships and social situations
- *inflexible:* not easily changed despite negative impact
- *lifelong:* at least adolescence or early adulthood
B.   Manifested in at least two of:
    (1) *cognition:* ways of perceiving and interpreting self, other people, and events
    (2) *affect:* the range, intensity, liability, and appropriateness of emotional response
    (3) *interpersonal functioning*
    (4) *impulse control*
C.   Not due to another disorder

Cluster A: "The Odd"
Paranoid Personality Disorder

A.   Unjustified distrust and suspiciousness of others with at least four of:

    (1)   Suspects that others are exploiting, harming, or deceiving him or her

    (2)   Is preoccupied with doubts about the trustworthiness of associates

    (3)   Is reluctant to confide in others because of unwarranted fear that the information will be used maliciously against him or her

    (4)   Reads hidden meaning or threatening meanings into benign remarks or events

    (5)   Bears grudges

    (6)   Perceives attacks to self that are not apparent to others

    (7)   Has recurrent suspicions of spouse's/partner's fidelity

Schizoid Personality Disorder

A.   Detachment from social relationships and a restricted emotional range with at least four of:

    (1)   Neither desires nor enjoys close relationships

    (2)   Almost always chooses solitary activities

    (3)   Has little interest in sexual experiences with another person

    (4)   Takes pleasure in few activities

    (5)   Lacks close friends or confidants other than first-degree relatives

    (6)   Appears indifferent to the praise or criticism of others

    (7)   Shows emotional detachment or flattened affect

Schizotypal Personality Disorder

A.   Discomfort with, and reduced capacity for, close relationships; cognitive or perceptual distortions; and eccentricities of behavior, with at least five of (see **Panels 1–3, Module 4** for definitions):

    (1)   Ideas of reference

    (2)   Odd beliefs or magical thinking that influence behavior and not consistent with subcultural norms

    (3)   Unusual perceptual experiences, including bodily illusions

    (4)   Vague, circumstantial, metaphoric, overelaborate, or stereotyped

    (5)   Suspiciousness or paranoia (see **Module 4**)

    (6)   Inappropriate or constricted affect

    (7)   Odd, eccentric, or peculiar appearance or behavior

    (8)   Lack of close friends or confidants other than first-degree relatives

    (9)   Paranoia in social situations that does not diminish with familiarity

Cluster B: "The Dramatic"
Antisocial Personality Disorder

A.   Violation of the rights of others since age 15 with at least five of:

    (1)   Failure to conform to social norms with respect to laws

    (2)   Deceitfulness, such as repeated lying, use of aliases, or conning others

    (3)   Impulsivity or failure to plan ahead

    (4)   Repeated physical fights or assaults

    (5)   Reckless disregard for safety of self or others

    (6)   Repeated failure to sustain consistent work behavior or honor financial obligations

(7) Lack of remorse, as indicated by being indifferent to or rationalizing having hurt, mistreated, or stolen from another

Note: Lack of remorse is a key. Not all illegal behavior is grounds for diagnosis.

Borderline Personality Disorder

A.   Instability of interpersonal relationships, self-image, and affects, and marked impulsivity with at least five of:

(1)   Frantic efforts to avoid real or imagined abandonment; not covered in (5)

(2)   Intense interpersonal relationships with unstable alternation between extremes of idealization and devaluation

(3)   Markedly unstable self-image or sense of self

(4)   Self-damaging impulsivity in at least two areas (e.g., spending, sex, substance abuse, reckless driving, binge eating); not covered in (5)

(5)   Recurrent suicidal behavior, threats, or self-mutilating behavior

(6)   Intense episodic dysphoria, irritability, or anxiety usually lasting a few hours and only rarely more than a few days

(7)   Chronic feelings of emptiness

(8)   Bouts of inappropriate, intense anger such as frequent displays of temper, constant anger, recurrent physical fights

(9)   Transient stress-related paranoia or dissociative symptoms

Narcissistic Personality Disorder

Grandiosity in fantasy or behavior, need for admiration, and lack of empathy, with at least five of:

(1)   Has a grandiose sense of self-importance, exaggerating achievements and talents, or expecting to be recognized as superior without commensurate achievements

(2)   Is preoccupied with fantasies of unlimited success, power, brilliance, beauty, or ideal love

(3)   Believes that he or she is "special" and unique and can only be understood by, or should associate with, other special or high-status people or institutions

(4)   Requires excessive admiration

(5)   Has a sense of entitlement: unreasonable expectations of especially favorable treatment or automatic compliance with his or her expectations

(6)   Takes advantage of others to achieve his or her own ends

(7)   Lacks empathy: is unwilling or unable to recognize or identify with the feelings and needs of others

(8)   Is often envious of others or believes that others are envious of him or her

(9)   Shows arrogant, haughty behavior or attitudes

Histrionic Personality Disorder

Excessive emotionality and attention seeking, in a variety of contexts, with at least five of:

(1)   Is uncomfortable in situations in which he or she is not the center of attention

(2)   Frequent inappropriate sexually seductive or provocative behavior

(3)   Displays rapidly shifting and shallow expression of emotions

(4) Consistently uses physical appearance to draw attention to self
(5) Has a style of speech that is excessively impressionistic and lacks detail
(6) Self-dramatization, theatricality, and exaggerated expression of emotion
(7) Easily influenced by others or circumstances
(8) Considers relationships to be more intimate than they actually are

Cluster C: "The Anxious"
Avoidant Personality Disorder

Social inhibition, feeling of inadequacy, and hypersensitivity to criticism, with at least four of:

(1) Avoids occupations with significant interpersonal contact, because of fears of criticism, disapproval, or rejection
(2) Is unwilling to get involved with people unless certain of being liked
(3) Shows restraint within intimate relationships because of the fear of being shamed or ridiculed
(4) Is preoccupied with being criticized or rejected in social situations
(5) Is inhibited in new interpersonal situations because of feelings of inadequacy
(6) Views self as socially inept, personally unappealing, or inferior to others
(7) Is unusually reluctant to take personal risks or to engage in any new activities because they may prove embarrassing

   Note: Although avoidant personality disorder shares some of the same behaviors with schizoid personality disorder, the key is motivation: the individual with avoidant personality disorder desires relationships, but abstains for fear of criticism. In contrast, the individual with schizoidal personality disorder has minimal or no motivation for relationships.

Dependent Personality Disorder

Need to be taken care of that leads to submissive or clinging behavior and fears of separation with at least five of:

(1) Has difficulty making everyday decisions without an excessive amount of advice and reassurance from others
(2) Needs others to assume responsibility for most major areas of his or her life
(3) Has difficulty expressing disagreement with others because of fear of loss of support or approval
(4) Has difficulty initiating projects or doing things on his or her own because of a lack of self-confidence
(5) Goes to excessive lengths to obtain nurturing and support
(6) Feels unable to care for himself or herself when alone
(7) Relationship ends and urgently seeks another as a source of care and support
(8) Is unrealistically preoccupied with fears of being left to take care of himself or herself

Obsessive-Compulsive Personality Disorder

Preoccupation with orderliness, perfectionism, and mental and interpersonal control, at the expense of flexibility, openness, and efficiency with at least four of:

(1) Is preoccupied with details, rules, lists, order, organization, or schedules to the extent that the major point of the activity is lost

239

(2) Shows perfectionism that interferes with task completion
(3) Is excessively devoted to work and productivity to the exclusion of leisure activities and friendships
(4) Is overconscientious, scrupulous, and inflexible about matters of morality, ethics, or values
(5) Is unable to discard worn-out or worthless objects with no sentimental value
(6) Is reluctant to delegate tasks or to work with others
(7) Miserly with a view of money as something to be hoarded for future catastrophes
(8) Shows rigidity and stubbornness

Note: Obsessive-compulsive personality disorder differs *substantially* from obsessive-compulsive disorder. Compare those criteria (page 182).

Clinical Highlights
Features

- The area of personality disorders is vast and complex—and fascinating. Many specifics are beyond the scope of this book, and clinicians are directed to several more detailed works in the **Key References** section.
- Personality disorders are listed in the DSM as "axis II" disorders, representing developmental conditions.
- The key to diagnosing and understanding personality disorders is to recall that their signs and symptoms derive from ways of interacting with the world that are:
  - *Pervasive*
  - *Inflexible*
  - *Lifelong*
- The origin of personality disorders, and generation of their signs and symptoms, is *biopsychosocial:*
  - Family studies indicate a familial, and perhaps genetic, component.
  - Several have substantial symptom overlap with axis I disorders that have a clear biologic component (e.g., cluster A and schizophrenia).
  - Biologically treatable comorbidities (e.g., major depressive disorder) are prevalent.
  - Years of psychotherapy research, description, and data-based theory indicate substantial impairment in *object relations* (the ability to form and maintain stable relationships with key persons in one's life, including one's self), and such deficits likely result in part from suboptimal development experiences.
  - Given that personality disorders have a familial component, it is likely that a child raised by a parent with a personality disorder will be at increased risk for suboptimal developmental experiences.
  - Once established, personality disorders typically lead to many unsuccessful interactions with others, leading to increased social stress, leading to additional symptoms and reinforcement of maladaptive coping responses.
  - Thus, there are likely both *nature* (genetic) and *nurture* (environmental) components to the development of personality disorders.
- Several key diagnostic features deserve highlighting:
  - Personality traits likely exist on a spectrum rather than categorically (either you have a personality disorder or you don't) as the DSM system assumes (see **Module 15**).

- Other disorders may mimic personality disorders (e.g., bipolar II leading to cluster B features; chronic medical illness leading to features of dependent personality disorder).
- These features do *not* represent personality disorders, which are lifelong.
- The dangers in overdiagnosing personality disorders includes:
  - Omission of efficacious treatment for axis I disorder
  - Labeling the condition as chronic when it may not be.
- Episodic symptoms suggest axis I disorder while chronic symptoms suggest personality disorder.
  - The diagnosis of a personality disorder cannot be made *cross-sectionally,* but depends on *longitudinal data* (see **Section I** on psychosocial assessment)
  - The diagnosis typically cannot be made during an acute episode of an axis I disorder unless there is compelling information from prior to the onset of the Axis I disorder.
- The diagnosis is not made on the basis of "counter-transference" (the "gut feeling" of the clinician toward the individual seeking treatment). In fact, reliance on the putative diagnostic capabilities of such one's own emotions typically dulls diagnostic acumen.
- It is a myth that suicidal behavior in individuals with personality disorders is trivial, or "a gesture" (see also **Module 6**). Suicide attempt rates are particularly high in:
  - Antisocial personality disorder
  - Borderline personality disorder

Gender Issues

Cluster A
- Schizoid: more common in males
- Schizotypal: more common in males

Cluster B
- Antisocial: more common in males
- Borderline: more common in females
- Histrionic: diagnosed more often in females in clinical settings; equal gender distribution outside of clinical settings

Cluster C
- Avoidant: equally common in males and females
- Dependent: more common in females
- Obsessive-compulsive: 2:1 males: females

Cultural Issues

- Schizoid: behaviors normal in different cultures may be labeled as "schizoid" or "schizotypal."
- Antisocial: associated with low socioeconomic status and urban settings.
- Dependent: norms vary across sociocultural groups.

Adult Life Cycle Issues

- By definition begin in childhood or early adult years
- Antisocial: reduction in severity with age
- Borderline: reduction in severity with age

241

Prevalence
Community
- Overall prevalence of personality disorders 6% to 9%

Cluster A
- Paranoid: 0.5% to 2.5%
- Schizotypal: 3%

Cluster B
- Antisocial: 3% males, 1% females
- Borderline: 2%
- Histrionic: 2% to 3%
- Narcissistic: less than 1%

Cluster C
- Avoidant: 0.5% to 1.0%
- Obsessive-compulsive: 1%

In Primary Care Practice
- N/A

In Outpatient Mental Health Practice
- Paranoid: 2% to 10%
- Borderline: 10% to 20%
- Histrionic: 10% to 15%
- Narcissistic: 2% to 16% in clinical populations
- Avoidant: 10%
- Obsessive-compulsive: 3% to 10%
- Antisocial: 3% to 30% in clinical settings
- Borderline: may represent up to 30% to 60% among those with a personality disorder

   Note: In clinical populations, individuals with a personality disorder frequently meet criteria for more than one.

Among Mental Health Admissions
- Personality disorders comprise approximately 0.3% of inpatient mental health admissions, although some studies cite a rate of 15% to 20%.

Course
- Personality disorders by definition have onset in adolescence or early adult life and are chronic.
- Antisocial: Cannot be diagnosed before age 18, although conduct disorder frequently precedes. Chronic course but reduction in severity as person ages.
- Borderline: Chronic instability in early adulthood, but reduction in severity as the person ages. Risk of suicide is greatest in young adults but decreases with age. Overall, impulsivity recedes, emptiness endures.
- Avoidant: May start in infancy and childhood with shyness, isolation, fear of strangers, and new situations. Increases during adolescence and early adulthood.

Common Comorbidities

Cluster A	Cluster B	Cluster C
• Schizophrenia	• Major depressive disorder	• Major depressive disorder
• Other psychotic disorders	• Dysthymia	• Anxiety disorders
	• Manic-depressive disorders	• Other cluster C disorders
	• Eating disorders	
	• Posttraumatic stress disorder	
	• Substance use disorders	
	• Somatoform disorders	
	• Other cluster B disorders	

Treatment considerations

Criteria for urgent intervention

- Suicidal ideation, plan, or attempt
- Psychosis
- Maladaptive substance use
- Inability to care for self
- Danger to others

Medication Options

- Treatment of comorbid disorders, (e.g., major depression, panic, delusional disorder) as indicated
- Treatment of focal high-morbidity symptoms (e.g., mood instability, impulsivity) is by extension from other disorders (e.g., lithium, antimanic or antidepressant agents, neuroleptics)

Psychotherapeutic Options

- Supportive care should focus on supporting medication management and role function. Where possible it should include education of the patient and his or her family.
- For formal psychotherapy options, see Psychotherapy in **Section IV.**
- Psychotherapeutic treatment of comorbid disorders (e.g., major depressive disorder) may be helpful if the individual is sufficiently stable to participate (see Psychotherapy in **Section IV** for specific disorders).

Considerations in Choosing Among Treatments

- As outlined under "Clinical Highlights: Features", personality disorders are best understood from the *biopsychosocial* perspective.
  - Treatment planning should include attention to aspects noted there.
- Accordingly, working with such individuals includes both psychosocial and medication intervention.
  - Medications are used aggressively to treat comorbid conditions and associated features such as impulsivity.
  - Psychosocial treatment is aimed at several aspects of the disorder:
    - Management of dysfunctional behaviors (e.g., avoidance in cluster C, self-harm in cluster B)

243

- Reinterpretation of misperceived of interpersonal cues and attendant affective response (all clusters)
- Minimization of interpersonal and functional difficulties by addressing social behaviors (all clusters)
- Although personality disorders are by definition chronic, they are not unmodifiable.
- Improvement may come in any of several domains (which may not change in unison):
  - Subjective symptoms
  - Maladaptive, especially dangerous, behaviors
  - Social role function
  - Utilization of health-care services or need for outside support
- The therapeutic approach to all is an *empathic, consistent* stance toward the individual. *Empathy* and *consistency* are two characteristics that have typically been sorely lacking in most of their own object relations.
  - In dealing with individuals with borderline personality disorder, the two-page first person account of having this personality disorder in the **Key References** section is required reading.
  - One may expect substantial—and often unstable—*transference* (feeling of the individual toward the clinician) when dealing with most individuals with personality disorders, especially cluster B.
  - *Counter-transference* (feelings of the clinician toward the individual) requires self-monitoring and modulation on the part of the clinician to support an *empathetic* and *consistent* stance toward the individual in treatment.
  - To reiterate: An *empathic* and *consistent* approach to the individual is most likely to lead to a stable treatment alliance and some measure of corrective emotional experience for them.

SECTION IV

Treatment

INTRODUCTION

This section supports the fourth of the four **Core Tasks of Assessment and Treatment Planning (Section I, Panel 3):**

1. Characterize symptoms and signs.
2. Build symptoms and signs into syndromes.
3. Build syndromes into disorders.
4. Treat the disorders.

The clinician may have arrived at an entry in this section by way of "Considerations in Choosing Among Treatments" in one of the entries in **Section III.** Alternately, he or she can easily use this section directly as a reference for choosing, initiating, and monitoring treatment in an already diagnosed disorder.

This section consists of the following:

- An outline of **psychotherapies** that includes:
  - An **overview of supportive psychotherapy** that should serve as the foundation for all clinical interactions, whether they are focused on medication treatment, psychotherapy, or watchful monitoring. It is based on the principles of the *Collaborative Practice Treatment Model* for treatment and the *Biopsychosocial Assessment and Treatment Model* for understanding psychiatric illnesses (see those sections in the **Key References**).
  - **A listing of formal, structured psychotherapies for specific disorders.** This section is organized by disorder and includes those treatments that have been shown in controlled trials to have efficacy for the disorders noted. The goal of this portion of the section is not to teach the clinician how, for example, to do cognitive-behavioral therapy for social phobia. Rather, it is to assist the clinician in making referral for, or choosing among, treatments for the disorder in question.
- An entry for each of the **medications** used in treating psychiatric disorders covered in this field guide.
- A brief outline of the **devices** currently used in treating psychiatric disorders covered in this Field Guide. This outline is brief because most of the devices either are not implemented by the general clinician but rather by the specialist [e.g., electroconvulsive therapy (ECT)] or are investigational (e.g., transcranial magnetic stimulation). Nonetheless, as for the formal psychotherapies, the informed clinician should know of their indications and their risks and benefits for the individual, so that appropriate referral can be made.

The overall orientation of this section reflects the fifth of the **five Principles of Assessment and Treatment Planning (Section I, Panels 2 and 3):**

- All treatments—*all* treatments—have costs and benefits.

The number and diversity of psychiatric treatments, both medical and psychotherapeutic, is proliferating rapidly. Thus, we have more and more options from which to choose. But, all of these treatments, however benign appearing, have costs and side effects, as well as benefits—true even of psychotherapy, as noted in that portion of this section. Consistent with the collaborative practice approach to treatment, specific treatment is chosen based on the relative preferences, priorities, and values of the individual in treatment. Our job is to provide

245

technical information, advice, and prioritized recommendations based on our specialized training and accumulated clinical experience. These two components—individual preference plus professional skill—provide the basis on which the choice of treatment is jointly made.

To aid in this endeavor with regard to psychopharmacologic agents, each medication entry is organized to provide key data of use to the clinician, whether he or she is prescribing the medication, or whether he or she is working with an individual who is being treated with medication prescribed by another clinician.

To assist the prescribing clinician in choosing among medications in a particular class, each class is preceded by a series of notes found in the panels entitled **"Introductory Notes."** These introductory notes summarize and highlight the major comparative information found within each individual medication entry.

The structure of each individual medication entry is as outlined below. As in the **Disorders** section, "N/A" indicates "Not available" or "Not applicable."

GENERIC AND TRADE NAMES, CHEMICAL CLASS, AND THERAPEUTIC/CLINICAL CLASS

This section lists this information, with trade names being primarily those available in the United States.

"ON-" AND "OFF-LABEL" INDICATIONS FOR USAGE

"On-label" uses reflect those approved by the U.S. Food and Drug Administration (FDA). "Off-label" uses reflect those in general clinical practice but not specifically approved by the FDA.

It has proven surprisingly difficult to get consistent information regarding which uses are on-label and which are off-label for many of the medications listed here. Repeated forays into the thicket that is the less-than-user-friendly FDA Web site did not reveal lists of agents with this basic information. Consultation of multiple drug reference books often gave conflicting information, and information was sometimes inconsistent *within* a single source. Where there were discrepancies regarding on- versus off-label use, the status listed in the *Red Book* of the American Society of Health System Pharmacists was listed, since this was the most consistent source (see **Key References**). Despite the difficulties in ascertaining on-/off-label indications precisely, the clinician can assume that the uses listed, whether in one subcategory or the other, are indeed encountered in general practice.

DOSAGE

Dosage guidelines include: standard dosages, in general those approved by the FDA, typical limits to higher doses often used in clinical practice, and dosing guidelines for the elderly. Of course, dosage will have to be adjusted based on drug interactions and other considerations. Where therapeutic serum levels are available, those levels take precedence over dosage.

TITRATION SCHEDULE

This section gives rough guidelines for starting dose and titration increment and schedule. The notation "as indicated" is shorthand for "if you need greater effect and side effects do not prevent further increase."

TAPER/SWITCH SCHEDULE

This provides the information necessary for discontinuation of a medication and, if necessary, initiation of an alternative agent.

LABORATORY MONITORING

This section designates laboratory studies to be done prior to or during treatment.

SIDE EFFECTS

Major side effects are listed here by organ system. Each is coded as to frequency of occurrence and severity. Frequency is coded from (+) for occasional to (+++) for frequently encountered. Those side effects in **bold** are considered life-threatening.

Assume that any medication can cause an allergic rash. Assume also that any medication can cause nausea. These are not repetitively listed under individual drugs unless the side effect is particularly frequent or particularly serious (e.g., rash with lamotrigine, Stevens-Johnson syndrome with carbamazepine).

PREGNANCY AND LACTATION

This section assigns the FDA pregnancy precaution class and notes whether the drug has been demonstrated to be secreted in breast milk. FDA Pregnancy Classes are:
- **Class A:** Adequate studies in pregnant women have not demonstrated fetal risk in the first trimester, and there is no evidence for risk in the second or third trimester.
- **Class B:** No adequate studies in women, but reproductive animal studies have demonstrated no risk; *or* adequate studies in women have shown no risk, but reproductive animal studies have.
- **Class C:** No adequate studies in women, but reproductive animal studies have shown a risk; *or* no adequate studies in women or animals. *Note:* The majority of psychotropics are Class C.
- **Class D:** Studies in women demonstrate fetal risk; but given the potential benefits of the drug, the risk of use may be acceptable in pregnant women.
- **Class X:** Studies in women demonstrate fetal risk, and the potential for harm outweighs any possible benefit in pregnant women.

OVERDOSE TOXICITY

This section summarizes toxicity in overdose. Most toxicities are dose-dependent, but also a function of individual factors (e.g., age, concomitant medications) so caution is the operative principle. Life-threatening toxicities (common or not) are listed in **bold.**

CONTRAINDICATIONS

This section lists those conditions or disorders in which the medication should not be used.

COMMON DRUG INTERACTIONS

This section lists the major or most frequent drug interactions. Most dangerous interactions are listed in **bold.**

Drug interactions can be *pharmacokinetic* or *pharmacodynamic.* Pharmacokinetic drug interactions are effects that are due to the alterations in the handling of the drug (e.g., its absorption, protein binding, metabolism, or excretion). The basis of pharmacokinetic interactions is frequently via the cytochrome P-450 system, as summarized in **Appendix 12** as described below. An example of a pharmacokinetic interaction is the increase in desipramine levels by the addition of fluvoxamine because of its ability to slow desipramine metabolism by inhibiting P-450 enzyme 1A2. Note that the drug interactions listed here typically reflect *clinical* experience, while the P-450 interactions summarized in **Appendix 12** reflect both clinical and *in vitro* data. Thus, some of the interactions in **Appendix 12** will be of more theoretical than clinical concern.

Pharmacodynamic interactions are those that take place at the level of drug effect, for instance at the receptor level or by effects at multiple receptors. An example of a pharmacodynamic interaction is the additive sedation produced by trazodone and benzodiazepines.

The drug interactions listed in this section are the most common, the most serious, or the most clinically relevant in other ways. The most obvious pharmacodynamic interactions are not listed—for example, the combination of typical neuroleptics and dopamine agonists resulting in reduced effectiveness of either, or the combination of ziprazadone and tricyclic antidepressants resulting in additive prolongation of the cardiac QTc interval.

Note that most psychotropics are highly protein-bound. Thus, co-treatment with other drugs that are highly protein-bound (e.g., warfarin) may lead to increased effect of either drug because of increased free drug, even though serum levels (= free + bound) are unchanged.

The **Key References** include print and electronic resources for more exhaustive coverage of drug interactions.

HINTS & TIPS

This section is similar in purpose and scope to the notations, "Considerations in Choosing Among Treatments" in each of the entries in **Section III.** Like those notations, these are based on a combination of empirical data and clinical experience that will help the clinician in choosing and in managing specific treatments.

RELEVANT APPENDICES

Note also that three **Appendices** are of particular relevance to medication treatment:
- An **equivalency table** (**Appendix 11**). This contains a listing of the drugs in each class with their approximate equivalent doses to others in their class. Listings are given for antidepressants in the classic imipramine-equivalents, for benzodiazepines in diazepam-equivalents, for typical neuroleptics in chlorpromazine-equivalents, and for atypical neuroleptics in risperidone-equivalents. They were derived by comparing the upper and lower limits of the typical dosage range. Note that these dosages are approximate, and do not necessarily indicate equivalent behavior in clinical usage in an individual. Nor do they imply that one should take *n* milligrams of chlorpromazine and immediately switch an individual over to *m* milligrams of haloperidol. These figures are for rough comparison only.
- A table of **cytochrome P-450 enzyme metabolism** (**Appendix 12**). Most psychotropic medications are metabolized by the liver, and most by the cytochrome P-450 system. Drug interactions are myriad, and only the most brilliant, or the most obsessive-compulsive, among us can memorize them all. This information is presented in a single table rather than being entered under each individual drug for ease of cross-referencing. Note, though, as stated above with respect to "Common Drug Interactions," pharmacodynamic as well as these pharmacokinetic interactions must also be considered when combining medications. This table reflects only P-450–based pharmacokinetic interactions.
- Basic information on **Alternative and Complementary Treatments** (**Appendix 14**). This includes a listing of common agents used for psychiatric symptoms, their uses, and their relevant impact on psychiatric symptoms and treatments.

A NOTE ON DRUG DOSING IN INDIVIDUALS WITH RENAL OR HEPATIC FAILURE

The initial plan was to include an entry for each medication regarding how to dose the drug in individuals with hepatic or renal failure. What we found, not surprisingly, is that relatively few drugs had been tested. The reports that we did find were case reports of individuals whose treatment had gone awry or were investigations that had been done on small numbers of volunteers. Sometimes results were inconsistent across studies with regard to the degree to which metabolism and excretion was impaired, and the clinical relevance of those impairments was often speculative. Only in the rare case had detailed nomograms been worked out. For instance, there exists such a calculation to reduce the dose of lithium in the face of renal failure, developed in the 1960s and 1970s. In the present day, we thankfully have several alternatives to lithium, so that the clinician's typical move with an individual who had developed or was beginning to develop renal failure would be to use a different medication. Nonetheless, several principles can be articulated for dosing in hepatic failure, and several specific recommendations can be made as well for dosing in renal failure.

Keep in mind, however, that not all drugs have been tested, so that the absence of concern does not equate to safety. *In all cases, the "bioassay" of individual response—side effects versus drug efficacy—is your most valuable guide. With individuals with renal or hepatic compromise, begin low and go slow!*

Drug Dosing in Individuals with Hepatic Compromise

In hepatic compromise, several things happen that potentially raise drug serum levels and lead to toxicity. For instance, in acute hepatitis, parenchymal function is reduced and biliary excretion is compromised. First-pass metabolism may be reduced. In chronic hepatic failure, such as cirrhosis, reduction in plasma protein synthesis and resultant reduction in protein-binding capacity for drugs also becomes relevant; with reduced protein-binding capacity, drug toxicity can increase even with normal total serum levels because free drug levels are increased. Moreover, such individuals are often frail or compromised for other reasons and may be more susceptible to cerebral toxicity of drugs, such as sedation. Frequently, they are on multiple medications that may contribute drug interactions as well.

With these physiologic principles as background, and the scattered drug studies that indicate reductions in clearance of one-third to two-thirds with varying degrees of hepatic impairment, it is reasonable to reduce initial doses of hepatically metabolized psychotropics by 25% to 50%, as most of the formal studies recommend.

Drug Dosing in Individuals with Renal Compromise

Similar clinical reasoning attends the use of psychotropics in individuals with varying degrees of acute or chronic renal failure. The kidney itself contains substantial amounts of P-450 enzyme activity in its epithelial cells, although it does not play a major role in metabolizing most psychotropic drugs. Of more relevance is renal elimination of drugs, including filtration by the glomeruli, and secretion and reabsorption by the tubules. Active drugs and their metabolites, both active and inactive, are subject to renal excretion, particularly in the free form not bound to plasma proteins.

Renal dosing is therefore based primarily on the glomerular filtration rate (**GFR**), as approximated by the creatinine clearance (C_{Cr}):

$$C_{Cr} = [(140 - age) \times (\text{ideal body weight in kilograms})]/72 \\ \times \text{serum creatinine in mg/dL}]$$

For women, the calculated value should be reduced by multiplying the result by 0.85. Note that C_{Cr} by this formula somewhat overestimates the actual GFR, so one should err on the side of caution.

Swann and Bennett (see **Key References,** Psychopharmacology Treatment Resources: General) do not recommend dose adjustments for GFR of greater than 50 mL/min. Based on the above calculation, they make specific recommendations for dose reductions for the psychotropics listed in the following table. They recommend reducing the dose first rather than increasing the interval between doses.

	GFR 10–50 mL/min	GFR <10 mL/min
Buspirone	No adjustment	50% of normal dose
Chlordiazepoxide	No adjustment	50% of normal dose
Gabapentin	50% of normal dose	10% of normal dose
Lithium[a]	50% of normal dose	25% of normal dose
Paroxetine	50% of normal dose	50% of normal dose

[a]As noted above, with renal impairment, alternative agents to lithium for mood stabilization are recommended. If it is necessary to use lithium, serum levels should serve as the most accurate guide for dose adjustment. Levels, electrolytes, and renal function should be checked no less than monthly.

Swann and Bennett indicate no need for dose adjustment in renal failure for carbamazepine, oxcarbazepine, valproate, tricyclics, phenelzine, bupropion, fluoxetine, fluvoxamine, sertraline, benzodiazepines other than those mentioned above, chlorpromazine, haloperidol, or clozapine. No information to the contrary was found in further literature review. However, caution is urged, with attention to the "bioassay" as noted above.

Psychotherapy: Supportive Psychotherapy Techniques and Referral Information for Formal, Disorder-Specific Psychotherapies

Orienting Notes

- Conceptually and clinically, there are 2 major categories of psychotherapy:
  - *Supportive psychotherapy:* Techniques to be woven into *all* clinical interactions for all mental health (and medical-surgical) conditions. The focus is on:
    - Collaborative disease management
    - Problem solving around life difficulties due to illness
  - *Formal psychotherapies:* Specific interventions for specific conditions. Typically:
    - Condition-specific
    - Manual-based
    - Require specialized training
    - Supported by research data
- What is the purpose of the section?
  - Outline of supportive therapy techniques
  - If you already know a formal psychotherapy for a given condition, you'll probably use it.
  - But if you don't, your question will be: "What type of formal psychotherapy do I look for to refer this individual who has condition X?"

- For an outline of supportive psychotherapy, continue to **Panel 1.**
- For formal psychotherapy options for specific conditions, go to **Panel 5.**

Panel 1: Outline of Supportive Psychotherapy: What, When, and for Whom?

- What? The major components:
  - Collaborative disease management
  - Problem solving around life difficulties due to illness
- When?
  - From the very first contact
  - Reiteration as needed in every contact
- For whom?
  - Individuals with *any* chronic illness—mental health, medical, or surgical
  - Identify the relevant "unit" of treatment. The relevant unit may be:
    - The individual
    - The individual within his or her family
    - The individual within a care-giving institution (e.g., nursing home, acute medical floor)
    - The individual and various "silent partners" who may or may not be immediately recognized, for example:
      - A key significant other or advisor (e.g., friend, trusted family pharmacist, masseuse, private therapist, healer)
      - The extended family or clan
      - A religious community

Note: Consult **Key References** on the Biopsychosocial Assessment and Treatment Model and Collaborative Practice Treatment Model for background.

Continue to **Panel 2.**

Panel 2: Outline of Supportive Psychotherapy:
The Major Components

- The major components of supportive psychotherapy:
  - *Collaborative disease management*
    - Establishing treatment alliance—a collaborative relationship
    - Bidirectional education:
      - Education by the professional regarding technical issues of illness, treatment
      - Education by the individual regarding his or her priorities, values, preferences
    - Joint problem identification, prioritization, goal setting
  - *Problem solving around life difficulties due to illness*
    - In technical terms:
      - Maximizing *functional outcome*
      - Improving *health-related quality of life*
- The overall orientation is *collaborative:* clinician and individual being treated are each expert in their own field:
  - The clinician on technical matters
  - The individual on what it means to live with the illness and on his or her own priorities, values, preferences
- Consider: "the clinician as *coach.*"
- Alternative, less successful approaches (with credit to Drs. Evette Ludman and Greg Simon for this pithy conceptualization):
  - *Paternalistic:* "I know what's best for you, so do what I say."
  - *Maternalistic:* "Give me all your problems, and I'll solve them for you."

Continue to **Panel 3.**

Panel 3: The Collaborative Disease Management Agenda for Supportive Psychotherapy

Note: The specific approach for generic supportive psychotherapy in *Panels 3* and *4* is derived from the Life Goals Program, developed for manic-depressive disorder, as outlined in the Bauer and McBride citation in the Collaborative Practice Treatment Model section of the **Key References.** The approach is consistent with the overall collaborative practice models elucidated in other citations in that section.

1. What is this disorder?
   a. What causes these symptoms?
   b. What treatments in general are used?
   c. What is the course and outcome with and without treatment?
2. What is *your* specific pattern of symptoms?
3. What are the most troublesome symptoms for you?
4. [For chronic illnesses]: What are your early warning signs for relapse?
5. What are your triggers that lead to new or worsening symptoms?
6. What are your methods of coping with symptoms? How do you cope with life despite your symptoms?
7. For your typical coping responses:
   a. What are the positive aspects (benefits)?
   b. What are the negative aspects (costs)?
8. What are the coping responses you want to emphasize:
   a. In your own self-management?
   b. By using significant others, family, other support systems?
   c. By activating your clinician?
9. What are the coping responses you want to replace?

Note: The work with coping responses is based on the assumption that *all* illness behaviors have self-perceived costs and benefits—*always both.* What is essential—before teaching, scolding, cajoling, motivating—is to determine this metric in the individual. What may seem ill advised, and may well be (i.e., use of substances, social isolation), has some intrinsic perceived benefit to the individual. Our task is to help the individual clarify both the benefits *and* the costs. The individual then chooses to emphasize, replace, or alter a coping response. Our professional judgment is used to guide them in this.

- In providing education to individuals and their families, be sure to provide access to reputable, collaborative support groups and related resources. Suggested resources for most major disorders can be found in **Appendix 10, Some Self-Help Resources.**
- Continue to **Panel 4.**

Panel 4: The Problem-Solving Agenda Around Life Difficulties for Supportive Psychotherapy

- This functional maximization agenda focuses on social role function issues (work role, family role, social activities, health-related subjective quality of life).
- The collaborative approach continues:
  - The individual identifies functional difficulties due to the illness that are of high priority to him or her.
  - Coping responses to address the difficulties are identified.
  - Costs and benefits of various strategies are made explicit.
  - The clinician serves as coach, advisor, supporter, educator.

1. How have your symptoms prevented you from doing what you want in your life?

2. Identify a goal that is:
    a. Important, yet . . .
    b. Realistic (success breeds success; failure, demoralization)

3. State the goal in explicit, behavioral terms—so that both the individual and you know when it has been achieved, and when not.

4. Break the goal down into manageable, behaviorally identifiable steps.
    a. Manageable: success breeds success
    b. Behavioral: to know when you've succeeded

5. Analyze and address "roadblocks":
    a. Strategize problem-solving.
    b. Consider personal costs and benefits of various options.
    c. Support.
    d. Destigmatize.

6. Process subsequent high-priority goals iteratively.

7. Recapitulate disease management skills issues (**Panel 3**) frequently—mastery takes time and practice, success and failure.

Panel 5: Formal Psychotherapies: Overview

- Recall that formal psychotherapies typically:
  - Are condition specific
  - Are manual based
  - Require specialized training
  - Are supported by controlled trial research data
- They are often not available in general clinical practice because of:
  - Insurance reimbursement
  - Lack of training and broad dissemination
- The following panels facilitate referral. They:
  - Are organized by disorder
  - List applicable types of formal psychotherapy with reasonable controlled trial data indicating improved clinical or functional outcome (acute or preventive)

Note: The reader will see below that certain types of therapy (e.g., "behavior therapy," "cognitive-behavior therapy") appear frequently and under quite diverse disorders. These represent broad categories of interventions. For instance, cognitive-behavior therapy for depression differs substantially from that for schizophrenia or eating disorders. An attempt has been made to follow the nomenclature of the investigators reporting the study. However, it should be kept in mind that the entries below denote broad categories rather than single, specific, cure-all treatments.

Panel 6: Formal Psychotherapies: Mood Disorders—Major Depressive Disorder and Dysthymia

- Behavior therapy
- Cognitive-behavioral therapy
- Cognitive-behavior analysis system of psychotherapy
- Interpersonal therapy
- Problem-solving therapy

Panel 7: Formal Psychotherapies: Mood Disorders–Manic-Depressive Disorder

- Cognitive-behavioral therapy
- Family therapy
- Interpersonal/social rhythms therapy
- Psychoeducation, individual
- Psychoeducation, group

Panel 8: Formal Psychotherapies: Anxiety Disorders—Panic Disorder With or Without Agoraphobia

- Behavior therapy
- Cognitive-behavior therapy

Panel 9: Formal Psychotherapies: Anxiety Disorders—Phobias

- Simple
  - Behavior therapy
- Social
  - Behavior therapy
  - Group cognitive-behavioral therapy

Panel 10: Formal Psychotherapies: Anxiety Disorders—Generalized Anxiety Disorder

- Behavior therapy
- Cognitive-behavioral therapy

Panel 11: Formal Psychotherapies: Anxiety Disorders—Obsessive-Compulsive Disorder

- Behavior therapy
- Cognitive-behavioral therapy

Panel 12: Formal Psychotherapies: Anxiety Disorders—Posttraumatic Stress Disorder

- Behavior therapy
  - Desensitization
  - Eye movement response desensitization
- Cognitive-behavioral therapy
- Multisession debriefing (single-session debriefing has been shown to do more harm than good and is contraindicated)

Panel 13: Formal Psychotherapies: Substance Use Disorders—Alcohol

Note: In alcohol treatment, psychotherapies have typically been investigated as additions to standard "drug counseling." This typically includes substance use monitoring, problem solving, and coping skills training administered by drug counselors (see "Considerations in Choosing Among Treatments" in the Substance Use Disorders entry in *Section III*). Programs may be administered on an outpatient basis or as part of inpatient or halfway house residence. The American Society for Addiction Medicine (ASAM) provides a guide to select level of care among these psychosocial structuring interventions (see *Key References*).
- 12-step programs (see also *Appendix 10*)
- Behavior therapy
- Social skills training
- Cognitive-behavioral therapy

Panel 14: Formal Psychotherapies: Substance Use Disorders—Drugs

Note: In drug treatment, psychotherapies have typically been investigated as additions to standard "drug counseling." This typically includes substance use monitoring, problem solving, and coping skills training administered by drug counselors (see "Considerations in Choosing Among Treatments" in the Substance Use Disorders entry in **Section III**). Programs may be given outpatient or as part of inpatient or halfway house residence. The ASAM provides a guide to select level of care among these psychosocial structuring interventions (see *Key References*).
- 12-step programs (see also *Appendix 10*)
- Behavior therapy
- Social skills training
- Cognitive-behavioral therapy
- Drug-specific investigations have shown some efficacy for the following:
  - Cocaine: family therapy
  - Opiates: supportive-expressive therapy (a psychodynamic derivative; see *Key References*)
  - Tobacco: individual/group behavior therapy

Note: For these drug-specific interventions, it does not mean that these interventions do *not* work with other dependence types, only that they may not have been studied.

Panel 15: Formal Psychotherapies: Gambling

- Behavior therapy
- Cognitive-behavioral therapy

Note: Gambling 12-step programs, similar to those for alcohol and drugs, also have been developed; however, we were unable to find specific studies supporting this use. See also *Appendix 10*.

Panel 16: Formal Psychotherapies: Schizophrenia

- Family therapy
- Psychoeducation
- Social skills training
- Cognitive-behavioral therapy

Panel 17: Formal Psychotherapies: Somatization Disorders

- Chronic fatigue syndrome (variably defined): cognitive-behavioral therapy

Panel 18: Formal Psychotherapies: Eating Disorders—Anorexia Nervosa

Note: Formal psychotherapies for anorexia nervosa have typically been studied as add-ons to basic management packages that include weight and dietary monitoring, assessment of physiologic complications, and education.

- Behavior therapy
- Cognitive-behavioral therapy
- Family therapy

**Panel 19: Formal Psychotherapies:
Eating Disorders—Bulimia**

Note: Formal psychotherapies for bulimia have typically been studied as add-ons to basic management packages that include weight and dietary monitoring, assessment of physiologic complications, and education.

- Behavior therapy
- Cognitive-behavioral therapy
- Group interpersonal therapy

Panel 20: Formal Psychotherapies: Sexual Disorders

- Most psychotherapies for sexual disorders use a multimodal approach that includes:
  - Psychoeducation
  - Behavioral techniques
  - Couples work
- This type of multimodal intervention was pioneered by Masters and Johnson.
- See *Module 12* for an overall approach that can be used by the general clinician.

Panel 21: Formal Psychotherapies: Personality Disorders

- Avoidant personality disorder
  - Behavior therapy
- Borderline personality disorder
  - Dialectical behavior therapy

ANTIDEPRESSANTS

Introductory Notes

- Antidepressants are to a first approximation equally efficacious (with some metanalyses showing tricyclics a bit more efficacious than serotonin reuptake inhibitors), and differ primarily in side effect profile (with some metanalyses showing tricyclics having a few more side effects than serotonin reuptake inhibitors) and toxicity [with tricyclics clearly more toxic in overdose than the others and monoamine oxidase inhibitors (MAOIs) with clearly more toxic drug interactions than the others].
- Therefore, choice among classes should be made on the basis of the side effects one desires (e.g., sedation) and those one wants to avoid (e.g., sexual dysfunction).

TRICYCLICS

Introductory Notes

- Among tricyclics, secondary amines (nortriptyline, desipramine, and protriptyline) are better tolerated than the older, more sedating tertiary amine tricyclics.
- Pretreatment screening for cardiac and anticholinergic risks is required.
- Dose titration is necessary.
- Serum levels are available to guide treatment.
- Among tricyclics, clomipramine may be unique in its obsessive-compulsive disorder (OCD) effects and protriptyline in its sleep apnea effects.

Amitriptyline

Trade Name:	Elavil
Chemical Class:	Tertiary amine tricyclic
Therapeutic/Clinical Class:	Antidepressant; anxiolytic
"On-Label" Indications:	Major depressive disorder
"Off-Label" Indications:	Panic disorder
	Bipolar-depressive episodes
	Dysthymia
Dosage:	Typical: 150 to 250 mg/day
	High range: 250 to 450 mg/day
	Geriatric: Avoid
Titration Schedule:	50 mg every 2 to 3 days to therapeutic serum levels

Taper/Switch Schedule:	Reverse of titration schedule
	May concurrently start other classes
	2-week washout going to/from MAOIs
Laboratory Monitoring:	Serum level at steady state (5–7 days)
Side Effects:	Central nervous system (CNS): dizziness (+++), sedation (+++), activation/mania (+)
	Cardiovascular (CV): tachycardia (+++), orthostatic hypotension (+++), quinidine-like slowing of cardiac conduction (e.g., prolongation of PR, QRS) (++)
	Eyes, ears, nose, throat (EENT): blurred vision (++), tinnitus (+), dry mouth (+++)
	Gastrointestinal (GI): nausea (+), constipation (++)
	Genitourinary (GU): urinary retention (++), impotence (+)
Overdose Toxicity:	**Arrhythmias,** stupor
Pregnancy and Lactation:	Category C: drug excreted into breast milk
Contraindications:	• Prostatic hypertrophy
	• Within 4 to 6 weeks of myocardial infarction
	• Narrow-angle glaucoma
	• Cardiac conduction abnormalities including sick sinus syndrome, second degree heart block (with caution in first degree heart block, PR interval > 200 msec), left bundle or fascicular block (with great caution in right bundle branch block), a QT interval > 500 msec.
Common Drug Interactions:	Barbiturates: reduce amitriptyline levels
	Bupropion: increases amitriptyline levels
	Carbamazepine: reduces amitriptyline levels
	Cimetidine: increases amitriptyline levels
	Diltiazem: increases amitriptyline levels
	Fluoxetine: increases amitriptyline levels
	Fluvoxamine: increases amitriptyline levels
	Galantamine: increases galantamine levels
	Indinavir: increases amitriptyline levels
	MAOIs: hypertensive crisis
	Paroxetine: increases amitriptyline levels
	Quinidine: increases amitriptyline levels
	Quinidine-like (type Ia) anti-arrhythmics: dysrhythmias
	Ritonavir: increases amitriptyline levels
	Sympathomimetics: hypertension and dysrhythmias
Hints & Tips:	• Dose at bedtime
	• Metabolized to nortriptyline
	• Probably the most anticholinergic of the tricyclics.
	• Therapeutic trial 4 weeks; typically some improvement by 2nd week.

- Treatment duration 6 months for first or second episode of major depression; chronic treatment for third episode.
- Abrupt discontinuation may cause withdrawal symptoms of headaches, vomiting.
- Use with caution with suicidal patients, as overdose may be lethal via **cardiac arrhythmias.**
- Not recommended in geriatric patients because of fall risk from sedation, hypotension.
- Tertiary amine tricyclics are second-line treatment among tricyclics (compared with the secondary amines nortriptyline and desipramine) unless sedation is specifically desired.

Clomipramine

Trade Name:	Anafranil
Chemical Class:	Tertiary amine tricyclic
Therapeutic/Clinical Class:	Antidepressant; anti-obsessional
"On-Label" Indications:	OCD
"Off-Label" Indications:	Major depressive disorder
	Panic disorder
	Bipolar depressive episodes
	Dysthymia
Dosage:	Typical: 150 to 250 mg/day
	High range: 250 to 450 mg/day
	Geriatric: 25 to 75 mg/day
Titration Schedule:	50 mg every 2 to 3 days to therapeutic serum levels
Taper/Switch Schedule:	Reverse of titration schedule
	May concurrently start other classes
	2-week washout going to/from MAOIs
Laboratory Monitoring:	Serum level at steady state (5–7 days)
Side Effects:	CNS: dizziness (+++), sedation (+++), activation/mania (+)
	CV: tachycardia (+++), orthostatic hypotension (+++), quinidine-like slowing of cardiac conduction (e.g., prolongation of PR, QRS) (++)
	EENT: blurred vision (++), tinnitus (+), dry mouth (+++)
	GI: nausea (+), constipation (++)
	GU: urinary retention (++), impotence (+)
Overdose Toxicity:	**Arrhythmias,** stupor
Pregnancy and Lactation:	Category C: drug excreted into breast milk
Contraindications:	• Prostatic hypertrophy
	• Hypersensitivity to tricyclic antidepressants
	• Within 4 to 6 weeks of myocardial infarction
	• Narrow-angle glaucoma
	• Cardiac conduction abnormalities including sick sinus syndrome, second degree heart

	block (with caution in first degree heart block, PR interval > 200 msec), left bundle or fascicular block (with great caution in right bundle branch block), or QT interval > 500 msec.
Common Drug Interactions:	Barbiturates: reduce clomipramine levels
	Bupropion: increases clomipramine levels
	Carbamazepine: reduces clomipramine serum levels
	Cimetidine: increases clomipramine levels
	Diltiazem: increases clomipramine levels
	Fluoxetine: increases clomipramine levels
	Fluvoxamine: increases clomipramine levels
	Galantamine: increases galantamine levels
	Indinavir: increases clomipramine levels
	MAOIs: hypertensive crisis
	Paroxetine: increases clomipramine levels
	Quinidine: increases clomipramine levels
	Quinidine-like (type Ia) anti-arrhythmics: dysrhythmias
	Ritonavir: increases clomipramine levels
	Sympathomimetics: hypertension and dysrhythmias

Hints & Tips:

- May be unique among tricyclics for its anti-OCD properties.
- Some reviews indicate somewhat better OCD efficacy than serotonin reuptake inhibitors.
- Therapeutic trial 4 weeks; typically some improvement by 2nd week.
- Treatment duration 6 months for first or second episode of major depression; chronic treatment for third episode.
- Abrupt discontinuation may cause withdrawal symptoms of headaches, vomiting.
- Use with caution with suicidal patients, as overdose may be lethal via **cardiac arrhythmias.**
- Dose at bedtime.

Desipramine

Trade Name:	Norpramin
Chemical Class:	Secondary amine tricyclic
Therapeutic/Clinical Class:	Antidepressant
"On-Label" Indications:	Major depressive disorder
"Off-Label" Indications:	Panic disorder
	Cocaine craving
	Bipolar depressive episodes
	Dysthymia
Dosage:	Typical: 75 to 150 mg/day
	High range: 150 to 250 mg/day
	Geriatric: 25 to 75 mg/day

Titration Schedule:	25 to 50 mg every 2 to 3 days to therapeutic serum levels
Taper/Switch Schedule:	Reverse of titration schedule
	May concurrently start other classes
	2-week washout going to/from MAOIs
Laboratory Monitoring:	Serum level at steady state (5–7 days)
Side Effects:	CNS: dizziness (++), activation/mania (+)
	CV: tachycardia (+), orthostatic hypotension (+), quinidine-like slowing of cardiac conduction (e.g., prolongation of PR, QRS) (++)
	EENT: blurred vision (+), tinnitus (+), dry mouth (+)
	GI: constipation (+)
	GU: urinary retention (+), impotence (+)
Overdose Toxicity:	**Arrhythmias,** stupor
Pregnancy and Lactation:	Category C: drug excreted into breast milk
Contraindications:	• Prostatic hypertrophy
	• Within 4 to 6 weeks of myocardial infarction
	• Narrow-angle glaucoma
	• Cardiac conduction abnormalities including sick sinus syndrome, second degree heart block (with caution in first degree heart block, PR interval > 200 msec), left bundle or fascicular block (with great caution in right bundle branch block), or QT interval > 500 msec.
Common Drug Interactions:	Barbiturates: reduce desipramine levels
	Bupropion: increases desipramine levels
	Carbamazepine: reduces desipramine levels
	Cimetidine: increases desipramine levels
	Diltiazem: increases desipramine levels
	Fluoxetine: increases desipramine levels
	Fluvoxamine: increases desipramine levels
	Galantamine: increases galantamine levels
	Indinavir: increases desipramine levels
	MAOIs: hypertensive crisis
	Paroxetine: increases desipramine levels
	Quinidine: increases desipramine levels
	Quinidine-like (type Ia) anti-arrhythmics: dysrhythmias
	Ritonavir: increases desipramine levels
	Sympathomimetics: hypertension and dysrhythmias
Hints & Tips:	• Probably least sedating of tricyclics.
	• Therapeutic trial 4 weeks; typically some improvement by 2nd week.
	• Treatment duration 6 months for first or second episode of major depression; chronic treatment for third episode.
	• May be given in divided doses over the day since it is not typically sedating.

- Abrupt discontinuation may cause withdrawal symptoms of headaches, vomiting.
- Use with caution with suicidal patients, as overdose may be lethal via **cardiac arrhythmias.**
- Secondary amines are first-line treatment among tricyclics because of less sedation and orthostatic hypotension.

Doxepin

Trade Name:	Sinequan
Chemical Class:	Tertiary amine tricyclic
Therapeutic/Clinical Class:	Antidepressant
"On-Label" Indications:	Major depressive disorder
"Off-Label" Indications:	Panic disorder
	Bipolar depressive episodes
	Dysthymia
Dosage:	Typical: 150 to 250 mg/day
	High range: 250 to 450 mg/day
	Geriatric: Avoid
Titration Schedule:	50 mg every 2 to 3 days to therapeutic serum levels
Taper/Switch Schedule:	Reverse of titration schedule
	May concurrently start other classes
	2-week washout going to/from MAOIs
Laboratory Monitoring:	Serum level at steady state (5–7 days)
Side Effects:	CNS: dizziness (+++), sedation (+++), activation/mania (+)
	CV: tachycardia (+++), orthostatic hypotension (+++), quinidine-like slowing of cardiac conduction (e.g. prolongation of PR, QRS) (++)
	EENT: blurred vision (++), tinnitus (+), dry mouth (+++)
	GI: nausea (+), constipation (++)
	GU: urinary retention (++), impotence (+)
Overdose Toxicity:	**Arrhythmias,** stupor
Pregnancy and Lactation:	Category C: drug excreted into breast milk
Contraindications:	• Prostatic hypertrophy
	• Within 4 to 6 weeks of myocardial infarction
	• Narrow-angle glaucoma
	• Cardiac conduction abnormalities including sick sinus syndrome, second degree heart block (with caution in first degree heart block, PR interval > 200 msec), left bundle or fascicular block (with great caution in right bundle branch block), or QT interval > 500 msec.
Common Drug Interactions:	Barbiturates: reduce doxepin levels
	Bupropion: increases doxepin levels

Carbamazepine: reduces doxepin levels
Cimetidine: increases doxepin levels
Diltiazem: increases doxepin levels
Fluoxetine: increases doxepin levels
Fluvoxamine: increases doxepin levels
Galantamine: increases galantamine levels
Indinavir: increases doxepin levels
MAOIs: hypertensive crisis
Paroxetine: increases doxepin levels
Quinidine: increases doxepin levels
Quinidine-like (type Ia) anti-arrhythmics: dysrhythmias
Ritonavir: increases doxepin levels
Sympathomimetics: hypertension and dysrhythmias.

Hints & Tips:
- Dose at bedtime.
- Frequently used in low doses (25–75 mg) as a hypnotic, as is probably the most sedating of the tricyclics.
- Therapeutic trial 4 weeks; typically some improvement by 2nd week.
- Treatment duration 6 months for first or second episode of major depression; chronic treatment for third episode.
- Abrupt discontinuation may cause withdrawal symptoms of headaches, vomiting.
- Use with caution with suicidal patients, as overdose may be lethal via **cardiac arrhythmias.**
- Not recommended in geriatric patients because of fall risk from sedation, hypotension.
- Tertiary amine tricyclics are second-line treatment among tricyclics (compared with the secondary amines nortriptyline and desipramine) unless sedation is specifically desired.

Imipramine

Common Trade Name:	Tofranil
Chemical Class:	Tertiary amine tricyclic
Therapeutic/Clinical Class:	Antidepressant
"On-Label" Indications:	Major depressive disorder
"Off-Label" Indications:	Panic disorder
	Bipolar depressive episodes
	Dysthymia
Dosage:	Typical: 150 to 250 mg/day
	High range: 250 to 450 mg/day
	Geriatric: Avoid
Titration Schedule:	50 mg every 2 to 3 days to therapeutic serum levels

Taper/Switch Schedule:	Reverse of titration schedule
	May concurrently start other classes
	2-week washout going to/from MAOIs
Laboratory Monitoring:	Serum level at steady state (5–7 days)
Side Effects:	CNS: dizziness (+++), sedation (+++), activation/mania (+)
	CV: tachycardia (+++), orthostatic hypotension (+++), quinidine-like slowing of cardiac conduction (e.g., prolongation of PR, QRS) (++)
	EENT: blurred vision (++), tinnitus (+), dry mouth (+++)
	GI: nausea (+), constipation (++)
	GU: urinary retention (++), impotence (+)
Overdose Toxicity:	**Arrhythmias,** stupor
Pregnancy and Lactation:	Category C: drug excreted into breast milk
Contraindications:	• Prostatic hypertrophy
	• Within 4 to 6 weeks of myocardial infarction
	• Narrow-angle glaucoma
	• Cardiac conduction abnormalities including sick sinus syndrome, second degree heart block (with caution in first degree heart block, PR interval > 200 msec), left bundle or fascicular block (with great caution in right bundle branch block), or QT interval > 500 msec.
Common Drug Interactions:	Barbiturates: reduce imipramine levels
	Bupropion: increases imipramine levels
	Carbamazepine: reduces imipramine levels
	Cimetidine: increases imipramine levels
	Diltiazem: increases imipramine levels
	Fluoxetine: increases imipramine levels
	Fluvoxamine: increases imipramine levels
	Galantamine: increases galantamine levels
	Indinavir: increases imipramine levels
	MAOIs: hypertensive crisis
	Paroxetine: increases imipramine levels
	Quinidine: increases imipramine levels
	Quinidine-like (type Ia) anti-arrhythmics: dysrhythmias
	Ritonavir: increases imipramine levels
	Sympathomimetics: hypertension and dysrhythmias
Hints & Tips:	• Metabolized to desipramine.
	• Strongest antipanic efficacy data among tricyclics.
	• Therapeutic trial 4 weeks; typically some improvement by 2nd week.
	• Treatment duration 6 months for first or second episode of major depression; chronic treatment for third episode.

269

- Abrupt discontinuation may cause withdrawal symptoms of headaches, vomiting.
- Use with caution with suicidal patients, as overdose may be lethal via **cardiac arrhythmias.**
- Not recommended in geriatric patients because of fall risk from sedation, hypotension.
- Tertiary amine tricyclics are second-line treatment among tricyclics (compared with the secondary amines nortriptyline and desipramine) unless sedation is specifically desired.

Nortriptyline

Trade Name:	Aventyl, Pamelor
Chemical Class:	Secondary amine tricyclic
Therapeutic/Clinical Class:	Antidepressant
"On-Label" Indications:	Major depressive disorder
"Off-Label" Indications:	Panic disorder
	Bipolar depressive episodes
	Dysthymia
Dosage:	Typical: 50 to 125 mg/day
	High range: N/A
	Geriatric: 25 to 50 mg/day
Titration Schedule:	25 mg every 2 to 3 days to therapeutic serum level
Taper/Switch Schedule:	Reverse of titration schedule
	May concurrently start other classes
	2-week washout going to/from MAOIs
Laboratory Monitoring:	Serum level at steady state (5–7 days)
Side Effects:	CNS: dizziness (++), activation/mania (+)
	CV: tachycardia (+), orthostatic hypotension (+), quinidine-like slowing of cardiac conduction (e.g., prolongation of PR, QRS) (++)
	EENT: blurred vision (+), tinnitus (+), dry mouth (+)
	GI: constipation (+)
	GU: urinary retention (+), impotence (+)
Overdose Toxicity:	**Arrhythmias,** stupor
Pregnancy and Lactation:	Category C: drug excreted into breast milk
Contraindications:	• Prostatic hypertrophy
	• Within 4 to 6 weeks of myocardial infarction
	• Narrow-angle glaucoma
	• Cardiac conduction abnormalities including sick sinus syndrome, second degree heart block (with caution in first degree heart block, PR interval > 200 msec), left bundle or fascicular block (with great caution in

right bundle branch block), or QT interval > 500 msec.

Common Drug Interactions:	Barbiturates: reduce nortriptyline levels
	Bupropion: increases nortriptyline levels
	Carbamazepine: reduces nortriptyline levels
	Cimetidine: increases nortriptyline levels
	Diltiazem: increases nortriptyline levels
	Fluoxetine: increases nortriptyline levels
	Fluvoxamine: increases nortriptyline levels
	Galantamine: increases galantamine levels
	Indinavir: increases nortriptyline levels
	MAOIs: hypertensive crisis
	Paroxetine: increases nortriptyline levels
	Quinidine: increases nortriptyline levels
	Quinidine-like (type Ia) anti-arrhythmics: dysrhythmias
	Ritonavir: increases nortriptyline levels
	Sympathomimetics: hypertension and dysrhythmias

Hints & Tips:

- Therapeutic trial 4 weeks; typically some improvement by 2nd week.
- Treatment duration 6 months for first or second episode of major depression; chronic treatment for third episode.
- Abrupt discontinuation may cause withdrawal symptoms of headaches, vomiting.
- Use with caution with suicidal patients, as overdose may be lethal via **cardiac arrhythmias.**
- Secondary amines are first-line treatment among tricyclics because of less sedation and orthostatic hypotension.
- Unique among tricyclics for having a therapeutic window that demonstrates efficacy reduction both below *and above* the therapeutic range.

Protriptyline

Trade Name:	Vivactil
Chemical Class:	Secondary amine tricyclic
Therapeutic/Clinical Class:	Antidepressant
"On-Label" Indications:	Major depressive disorder
	Obstructive sleep apnea
"Off-Label" Indications:	Bipolar depressive episodes
	Dysthymia
Dosage:	Typical: 5 to 10 mg three times daily
	High range: 10 to 20 mg three times daily
	Geriatric: 5 mg three times daily
Titration Schedule:	10 mg every 2 to 3 days to therapeutic serum level

Taper/Switch Schedule:	Reverse of titration schedule
	May concurrently start other classes
	2-week washout going to/from MAOIs
Laboratory Monitoring:	Serum level at steady state (5–7 days)
Side Effects:	CNS: dizziness (++), activation/mania (+)
	CV: tachycardia (+), orthostatic hypotension (+), quinidine-like slowing of cardiac conduction (e.g., prolongation of PR, QRS) (++)
	EENT: blurred vision (++), tinnitus (+), dry mouth (+++)
	GU: urinary retention (+), impotence (+)
Overdose Toxicity:	**Arrhythmias,** stupor
Pregnancy and Lactation:	Category C: drug excreted into breast milk
Contraindications:	• Prostatic hypertrophy
	• Within 4 to 6 weeks of myocardial infarction
	• Narrow-angle glaucoma
	• Cardiac conduction abnormalities including sick sinus syndrome, second degree heart block (with caution in first degree heart block, PR interval > 200 msec), left bundle or fascicular block (with great caution in right bundle branch block), or QT interval > 500 msec.
Common Drug Interactions:	Barbiturates: reduce protriptyline levels
	Bupropion: increases protriptyline levels
	Carbamazepine: reduces protriptyline levels
	Cimetidine: increases protriptyline levels
	Diltiazem: increases protriptyline levels
	Fluoxetine: increases protriptyline levels
	Fluvoxamine: increases protriptyline levels
	Galantamine: increases galantamine levels
	Indinavir: increases protriptyline levels
	MAOIs: hypertensive crisis
	Paroxetine: increases protriptyline levels
	Quinidine: increases protriptyline levels
	Quinidine-like (type Ia) anti-arrhythmics: dysrhythmias
	Ritonavir: increases protriptyline levels
	Sympathomimetics: hypertension and dysrhythmias
Hints & Tips:	• Unique among tricyclics for efficacy in obstructive sleep apnea; mechanism and efficacy in other forms of sleep apnea are unclear.
	• Therapeutic trial 4 weeks; typically some improvement by 2nd week.
	• Treatment duration 6 months for first or second episode of major depression; chronic treatment for third episode.
	• Abrupt discontinuation may cause withdrawal symptoms of headaches, vomiting.

- Use with caution with suicidal patients, as overdose may be lethal via **cardiac arrhythmia.**
- Somewhat activating, as is desipramine; if not, may be given in single daily dose.

SELECTIVE SEROTONIN REUPTAKE INHIBITORS

Introductory Notes

- SSRIs have taken the antidepressant world by storm primarily because of their ease of use for providers and safety in overdose.
- Sexual side effects tend to be silent compliance killers (individuals tend toward the don't-ask-don't-tell approach to such "private" matters).
- P-450–based drug interactions are tricky, particularly fluoxetine and fluvoxamine.
- Antianxiety spectrum appears to be good and there are several FDA indications for anxiety disorders.
- Lack of sedative effect can be good in some cases, but can require adjuvant hypnotic treatment in others.

Citalopram

Trade Name:	Cylexa
Chemical Class:	SSRI
Therapeutic/Clinical Class:	Antidepressant
"On-Label" Indications:	Major depressive disorder
"Off-Label" Indications:	Bipolar depressive episodes
	Dysthymia
	Posttraumatic stress disorder (PTSD)
	OCD
	Social phobia
	Generalized anxiety disorder
	Panic disorder
	Poststroke emotional lability and agitation in dementia
	Bulimia
	Premenstrual dysphoric disorder
Dosage:	Typical: 20 to 30 mg/day
	High range: 40 to 80 mg/day
	Geriatric: 10 to 20 mg/day
Titration Schedule:	Standard first course of treatment is 20 mg/day. Dose can be increased after 2 to 4 weeks for complete or partial nonresponse.
Taper/Switch Schedule:	Over 1 to 2 weeks while initiating other therapy except MAOIs
Laboratory Monitoring:	N/A

Side Effects:	CNS: agitation/mania (+), migraine (++), somnolence (+), agitation (+), insomnia (+), parkinsonian symptoms (+ in the elderly)
	CV: postural hypotension, conduction abnormalities similar to tricyclics (+), **bradycardia** (+)
	EENT: dry mouth (+)
	GI: nausea (+), vomiting (+), diarrhea (+)
	GU: decreased libido and anorgasmia in men and women (+++), erectile dysfunction in men (+++)
	Metabolism: hyponatremia (+)
	Musculoskeletal: myalgia (+)
Overdose Toxicity:	**Serotonin syndrome,** bradycardia, **arrhythmias**
Pregnancy and Lactation:	Category C: drug excreted into breast milk
Contraindications:	• Use of MAOIs within 2 weeks
Common Drug Interactions:	Cimetidine: increases levels of citalopram active metabolite
	MAOIs: serotonin syndrome
Hints & Tips:	• Has been reported to have tricyclic-like dysrhythmia effects in overdose.
	• Among SSRIs, has some evidence for efficacy as monotherapy for agitation in dementia in place of neuroleptics.
	• High doses (e.g., 80 mg/day) may be needed for panic disorder or OCD.

Escitalopram Oxalate

Trade Name:	Lexapro
Chemical Class:	S-enantiomer of citalopram
Therapeutic/Clinical Class:	SSRI
"On-Label" Indications:	Major depressive disorder
"Off-Label" Indications:	Probably as for citalopram
Dosage:	Typical: 10 to 20 mg/day
	High range: 30 mg/day
	Geriatric: 10 mg/day
Titration Schedule:	Standard first course is 10 mg/day. Dose can be raised after 2 to 4 weeks for complete or partial nonresponse.
Taper/Switch Schedule:	Over 1 to 2 weeks while initiating other therapy except MAOIs
Laboratory Monitoring:	N/A
Side Effects:	CNS: dizziness (+), mania (+), parkinsonian symptoms (+ in the elderly)
	EENT: dry mouth (+), sweating (+)
	GU: decreased libido and anorgasmia in men and women (+++), erectile dysfunction in men (+++)
	Metabolism: hyponatremia (+)

Overdose Toxicity:	Probably the same as citalopram
Pregnancy and Lactation:	Category C: drug excreted into breast milk
Contraindications:	• Concomitant use of MAOIs
Common Drug Interactions:	Probably the same as citalopram
Hints & Tips:	• 10 mg/day reported to have equivalent effects to 20 mg/day citalopram
	• Advantages over citalopram unclear

Fluoxetine

Trade Name:	Prozac, Sarafem
Chemical Class:	SSRI
Therapeutic/Clinical Class:	Antidepressant
"On-Label" Indications:	Bulimia
	Major depressive disorder
	OCD
	Premenstrual dysphoric disorder
"Off-Label" Indications:	Bipolar depressive episodes
	Dysthymia
	PTSD
	Panic disorder
	Social phobia
	Generalized anxiety disorder
Dosage:	Typical: 20 mg/day
	High: 40 to 100 mg/day
	Geriatric: 10 to 20 mg/day
Titration Schedule:	Standard first course of treatment is 20 mg/day. Dose can be increased after 2 to 4 weeks for complete or partial nonresponse.
Taper/Switch Schedule:	Because of long half-life (5 days), 20 to 40 mg doses can be stopped; higher doses can be tapered over 2 weeks
Laboratory Monitoring:	N/A
Side Effects:	CNS: agitation/mania (+), anxiety (++), headache (+), insomnia (+), parkinsonian symptoms (+ in the elderly)
	EENT: dry mouth (+)
	GI: diarrhea (+), anorexia (++)
	GU: decreased libido and anorgasmia in men and women (+++), erectile dysfunction in men (+++)
	Metabolism: hyponatremia (+)
Overdose Toxicity:	**Serotonin syndrome,** bradycardia
Pregnancy and Lactation:	Category C: drug excreted into breast milk
Contraindications:	• Use of MAOIs within 2 weeks
Common Drug Interactions:	Alprazolam: increases alprazolam levels
	Antihistamines, nonsedating: increase antihistamine levels and potential QT prolongation
	Beta-blockers (except atenolol): increase beta-blocker levels

275

Carbamazepine: decreases fluoxetine levels
and increased levels of carbamazepine's
active metabolite

Chlordiazepoxide: increases chlordiazepoxide
levels

Clonazepam: increases clonazepam levels

Clozapine: increases clozapine levels

Diazepam: increases diazepam levels

Haloperidol: increases haloperidol
concentrations

HMG-CoA reductase inhibitors (statins):
increase statin levels

Loop diuretics: additive hyponatremic effect

MAOI inhibitors: serotonin syndrome

Phenytoin: increases phenytoin levels

Theophylline: increases theophylline levels

Trazodone: increases trazodone concentrations

Triazolam: increases triazolam levels

Tricyclics: increases tricyclic levels

Hints & Tips:
- With fluoxetine, more P-450 interactions than most antidepressants.
- Once-a-week 90-mg pill available, though recommended only for maintenance; 90 mg is calibrated to 20 mg/day dose.
- Among SSRIs most likely to reduce appetite and cause weight loss.
- Perhaps the most activating of SSRIs.
- 5-day half-life makes use in bipolar depression less desirable since if a manic switch occurs, fluoxetine remains in body longer.
- Requires 5-week washout prior to MAOI use.
- High doses (e.g., 80 mg/day) may be needed for panic disorder or OCD.
- Lower doses (10–20 mg) and premenstrual dosing alone may be sufficient for premenstrual dysphoric disorder.

Fluvoxamine

Trade Name:	Luvox
Chemical Class:	SSRI
Therapeutic/Clinical Class:	Antidepressant
"On-Label" Indications:	OCD
"Off-Label" Indications:	Major depressive disorder
	Bipolar depressive episodes
	Dysthymia
	PTSD
	Panic disorder
	Bulimia
	Premenstrual dysphoric disorder

Dosage:	Typical: 50 to 100 mg/day
	High: 100 to 300 mg/day (divide doses at >100 mg/day)
	Geriatric: 25 to 50 mg/day
Titration Schedule:	50 mg for 2 days then 100 mg for up to 4 weeks and increase as necessary
Taper/Switch Schedule:	Over 1 to 2 weeks while initiating other therapy except MAOIs
Laboratory Monitoring:	N/A
Side Effects:	CNS: agitation/mania (+), somnolence (+), parkinsonian symptoms (+ in the elderly)
	CV: hypotension (+)
	EENT: dry mouth (+)
	GU: decreased libido and anorgasmia in men and women (+++), erectile dysfunction in men (+++)
	Metabolism: hyponatremia (+)
Overdose Toxicity:	**Serotonin syndrome,** bradycardia
Pregnancy and Lactation:	Category C: drug excreted into breast milk
Contraindications:	• MAOIs within 2 weeks
Common Drug Interactions:	Alprazolam: increases alprazolam levels
	Antihistamines, nonsedating: increase antihistamine levels and potential QT prolongation
	Beta-blockers (except atenolol): increase beta-blocker levels
	Carbamazepine: decreases fluvoxamine levels and increases levels of carbamazepine's active metabolite
	Chlordiazepoxide: increases chlordiazepoxide levels
	Clonazepam: increases clonazepam levels
	Clozapine: increases clozapine levels
	Diazepam: increases diazepam levels
	Haloperidol: increases haloperidol concentrations
	HMG-CoA reductase inhibitors (statins): increase statin levels
	Loop diuretics: additive hyponatremic effect
	MAOI inhibitors: serotonin syndrome
	Olanzapine: increases olanzapine levels
	Phenytoin: increases phenytoin levels
	Theophylline: increases theophylline levels
	Trazodone: increases trazodone concentrations
	Triazolam: increases triazolam levels
	Tricyclics: increase tricyclic levels
Hints & Tips:	As with fluoxetine, more P-450 interactions than most antidepressants.
	Most studied SSRI for OCD. Doses up to 200 mg/day frequently needed.

Paroxetine

Trade Name:	Paxil
Chemical Class:	SSRI
Therapeutic/Clinical Class:	Antidepressant
"On-Label" Indications:	Major depressive disorder
	OCD
	Panic disorder
	Social phobia
"Off-Label" Indications:	Generalized anxiety disorder
	PTSD
	Bulimia
	Dysthymia
	Premenstrual dysphoric disorder
	Bipolar depressive episodes
Dosage:	Typical: 20 to 30 mg/day
	High range: 40 to 80 mg/day
	Geriatric: 10 to 20 mg/day
Titration Schedule:	Standard first course of treatment is 20 mg/day. Dose can be increased after 2 to 4 weeks for complete or partial nonresponse.
Taper/Switch Schedule:	Over 1 to 2 weeks while initiating other therapy except MAOIs
Laboratory Monitoring:	N/A
Side Effects:	CNS: agitation/mania (+), somnolence (+), insomnia (+), parkinsonian symptoms (+ in the elderly)
	CV: postural hypotension,
	GI: diarrhea (+)
	GU: decreased libido and anorgasmia in men and women (+++), erectile dysfunction in men (+++)
	Metabolism: hyponatremia (+)
Overdose Toxicity:	**Serotonin syndrome,** bradycardia
Pregnancy and Lactation:	Category C: drug excreted into breast milk
Contraindications:	• Use of MAOIs within 2 weeks
Common Drug Interactions:	Alprazolam: increases alprazolam levels
	Antihistamines, nonsedating: increase antihistamine levels and potential QT prolongation
	Beta-blockers (except atenolol): increase beta-blocker levels
	Carbamazepine: decreases paroxetine levels and increases levels of carbamazepine's active metabolite
	Clozapine: increases clozapine levels
	Diazepam: increases diazepam levels
	Haloperidol: increases haloperidol concentrations
	HMG-CoA reductase inhibitors (statins): increase statin levels

Loop diuretics: additive hyponatremic effect
MAOI inhibitors: serotonin syndrome
Phenytoin: increases phenytoin levels
Theophylline: increases theophylline levels
Trazodone: increases trazodone concentrations
Triazolam: increases triazolam levels
Tricyclics: increase tricyclic levels

Hints & Tips:
- Among SSRIs, considered to be less activating and may need to be dosed at bedtime in case of somnolence.
- Higher doses may be needed for panic disorder, OCD.
- See **Introduction** for note on dosing in renal compromise.

Sertraline

Trade Name:	Zoloft
Chemical Class:	SSRI
Therapeutic/Clinical Class:	Antidepressant
"On-Label" Indications:	Major depressive disorder
	Panic disorder
	PTSD
"Off-Label" Indications:	Bipolar depressive episodes
	Bulimia nervosa
	OCD
	Premenstrual dysphoric disorder
Dosage:	Typical: 50 to 100 mg/day
	High range: 100 to 200 mg/day
	Geriatric: 25 to 50 mg/day
Titration Schedule:	Standard first course of treatment is 50 mg/day. Dose can be increased after 2 to 4 weeks for complete or partial nonresponse.
Taper/Switch Schedule:	Over 1 to 2 weeks while initiating other therapy except MAOIs
Laboratory Monitoring:	N/A
Side Effects:	CNS: somnolence (+), insomnia (+), parkinsonian symptoms (+ in the elderly)
	CV: hypotension (+)
	EENT: dry mouth (+)
	GI: diarrhea (+)
	GU: decreased libido and anorgasmia in men and women (+++), erectile dysfunction in men (+++)
	Metabolism: hyponatremia (+)
	MS: myalgia (+)
Overdose Toxicity:	**Serotonin syndrome,** bradycardia
Pregnancy and Lactation:	Category C: drug excreted into breast milk
Contraindications:	• Concurrent use of MAOIs or discontinuing action within 2 weeks

Common Drug Interactions:	Carbamazepine: decreases sertraline levels and increases levels of carbamazepine active metabolite
	MAOIs: serotonin syndrome
	Pimozide: increases QT interval by unclear mechanism
	Tricyclics: increase tricyclic levels
Hints & Tips:	• In studies of PTSD, differs from placebo only in women.
	• Among SSRIs, relatively few drug interactions.
	• High doses may be needed for panic disorder, OCD.

MONOAMINE OXIDASE INHIBITORS

Introductory Notes:

• These are clearly efficacious antidepressant and antipanic medications, but stringent dietary and drug interaction requirements limit utility.
• They are typically fairly well tolerated in terms of side effects.
• There are few differences between the two most commonly used agents.

Phenelzine

Trade Name:	Nardil
Chemical Class:	Hydrazine derivative
Therapeutic/Clinical Class:	MAOI antidepressant
"On-Label" Indications:	Major depressive disorder
"Off-Label" Indications:	Panic disorder
	Bipolar depressive episode
	Dysthymia
	Social phobia
Dosage:	Typical: 15 mg in the morning to 45 mg/day
	High range: 60 to 90 mg/day in two to three divided doses
	Geriatric: 15 mg/day
Titration Schedule:	15 mg/day for 2 days, then 30 mg/day, and adjust as needed after 2 to 4 weeks for complete or partial nonresponse
Taper/Switch Schedule:	Taper 25% per day each 2 to 7 days. MAO is irreversibly inhibited and does not regenerate for up to 2 weeks

Laboratory Monitoring:	Percentage of MAO inhibited more than 80% is sometimes used to confirm adequate treatment, but blood test not widely available
Side Effects:	CNS: dizziness (+++), sedation (+), agitation/mania (+), insomnia (++)
	CV: orthostatic hypotension (++)
	EENT: blurred vision (++)
	GI: diarrhea (+), dry mouth (+), increased liver transaminases (+)
	GU: urinary retention (+), incontinence (+), erectile dysfunction (++)
	Hematologic: thrombocytopenia (+), anemia (+), leukopenia (+)
	Metabolic: syndrome of inappropriate anti-diuretic hormone (SIADH)
	MS: myoclonic jerks (+)
Overdose Toxicity:	Hypotension, stupor
Contraindications:	• Concurrent treatment or use within 2 weeks of other antidepressants—5 weeks for fluoxetine, concurrent use of sympathomimetics, concurrent use of meperidine (Demerol)
	• Pheochromocytoma
Pregnancy and Lactation:	Category C: drug excreted into breast milk
Common Drug Interactions:	**Bupropion: hypertensive crisis**
	Dexfenfluramine: increases risk for serotonin syndrome
	HMG-CoA reductase inhibitors: may lead to rhabdomyolysis
	L-Dopa: hypertensive crisis
	Meperidine (Demerol): hyperpyrexia and shock
	Mirtazapine, venlafaxine: hypertensive crisis
	SSRIs, nefazodone, trazodone, serotonin syndrome
	Sympathomimetics: hypertensive crisis
	Tricyclics: hypertensive crisis
Hints & Tips:	• In standard usage, the most common side effects are dizziness or hypotension and secondary tachycardia.
	• With untoward drug or food interaction, **hypertensive crisis** is a life-threatening concern.
	• Dose morning, morning and noon, or morning, noon, and midafternoon to avoid insomnia.
	• Must be on MAOI (low tyramine) diet for at least 3 days before initiating and for 2 weeks after discontinuation (see **Appendix 13** for diet and drug instructions).

Tranylcypromine

Trade Name:	Parnate
Chemical Class:	Nonhydrazine derivative
Therapeutic/Clinical Class:	MAOI antidepressant
"On-Label" Indications:	Major depressive disorder
"Off-Label" Indications:	Panic disorder
	Bipolar depressive episodes
	Dysthymia
	Social phobia
Dosage:	Typical: 10 mg every morning to 30 mg/daily
	High range: 40 to 60 mg/day in two to three divided doses
	Geriatric: 10 mg/day
Titration Schedule:	10 mg/day for 2 days, then 20 mg/day, and adjust as needed after 2 to 4 weeks for complete or partial nonresponse
Taper/Switch Schedule:	Taper 25% per day each 2 to 7 days. MAO is irreversibly inhibited and does not regenerate for up to 2 weeks.
Laboratory Monitoring:	Percentage of MAO inhibited greater than 80% is sometimes used to confirm adequate treatment, but blood test not widely available
Side Effects:	CNS: dizziness (+++), sedation (+), agitation/mania (+), insomnia (++)
	CV: orthostatic hypotension (++)
	EENT: blurred vision (++)
	GI: diarrhea (+), dry mouth (+), increased liver transaminases (+)
	GU: urinary retention (+), incontinence (+), erectile dysfunction (++)
	HEME: thrombocytopenia (+), anemia (+), leukopenia (+)
	METAB: SIADH
	MS: myoclonic jerks (+)
Overdose Toxicity:	Hypotension, stupor
Contraindications:	• Concurrent treatment or use within 2 weeks of other antidepressants: 5 weeks for fluoxetine, concurrent use of sympathomimetics, concurrent use of meperidine (Demerol)
	• Pheochromocytoma
Pregnancy and Lactation:	Category C: drug excreted into breast milk
Common Drug Interactions:	**Bupropion: hypertensive crisis**
	Dexfenfluramine: increases risk for serotonin syndrome
	HMG-CoA reductase inhibitors: may lead to rhabdomyolysis
	L-Dopa: hypertensive crisis
	Meperidine (Demerol): hyperpyrexia and shock

Mirtazapine, venlafaxine: **hypertensive crisis**
SSRIs, nefazodone, trazodone, **serotonin**
syndrome
Sympathomimetics: **hypertensive crisis**
Tricyclics: **hypertensive crisis**

Hints & Tips:
- In standard usage, the most common side effects are dizziness or hypotension and secondary tachycardia.
- With untoward drug or food interaction, **hypertension crisis** is a life-threatening concern.
- Dose morning, morning and noon, or morning, noon, and midafternoon to avoid insomnia.
- Must be on MAOI (low tyramine) diet for at least 3 days before initiating and for 2 weeks after discontinuation (see **Appendix 13** for diet and drug instructions).

OTHER ANTIDEPRESSANTS

Introductory Notes

- This heterogeneous group includes agents whose main effects are as serotonin-norepinephrine reuptake inhibitors (SNRIs; venlafaxine and mirtazapine), serotonin-2 receptor blockers (trazodone and nefazodone), or dopamine reuptake inhibitors (bupropion).
- As with other classes, a choice can be made based on the side effects desired and not desired.

Bupropion

Trade Name:	Wellbutrin, Zyban
Chemical Class:	Aminoketone derivative dopamine reuptake inhibitor
Therapeutic/Clinical Class:	Antidepressant
"On-Label" Indications:	Major depressive disorder
	Smoking cessation (with psychosocial program)
"Off-Label" Indications:	Attention deficit hyperactivity disorder
	Bipolar depressive episodes
	Dysthymia
Dosage:	Typical: 150 to 300 mg/day
	High range: 450 to 600 mg/day
	Geriatric: 75 to 150 mg/day
Titration Schedule:	75 mg q.d. to b.i.d. and increase optional to 150 mg twice daily for 2 to 4 weeks then increase for complete or partial nonresponse
Taper/Switch Schedule:	Over 1 to 2 weeks while initiating other therapy except MAOIs

Laboratory Monitoring:	N/A
Side Effects:	CNS: dizziness (+), **seizures (+),** confusion (+), agitation/mania (+), insomnia (++)
	CV: arrhythmias (+), hypertension (+), edema (+)
	EENT: blurred vision (+)
	MS: arthritis (+)
Overdose Toxicity:	**Seizures**
Pregnancy and Lactation:	Category B: excretion into breast milk unknown
Contraindications:	• Seizure disorder
	• Prior or current diagnosis of bulimia (increased risk of seizure)
	• Use of MAOIs within 2 weeks
Common Drug Interactions:	Beta-blockers: increase beta-blocker levels
	Barbiturates: decrease bupropion levels
	Carbamazepine: decreases bupropion levels
	Cimetidine: increases bupropion levels
	MAOIs: hypertensive crisis
	Phenytoin: decreases bupropion levels
	Tricyclics: increase tricyclic levels
Hints & Tips:	• Limit to no more than 150 mg/dose to minimize seizure.
	• Dose morning or morning and noon, to avoid insomnia.
	• Often added to SSRI to reduce sexual dysfunction (75–300 mg/day), but it is probably more sensible just to switch to a different single agent.
	• A sustained release preparation is available for single daily dosing.
	• Smoking cessation efficacy (150 mg/day) has only been shown in conjunction with a behavioral stop-smoking program.

Mirtazapine

Trade Name:	Remeron
Chemical Class:	SNRI
Therapeutic/Clinical Class:	Antidepressant
"On-Label" Indications:	Major depressive disorder
"Off-Label" Indications:	Bipolar depressive episodes
	Dysthymia
Dosage:	Typical: 15 to 30 mg at bedtime
	High range: 45 to 60 mg at bedtime
	Geriatric: 7.5 to 15 mg at bedtime
Titration Schedule:	7.5 to 15 mg at bedtime for 2 to 4 weeks and increase as needed
Taper/Switch Schedule:	Standard first course of treatment is 30 mg/day. Dose can be increased after 2 to 4 weeks for complete or partial nonresponse.
Laboratory Monitoring:	N/A

Side Effects:	CNS: dizziness (+), confusion (+), somnolence (++), agitation/mania (+)
	CV: bradycardia (+)
	EENT: dry mouth (++)
	GI: constipation (+), increased appetite (+++)
	HEME: thrombocytopenia (+), leukopenia (+)
	METAB: elevated cholesterol (+), weight gain (+++)
Overdose Toxicity:	(++) stupor, hypotension, bradycardia
Pregnancy and Lactation:	Category C
Contraindications:	• Use of MAOIs within 2 weeks
Common Drug Interactions:	**MAOIs: serotonin syndrome**
Hints & Tips:	• Weight gain is a significant issue.
	• Somnolence more common at lower doses (7.5–15 mg) than at higher doses.
	• Sometimes used as a hypnotic, but only about 50% reported sedation in trials for depression. Particularly given its expense, other agents have more to recommend them if a non-GABA hypnotic is desired (e.g., diphenhydramine, hydroxyzine, tertiary amine tricyclics, trazodone).

Nefazodone

Trade Name:	Serzone
Chemical Class:	Phenylpiperazine derivative serotonin 2A/2C antagonist
Therapeutic/Clinical Class:	Antidepressant
"On-Label" Indications:	Major depressive disorder
"Off-Label" Indications:	Panic disorder
	Generalized anxiety disorder
	PTSD
	Bipolar depressive episodes
	Dysthymia
Dosage:	Typical: 100 to 150 mg twice daily
	High range: 150 to 300 mg twice daily
	Geriatric: 75 to 100 mg twice daily
Titration Schedule:	Begin 50 to 100 mg b.i.d.; 100 to 150 mg twice daily for initial trial and after 2 to 4 weeks increase for complete or partial nonresponse
Taper/Switch Schedule:	Over 1 to 2 weeks while initiating other therapy except MAOIs
Laboratory Monitoring:	Consider SGPT, GGT as baseline and steady state
Side Effects:	CNS: dizziness (+), confusion (+), sedation (+), agitation/mania (+)
	CV: peripheral edema (+), sinus bradycardia (+), postural hypotension (+)
	EENT: blurred vision (+)

	GI: diarrhea (+), **liver failure** (FDA: "Black Box" warning) **(+)**
	GU: urinary frequency (+), impotence (+)
Overdose Toxicity:	Stupor, **serotonin syndrome**
Pregnancy and Lactation:	Category C
Contraindications:	• Use of MAOIs within 2 weeks
	• Hepatitis or cotreatment with other medications that may cause hepatic inflammation
Common Drug Interactions:	Benzodiazepines: increases levels of those metabolized by P-450 enzyme 3A4 (alprazolam, diazepam, triazolam)
	Buspirone: increases buspirone levels
	MAOIs: serious hyperthermia, rigidity, myoclonus, seizures
	Simivastatin: increases simivastatin levels
Hints & Tips:	• Generally well-tolerated
	• Good antianxiety spectrum
	• Black Box warning unfortunately renders nefazodone as a second- or third-line treatment.

Trazodone

Trade Name:	Deseryl
Chemical Class:	Triazolopyridine derivative serotonin 2A/2C antagonist
Therapeutic/Clinical Class:	Antidepressant
"On-Label" Indications:	Major depressive disorder
"Off-Label" Indications:	Panic disorder
	Bipolar depressive episodes
	Insomnia
	Agitation in dementia
Dosage:	Typical: 150 to 300 mg at bedtime
	High range: 300 to 600 mg at bedtime
	Geriatric: 25 to 100 mg at bedtime
Titration Schedule:	Start at 75 to 100 mg at bedtime and increase by 50 mg every 2 to 3 days. May increase after 2 to 4 weeks for complete or partial nonresponse.
Taper/Switch Schedule:	Reverse of titration schedule
	May concurrently start other classes
	2-week washout going to/from MAOIs
Laboratory Monitoring:	Serum level at steady state (5–7 days) may provide some dosage guidance.
Side Effects:	CNS: dizziness (++), sedation (+++)
	CV: tachycardia (++), orthostatic hypotension (++), quinidine-like slowing of cardiac conduction (e.g., prolongation of PR, QRS) (++)
	EENT: blurred vision (++), tinnitus (+), dry mouth (++)
	GI: constipation (++)
	GU: urinary retention (++), impotence (+), **priapism** (+)
Overdose Toxicity:	Stupor, hypotension

Pregnancy and Lactation:	Category C: drug excreted into breast milk
Contraindications:	• Use of MAOIs within 2 weeks
	• Prostatic hypertrophy
	• Hypersensitivity to tricyclic antidepressants
	• Recovery phase of myocardial infarction
	• Narrow-angle glaucoma
	• Intraventricular conduction delays
	• First-degree or greater heart block
Common Drug Interactions:	Fluoxetine: increases trazodone concentrations
	MAOIs: hypertensive crisis
Hints & Tips:	• Therapeutic trial 4 weeks; typically some improvement by 2nd week.
	• Treatment duration 6 months for first or second episode of major depression; chronic treatment for third episode.
	• Abrupt discontinuation may cause withdrawal symptoms of headaches, vomiting.
	• Effective antidepressant at standard to high doses, but sedation often prevents dosing fully.
	• A good choice for anxious, insomniac depression.
	• Sometimes a small amount (10–25 mg) several times a day can reduce anxiety.
	• Occasionally used in low doses (e.g., 10 mg three times daily) to reduce agitation in dementia.
	• Often used as nonaddictive hypnotic at 25 to 150 mg at bedtime
	• Always caution about **priapism**—most is reversible with cessation of trazodone. Occasionally, surgical correction is necessary, and permanent impotence may result.
	• Clitoral priapism has been reported.

Venlafaxine

Trade Name:	Effexor
Chemical Class:	SNRI
Therapeutic/Clinical Class:	Antidepressant
"On-Label" Indications:	Major depressive disorder
	Bipolar depressive episode
	Generalized anxiety disorder
"Off-Label" Indications:	N/A
Dosage:	Typical: 150 to 300 mg/day
	High range: 300 to 600 mg/day
	Geriatric: 75 to 150 mg/day
Titration Schedule:	Start at 75 mg in the morning for 1 to 2 days, then 150 mg/day. Continue for 2 to 4 weeks, then increase for complete or partial nonresponse.
Taper/Switch Schedule:	Over 1 to 2 weeks while initiating other therapy except MAOIs

287

Laboratory Monitoring:	N/A
Side Effects:	CNS: dizziness (+), agitation/mania (+), **seizures** (+), insomnia (++)
	CV: hypertension (++), vasodilation (+), tachycardia (+)
	GI: anorexia (+)
	RESP: yawning (+)
	SKIN: sweating (+)
Overdose Toxicity:	Hypertension, stupor
Pregnancy and Lactation:	Category C
Contraindications:	• Use of MAOIs within 2 weeks
Common Drug Interactions:	**MAOIs: hypertensive crisis**
Hints & Tips:	• Dose morning or morning and noon to minimize insomnia.
	• Use caution with hypertension, seizures.
	• Sustained release preparation allows single daily dosing.

ANTIMANICS AND PUTATIVE MOOD STABILIZERS

Introductory Notes

* *Mood stabilizer* is not an FDA-recognized term, although a number of medications with clear antimanic effects have acquired that colloquial designation.
* Using a strict definition of mood stabilizer as an agent that (a) treats acute manic and depressive symptoms and (b) has prophylactic effects that reduce the likelihood of future manic and depressive symptoms, the strongest current evidence is for lithium. Thus, lithium may be considered a first-line agent for long-term treatment of manic-depressive disorder.
* Lithium and lamotrigine appear to be efficacious in acute depressive episodes and prophylaxis.
* Other agents have evidence primarily as acute antimanics.

Carbamazepine

Trade Name:	Tegretol
Chemical Class:	Iminostilbene derivative
Therapeutic/Clinical Class:	Anticonvulsant; antimanic
"On-Label" Indications:	Seizures
"Off-Label" Indications:	Manic-depressive disorder (mania, prophylaxis)
	Neuropathic pain
Dosage:	Typical: 200 to 400 mg twice daily
	High range: 600 to 800 mg twice daily
	Geriatric: 100 to 200 mg twice daily

Titration Schedule:	Begin 200 mg twice daily and titrate every 2 days to therapeutic serum levels. If no response at 2 to 3 weeks, switch agents.
Taper/Switch Schedule:	25% per week. May initiate other agents.
Laboratory Monitoring:	Check electrolytes, complete blood count (CBC), serum glutamic pyruvic transaminase (SGPT), γ-glutamyl transferase (GGT), prior to initiating and with serum levels.
	Levels every 3 to 7 days during titration, monthly for 3 months, then every 6 months.
Side Effects:	CNS: dizziness (++), confusion (+), lethargy (++), ataxia(++)
	EENT: blurred vision (+)
	GI: anorexia (+), nausea (++), diarrhea (+), increased liver function tests (+)
	GU: jaundice (+), urinary retention
	Endocrine: decreased levothyroxine (T$_4$) with normal thyroid-stimulating hormone (TSH) and no hypothyroid symptoms
	HEME: **agranulocytosis (+),** leukopenia (++), thrombocytopenia (+)
	METAB: hyponatremia (++)
	Skin: **Stevens-Johnson syndrome and toxic epidermal necrolysis (1.4/10,000)**
Overdose Toxicity:	Stupor
Pregnancy and Lactation:	Category D: transferred to breast milk, neural tube defects, maximum risk in first trimester
Contraindications:	• History of bone marrow suppression and leukopenia
	• Concomitant use of clozapine or other leukopenia-inducing medications
Common Drug Interactions:	Anticoagulants: decrease anticoagulant levels
	Benzodiazepines: decrease levels of those metabolized by P-450 enzyme 3A4 (alprazolam, diazepam, triazolam)
	Buspirone: decreases buspirone levels
	Corticosteroids: decrease steroid levels
	Diltiazem: increases carbamazepine levels and decreases diltiazem levels
	Doxycycline: decreases doxycycline levels
	Erythromycin/clarithromycin: increases carbamazepine levels
	Estrogen and oral contraceptives: decreases estrogen levels
	Fluoxetine: decreases fluoxetine levels and increases levels of carbamazepine active metabolite
	Fluvoxamine: decreases fluvoxamine levels and increases levels of carbamazepine active metabolite

289

Lamotrigine: decreases lamotrigine levels and increases carbamazepine levels

Methadone: decreases methadone levels

Neuroleptics: decrease neuroleptic levels

Omeprazole: increases carbamazepine levels

Paroxetine: decreases levels and increases levels of carbamazepine active metabolite

Phenytoin: decreases levels of phenytoin and carbamazepine

Propoxyphene: increases carbamazepine levels

Theophylline: decreases theophylline levels

Topiramate: decreases topiramate levels

Valproate: decreases valproate levels, increases or decreases carbamazepine levels

Verapamil: increases carbamazepine levels and decreases verapamil levels

Hints & Tips:

- Well tolerated at steady-state levels, although speed of titration limited by GI symptoms and ataxia, lethargy.
- Well-established antimanic efficacy.
- Reasonable data for prophylactic efficacy.
- Few data supporting use as acute antidepressant.
- Drug interactions (is strong P-450 inducer) somewhat complicate management.
- Leukophenia to 50% to 75% of baseline values is not uncommon, is benign, is dose-dependent, and occurs mainly in first 3 months.
- Agranulocytosis is rare (<1 in 200,000), is not dose dependent, and occurs mainly in first 3 months.
- Oxcarbazepine (see entry) has similar spectrum of effects and side effects, but without agranulocytosis and without applicable serum levels.
- Although has a "tricyclic" structure, may be used with MAOIs.
- Induces own metabolism, so that levels may decrease over 1 to 3 months despite consistent compliance.

Lamotrigine

Common Trade Name:	Lamictal
Chemical Class:	Phenyltriazine derivative
Therapeutic/Clinical Class:	Anticonvulsant
"On-Label" Indications:	Partial seizures
"Off-Label" Indications:	Manic-depressive disorder (depressive episodes, prophylaxis)
Dosage:	Typical: 25 to 100 mg twice daily

	High range: up to 150 to 300 mg three times daily
	Geriatric: 25 to 100 mg twice daily
Titration Schedule:	Begin 25 mg daily for 1 to 2 days then 25 mg twice daily. Then each week increase by 25 to 50 mg/day. Risk of rash increases with speed of titration.
Taper/Switch Schedule:	25% per week. May initiate other agents.
Laboratory Monitoring:	Serum levels are broad (e.g., 2–20 ng/mL) and of unclear clinical relevance. However, some individuals appear to be fast metabolizers; if levels are low at doses of 200 mg/day, increase until levels reach midtherapeutic (e.g., 5–10 ng/mL).
Side Effects:	CNS: ataxia (+), headache (++), dizziness (+)
	EENT: diplopia (+), tinnitus (+)
	GU: amenorrhea (+)
	Respiratory (RESP): pharyngitis (+)
	Skin: **Stevens-Johnson syndrome and toxic epidermal necrolysis (2/10,000),** rash (depends on speed of dose titration) (+++)
Overdose Toxicity:	Stupor, rash
Pregnancy and Lactation:	Category C: transferred to breast milk
Common Drug Interactions:	Carbamazepine: increases carbamazepine levels and decreases lamotrigine levels
	Phenobarbital: decreases lamotrigine levels
	Phenytoin: decreases lamotrigine levels
	Valproate: doubles lamotrigine levels (use 50% of above doses), decreases valproate levels. Synergistic risk of Stevens-Johnson syndrome
Hints & Tips:	• Only putative mood stabilizer besides lithium with well-established efficacy as an acute antidepressant in manic-depressive disorder.
	• Some data for acute antimanic efficacy, but slow speed of titration limits use.
	• Reasonable data for prophylactic efficacy, especially rapid cycling.

Lithium

Trade Name:	Lithane, Eskalith, Lithobid
Chemical Class:	Monovalent cation
Therapeutic/Clinical Class:	Mood stabilizer
"On-Label" Indications:	Manic-depressive disorder (mania, prophylaxis)
"Off-Label" Indications:	Adjuvant treatment for major depressive disorder
	Bipolar depressive episodes
Dosage:	Typical: 900 to 1,200 mg at bedtime
	High range: 1,800 to 2,100 mg q.h.s. to 1,200 mg twice daily
	Geriatric: 150 to 600 mg at bedtime

Titration Schedule:	300 mg three times daily and increase every 1 to 2 days to therapeutic levels, then convert to single daily bedtime dose to minimize polyuria and impact of tremors. If no response at 2 to 3 weeks, switch agents.
Taper/Switch Schedule:	25% per week. May initiate other agents.
Laboratory Monitoring:	Check TSH, urinalysis, electrolytes, blood urea nitrogen, creatinine prior to initiation. Check these and check lithium levels every 3 to 7 days until at steady state, then at 1 month, and every 6 months.
Side Effects:	CNS: lethargy (+), memory problems (+)
	GI: diarrhea (++)
	GU: nephrogenic diabetes insipidus and polyuria/polydipsia (+++)
	HEME: leukocytosis up to 20,000 (++)
	METAB: hypothyroidism (+), weight gain (++)
	MS: tremor (+++), myoclonus (++)
	Skin: psoriasis (+)
Overdose Toxicity:	**Stupor,** dehydration, **electrolyte imbalances, renal failure**
Pregnancy and Lactation:	Category D: Ebstein anomaly and "floppy baby" syndrome; maximum risk during first and third trimesters, respectively. Transferred to breast milk.
Contraindications:	• Severe renal disease
Common Drug Interactions:	ACE inhibitors: increase lithium levels
	Calcium channel blockers: rare reports of delirium
	Neuroleptics: rare reports of delirium
	Nonsteroidal antiinflammatory agents (NSAIDs; including both COX-nonselective and COX-2 inhibitors) increase lithium levels up to 200% (sulindac has least effect)
	Theophylline: decreases lithium levels
	Thiazide diuretics: increase lithium levels up to 200% (lithium can be used with loop diuretics)
Hints & Tips:	• Well-established acute antimanic efficacy, better in classic euphoric than mixed episodes.
	• Well-established acute antidepressant efficacy, though less robust effects than for mania.
	• Best data for prophylactic efficacy among putative mood stabilizers.
	• Data also support efficacy in unipolar major depressive disorder, though less robust than for depression during manic-depressive disorder. Probably best effects in highly recurrent major depressive disorder.

- Strong evidence for efficacy as adjuvant agent for refractory acute episodes, major depressive disorder: 300 mg three times daily or 600 mg b.i.d. in addition to antidepressant agent, with response in 2 days to 2 weeks.
- Long-term studies (10–20 years) show no increased rates of renal failure, although long-term treatment with other concomitant risk factors (e.g., hypertension, diabetes) may lead to renal compromise.
- Overdose (purposeful or via drug interactions) can be particularly pernicious: increased levels lead to polyuria, diarrhea, vomiting, and volume contraction, which lead to increased renal resorption of lithium, which lead to increased lithium level, which leads to a continuation of this vicious cycle.
- See Introduction for note on dosing in renal compromise.

Oxcarbazepine

Trade Name:	Trileptal
Chemical Class:	Iminostilbene derivative
Therapeutic/Clinical Class:	Anticonvulsant
"On-Label" Indications:	Seizures
"Off Label" Indications:	Manic-depressive disorder (mania, prophylaxis)
Dosage:	Typical: 400 to 800 mg twice daily
	High range: 800 to 1,200 mg twice daily
	Geriatric: 200 to 400 mg twice daily
Titration Schedule:	Begin 200 mg twice daily and titrate 200 to 400 mg/day every 2 days to therapeutic dose. May increase as tolerated at 2 weeks for partial response; if no response at 2 to 3 weeks, switch agents.
Taper/Switch Schedule:	25% per week. May initiate other agents.
Laboratory Monitoring:	Unlike carbamazepine, therapeutic serum levels not established. Check electrolytes, SGPT, GGT prior to initiation and at 1 week, 1 month, and every 6 months.
Side Effects:	CNS: dizziness (++), confusion (+), lethargy (++), ataxia (++)
	EENT: blurred vision (+)
	GI: increased liver transaminases
	HEME: leukopenia (++), thrombocytopenia (+)
	METAB: hyponatremia (++)
	MS: peripheral edema
Overdose Toxicity:	Stupor
Pregnancy and Lactation:	Category D: transferred to breast milk, neural tube defects, maximum risk in first trimester
Contraindications:	N/A

Common Drug Interactions:	Probably similar to carbamazepine
Hints & Tips:	• Older drug developed concurrently; with carbamazepine however, not released in United States until 2001 for seizures
	• Reasonable data for acute antimanic efficacy
	• Likely similar efficacy to carbamazepine for other uses in manic-depressive disorder, but no supporting data
	• Advantage versus carbamazepine: no agranulocytosis
	• Disadvantage versus carbamazepine: no therapeutic serum levels

Topiramate

Trade Name:	Topamax
Chemical Class:	Sulfamate-substituted monosaccharide derivative
Therapeutic/Clinical Class:	Anticonvulsant
"On-Label" Indications:	Seizures
"Off Label" Indications:	Manic-depressive disorder (mania)
Dosage:	Typical: 50 to 300 mg twice daily
	High range: 400 to 800 mg twice daily
	Geriatric: 25 to 100 mg twice daily
Titration Schedule:	Begin 50 mg twice daily and increase to 200 mg twice daily over first week. May increase as tolerated at 2 weeks for partial response; if no response at 2 to 3 weeks, switch agents.
Taper/Switch Schedule:	25% per week. May initiate other agents.
Laboratory Monitoring:	N/A
Side Effects:	CNS: ataxia (+), dizziness (+), cognitive slowing (+++)
	GI: anorexia and weight loss (++)
	GU: kidney stones (+)
	HEME: leukopenia (+)
Overdose Toxicity:	Stupor
Pregnancy and Lactation:	Category C
Contraindications:	N/A
Common Drug Interactions:	Carbamazepine: decreases topiramate levels
	Carbonic anhydrase inhibitors: increase the risk of kidney stone formation.
	Phenytoin: decreases topiramate levels
	Valproate: decreases topiramate levels
Hints & Tips:	• Early but promising data as acute antimanic.
	• Almost unique among psychiatric medications, may cause weight loss.
	• Cognitive slowing may limit utility in some individuals; appears dose-dependent.
	• Anecdotal data only for other uses in manic-depressive disorder.

Valproate

Trade Name:	Depakote, Divalproex, Depakene
Chemical Class:	Carboxylic acid derivative
Therapeutic/Clinical Class:	Anticonvulsant
"On-Label" Indications:	Mania
	Seizures
"Off-Label" Indications:	Neuropathic pain
	Manic-depressive disorder (prophylaxis)
Dosage:	Typical: 1,000 to 2,000 mg/day
	High range: 2,500 to 4,000 mg/day
	Geriatric: 250 to 500 mg twice daily
Titration Schedule:	Can be loaded for acute mania, about 20 mg/kg or 10 mg/pound
Taper/Switch Schedule:	25% per week. May initiate other agents.
Laboratory Monitoring:	Prior to initiation check CBC, electrolytes, SGPT, GGT. Serum levels at 4 and 7 days until steady state, then 1 and 3 months and every 6 months thereafter. Therapeutic level for mania is 45 to 125 ng/mL, broader than for seizures.
Side Effects:	CNS: depression (+), lethargy (+), ataxia (+)
	GI: nausea (++), some reports of polycystic ovaries in epileptic women
	GU: **hepatic necrosis (+),** jaundice (+)
	HEME: anemia, leukopenia, **thrombocytopenia (++)**
	METAB: weight gain (++)
	MS: back pain (+), tremor (++)
	Skin: alopecia (++); hair often grows back curly in 1 to 6 months
Overdose Toxicity:	Stupor
Pregnancy and Lactation:	Category D: transferred to breast milk, neural tube defects and orofacial malformations, maximum risk during first trimesters
Contraindications:	• Hepatic disease
	• Thrombocytopenia
Common Drug Interactions:	Barbiturates: increase barbiturate levels
	Carbamazepine: decreases valproate levels; carbamazepine levels increases or decreases
	Clozapine: decreases clozapine levels
	Lamotrigine: doubles lamotrigine levels and increases risk of rash; decrease lamotrigine dose by 50%; increases valproate levels. Synergistic risk of Stevens-Johnson syndrome.
	Phenytoin: increase or decrease in phenytoin and valproate levels
	Topiramate: decreases topiramate levels
	Zidovudine: increases zidovudine levels

295

Hints & Tips:	• Well-established antimanic efficacy.
	• May have greater efficacy than lithium for mixed episodes.
	• No data supporting acute antidepressant efficacy.
	• Equivocal data regarding prophylactic efficacy.
	• Weight gain can be substantial.
	• Thrombocytopenia is dose-dependent. Clinically significant coagulopathies occur with platelet counts of less than 20,000. If thrombocytopenia occurs, risk of coagulopathy increases with other anticoagulants (e.g., aspirin).
	• Hepatic necrosis is rare but may be irreversible.

Verapamil

Trade Name:	Calan
Chemical Class:	Phenylalkylamine, calcium channel blocker
Therapeutic/Clinical Class:	Antihypertensive; antianginal
"On-Label" Indications:	Angina pectoris
	Hypertension
	Dysrhythmias
"Off-Label" Indications:	Mania
Dosage:	Typical: 80 to 120 mg three times daily
	High range: up to 240 mg twice daily
	Geriatric: Avoid
Titration Schedule:	Start 40 to 80 mg three times daily and increase every 1 to 2 days. If partial response at 1 to 2 weeks, continue titration as tolerated. For nonresponse at 2 to 3 weeks, switch agents.
Taper/Switch Schedule:	25% per week. May initiate other agents.
Laboratory Monitoring:	Electrocardiography (EKG) prior to initiation, at 1 week and at steady state
Side Effects:	CNS: asthenia, dizziness, headache
	CV: **atrioventricular block (+), bradycardia, (++) hypotension (++)**
	GI: constipation
	GU: nocturia, polyuria
Overdose Toxicity:	**Hypotension**
Pregnancy and Lactation:	Category C: excreted in breast milk
Contraindications:	• Bradycardia
	• Cardiac conduction abnormalities including any heart block
	• Hypotension
Common Drug Interactions:	Barbiturates: decrease verapamil levels
	Beta-blockers: increase risk for bradycardia, hypotension, heart block

Carbamazepine: increases carbamazepine
levels and decreases verapamil levels
Cimetidine: increases verapamil level
Lithium: rare reports of delirium

Hints & Tips:
- Older, but reasonable, data for acute anti-manic efficacy
- Efficacy for other uses in manic-depressive disorder not established
- Hypotension and heart block are particular concern

ADJUVANT MOOD DISORDER AGENTS

Introductory Notes

- For adjuvant treatment of acute depressive episodes, agents include:
  - Lithium in doses of 300 mg three times daily or 600 mg twice daily
  - Triiodothyronine (T_3, liothyronine) in replacement doses (25 to 50 mcg/day)
- For adjuvant treatment of rapid cycling manic-depressive disorder, T_4 (levothyroxine) is used in high doses.
- There is some evidence that high-dose T_4 also may be effective in refractory bipolar depressive episodes.

Levothyroxine (Thyroxine, L-Thyroxine)

Common Trade Name:	Synthroid
Chemical Class:	Thyroid hormone levothyroxine (T_4)
Therapeutic/Clinical Class:	Hormone adjuvant for mood disorders
"On-Label" Indications:	Hypothyroidism
"Off-Label" Indications:	Adjuvant treatment for rapid cycling manic-depressive disorder
Dosage:	Typical replacement doses for hypo-thyroidism: enough to bring TSH levels into normal range (about 0.75–1.0 mg per pound body weight. Given in single morning dose)
	High doses for rapid cycling: enough to bring free T_4 levels to about 150% of top-normal range (0.2–0.6 mg/day) given in single morning dose
	Geriatric: Avoid
Titration Schedule:	Begin with 0.05 to 0.10 mg/day. Increase 0.05 mg/day each week until 0.2 to 0.3 mg/day and assess response and check level in 2 to 4 weeks. Increase at same rate as indicated. Reduce dose for symptoms of hyperthyroidism.

Taper/Switch Schedule:	Reduce 50% first week, 25% each of next 2 weeks
Laboratory Monitoring:	As noted above and every 6 months and with T_3 level for symptoms of hyperthyroidism. T_3 level should remain within normal range despite high free levothyroxine level; otherwise, hyperthyroid symptoms may occur.
Side Effects:	CNS: headache (+), tremors (++) CV: tachycardia (++) GI: diarrhea (+), increased liver transaminases (+) ENDO: other symptoms of **hyperthyroidism** (+)
Overdose Toxicity:	**Thyrotoxicosis, arrhythmias**
Pregnancy and Lactation:	Category B
Contraindications:	• Cardiac disease • Liver disease
Common Drug Interactions:	• Anticoagulants: thyroid hormones increase breakdown of vitamin K–dependent clotting factors, so that oral anticoagulants may need to be increased. • Beta-agonists: tachycardia • Stimulants: tachycardia
Hints & Tips:	• T_4 is an inactive prohormone, and high doses do not typically result in hyperthyroidism because most T_4 is converted to the inactive reverse T_3 (rT_3) not to T_3. • Mechanism of adjuvant mood stabilizer action is unknown. • Response does not depend on current or past hypothyroidism. • Appears to work best in rapid cycling with discrete switches between depression and euphoria rather than with mixed or labile states. • Should not be confused with adjuvant, standard dose T_3 for refractory depression (see Triiodothyronine entry). • However, some studies also have shown efficacy of high dose T_4 in refractory bipolar depression without rapid cycling.

Triiodothyronine (Liothyronine)

Common Trade Name:	Cytomel
Chemical Class:	Thyroid hormone triiodothyronine (T_3)
Therapeutic/Clinical Class:	Hormone adjuvant for mood disorders
"On-Label" Indications:	Hypothyroidism
"Off-Label" Indications:	Adjuvant treatment for refractory major depressive disorder

Dosage:	Typical: for replacement for hypothyroidism, sufficient to bring TSH into normal range (about 25–50 µg/day) in a single morning dose
	For adjuvant depression treatment 25 to 50 µg in a single morning dose
	High range: N/A
	Geriatric: N/A
Titration Schedule:	25 µg/day for 4 days, then 50 µg/day if no response
Taper/Switch Schedule:	1 day
Laboratory Monitoring:	N/A. Thyroid function typically remains normal; check T_3 level if symptoms of hyperthyroidism.
Side Effects:	CNS: headache (+), tremors (++)
	CV: tachycardia (++)
	GI: diarrhea (+), increased liver transaminases (+)
	ENDO: other symptoms of **hyper-thyroidism** (+)
Overdose Toxicity:	**Thyrotoxicosis, arrhythmias**
Pregnancy and Lactation:	Category B
Contraindications:	• Heart disease
	• Concurrent treatment with MAOIs
Common Drug Interactions:	Beta-agonists: tachycardia
	MAOIs: tachycardia, arrhythmias
	Stimulants: tachycardia
Hints & Tips:	• Use is in standard replacement doses and is not to be confused with use of high doses of T_4 for rapid cycling (see Levothyroxine entry).
	• Most experience is in combination with tricyclics, but may be effective with any antidepressant.
	• Because exogenous T_3 turns off endogenous T_3 production, hyperthyroidism typically does not occur.
	• Response can be dramatic, in 2 to 4 days.
	• Adequate trial is 2 weeks.

ANTIPSYCHOTICS/NEUROLEPTICS

Introductory Notes

- Antipsychotics are primarily divided into *typical* and *atypical* agents.
- *Typical* agents are divided into:
  - High potency: relatively less sedating, less anticholinergic effects, less hypotension, more propensity to cause extrapyramidal symptoms (EPS; see *Module 17*)
  - Low potency: relatively more sedating, more anticholinergic effects, more hypotension, less propensity to cause EPS
  - Medium potency: midway in all respects between high- and low-potency agents
- *Atypical* agents are newer and:
  - Do not have a clear high-/low-potency profile.
  - Appear to have less propensity to cause tardive dyskinesia.
  - Olanzapine, quetiapine, and clozapine have particular propensity to cause substantial weight gain, type II diabetes mellitus, and hyperlipidemia.
  - Ziprasidone (along with the typical agents thioridazine and mesoridazine) has EKG QT-prolongation effects.
- Atypical agents are considered first-line treatment, but the health and disfiguring effects of obesity must be considered.
- Atypical agents may be considered "doing and undoing" agents with regard to dopamine neurotransmission (see Hints & Tips for those entries). Thus, in some cases of severe agitation or psychosis, the purer dopamine-2 receptor blockade of the typical agents may be necessary.
- See *Module 17* for more details regarding neuroleptic-associated movement disorders.

TYPICAL NEUROLEPTICS

Introductory Notes

- Agents are equally efficacious and equally likely to cause tardive dyskinesia.
- Choose among them based on side effects desired and not desired (see Introductory Notes for Neuroleptics above and individual agent profiles).

Chlorpromazine

Common Trade Name:	Thorazine
Chemical Class:	Aliphatic phenothiazine derivative
Therapeutic/Clinical Class:	Typical antipsychotic (low potency)
"On-Label" Indications:	Schizophrenia
"Off-Label" Indications:	Mania
	Other psychotic symptoms
Dosage:	Typical: 100 to 600 mg/day with bulk of dose at bedtime to minimize daytime sedation
	High range: 800 to 2,000 mg/day with bulk of dose at bedtime to minimize daytime sedation
	Geriatric: 25 to 75 mg/day
	Intramuscular form: 25 to 50 mg/dose
Titration Schedule:	Start 50 to 100 mg twice daily and increase every 1 to 2 days as indicated.
Taper/Switch Schedule:	25% per week. May initiate other agents.
Laboratory Monitoring:	N/A
Side Effects:	CNS: somnolence (+++), **neuroleptic malignant syndrome** (+), EPS (+), **tardive dyskinesia** (++ with use over years)
	CV: hypotension (+++), tachycardia (+++)
	EENT: blurred vision (++), dry eyes (++), dry mouth (++)
	GI: constipation (++), increased appetite (++)
	GU: urinary retention (++), menstrual irregularities (++), gynecomastia (++), lactation (++)
	HEME: leukopenia (++)
	METAB: weight gain (++)
	Skin: photosensitivity (+)
Overdose Toxicity:	Hypotension, stupor
Pregnancy and Lactation:	Category C: excreted in breast milk
Contraindications:	N/A
Common Drug Interactions:	Barbiturates: decreases chlorpromazine levels
	Beta-blockers: increase chlorpromazine levels and increase beta-blocker levels
	Carbamazepine: decreases chlorpromazine levels
	Fluvoxamine: increases level of chlorpromazine and increases level of fluvoxamine
	Lithium: rare reports of delirium with high- and low-potency neuroleptics
	Opiates: hypotension
Hints & Tips:	• Injectable form available.
	• Liquid form available.
	• Low-potency typical neuroleptics have lower rates of EPS but higher rates of sedation and hypotension than high-potency agents.
	• May be preferable to use a low-potency neuroleptic than to combine a high-potency

agent plus an anti-EPS agent plus a benzodiazepine for sedation.
* All neuroleptics may lower seizure threshold.

Fluphenazine

Trade Name:	Prolixin
Chemical Class:	Piperazine, phenothiazine derivative
Therapeutic/Clinical Class:	Typical antipsychotic (high potency)
"On-Label" Indications:	Schizophrenia
"Off-Label" Indications:	Mania
	Other psychotic disorders
Dosage:	Typical: 1 to 10 mg twice daily with conversion to single daily dosing for convenience at steady state
	High range: 10 to 20 mg twice daily with conversion to single daily dosing for convenience at steady state
	Geriatric: 0.5 to 1 mg twice daily with conversion to single daily dosing for convenience at steady state
	Acute intravenous form: 0.25 to 1.0 mg/dose
	Acute intramuscular form: 1 to 5 mg/dose
	Depot intramuscular form: 12.5 to 37.5 mg every 2 to 3 weeks
Titration Schedule:	Start 1 to 2 mg twice daily and increase every 1 to 2 days as indicated.
Taper/Switch Schedule:	25% per week. May initiate other agents.
Laboratory Monitoring:	N/A
Side Effects:	CNS: drowsiness (+), **neuroleptic malignant syndrome** (+), EPS (+++), **tardive dyskinesia** (++ with use over years)
	EENT: dry eyes (+), dry mouth (+)
	GI: constipation (+), increased appetite (+), menstrual irregularities (++), gynecomastia (++), lactation (++)
	GU: urinary retention (+)
	HEME: leukopenia (+)
	METAB: weight gain (+)
	Skin: photosensitivity (+)
Overdose Toxicity:	Stupor, EPS
Pregnancy and Lactation:	Category C: excreted in breast milk
Contraindications:	N/A
Common Drug Interactions:	Barbiturates: decrease fluphenazine levels
	Beta-blockers: increase fluphenazine levels and increase beta-blocker levels
	Carbamazepine: decreases fluphenazine levels
	Fluvoxamine: increases level of fluphenazine and increases level of fluvoxamine
	Lithium: rare reports of delirium with high- and low-potency neuroleptics
	Opiates: hypotension

Hints & Tips:	• Injectable form available.
	• Liquid form available.
	• Depot preparation provides substantial benefits if compliance problems exist.
	• High-potency typical neuroleptics have lower rates of hypotension and sedation but higher rates of EPS than low-potency agents.
	• All neuroleptics may lower seizure threshold.

Haloperidol

Trade Name:	Haldol
Chemical Class:	Butyrophenone derivative
Therapeutic/Clinical Class:	Typical antipsychotic (high potency)
"On-Label" Indications:	Schizophrenia
"Off-Label" Indications:	Mania
	Other psychotic disorders
Dosage:	Typical: 1 to 10 mg twice daily with conversion to single daily dosing for convenience at steady state
	High range: 10 to 20 mg twice daily with conversion to single daily dosing for convenience at steady state
	Geriatric: 0.5 to 1 mg twice daily with conversion to single daily dosing for convenience at steady state
	Acute intravenous form: 0.25 to 1.0 mg/dose
	Acute intramuscular form: 1 to 5 mg/dose
	Depot intramuscular form: 25 to 100 mg every 3 to 4 weeks
Titration Schedule:	Start 1 to 2 mg twice daily and increase every 1 to 2 days as indicated.
Taper/Switch Schedule:	25% per week. May initiate other agents.
Laboratory Monitoring:	N/A
Side Effects:	CNS: drowsiness (+), **neuroleptic malignant syndrome** (+), EPS (+++), **tardive dyskinesia** (++ with use over years)
	EENT: dry eyes (+), dry mouth (+)
	GI: constipation (+), increased appetite (+), menstrual irregularities (++), gynecomastia (++), lactation (++)
	GU: urinary retention (+)
	HEME: leukopenia (+)
	METAB: weight gain (+)
	Skin: photosensitivity (+)
Overdose Toxicity:	Stupor, EPS
Pregnancy and Lactation:	Category C: excreted in breast milk
Contraindications:	N/A
Common Drug Interactions:	Barbiturates: decrease haloperidol levels
	Beta-blockers: increase haloperidol levels and increase beta-blocker levels

Carbamazepine: decreases haloperidol levels

Clonidine: hypotension

Fluoxetine: increases haloperidol concentrations

Fluvoxamine: increases level of haloperidol
and increases level of fluvoxamine

Lithium: rare reports of delirium with high-
and low-potency neuroleptics

Opiates: hypotension

Paroxetine: increased haloperidol concentrations

Quinidine: increases haloperidol concentration

Hints & Tips:
- Injectable form available.
- Liquid form available.
- Depot preparation provides substantial bene-
fits if compliance problems exist.
- High-potency typical neuroleptics have lower
rates of hypotension and sedation but higher
rates of EPS than low-potency agents.
- All neuroleptics may lower seizure threshold.

Loxapine

Trade Name:	Loxitane
Chemical Class:	Dibenzoxazepine derivative
Therapeutic/Clinical Class:	Typical antipsychotic (medium potency)
"On-Label" Indications:	Schizophrenia
"Off-Label" Indications:	Mania
	Other psychotic symptoms

Dosage: Typical: 25 to 50 mg twice daily, with single
daily dosing at steady state for
convenience

High range: 75 to 125 mg twice daily with
single daily dosing at steady state for
convenience

Geriatric: 10 to 20 mg twice daily

Intramuscular form: 12.5 to 50 mg/dose

Titration Schedule: 2 to 4 mg twice daily and increase every 1 to
2 days as indicated

Taper/Switch Schedule: 25% per week. May initiate other agents

Laboratory Monitoring: N/A

Side Effects: CNS: drowsiness (+), **neuroleptic malignant
syndrome** (+), EPS (++), **tardive dyskine-
sia** (++ with use over years)

CV: hypotension (+), tachycardia (+)

EENT: blurred vision (+), dry eyes (+),
dry mouth (+)

GI: constipation (+), increased appetite (++)

GU: urinary retention (+), menstrual irregularities (++), gynecomastia (++), lactation (++),

HEME: leukopenia (+)

METAB: weight gain (+)

Skin: photosensitivity (+)

Overdose Toxicity:	Stupor, EPS
Pregnancy and Lactation:	Category C: breast milk excretion unclear
Contraindications:	N/A
Common Drug Interactions:	Barbiturates: decrease loxapine levels

Beta-blockers: increase loxapine levels and increase beta-blocker levels

Carbamazepine: decreases loxapine levels

Fluvoxamine: increases level of loxapine and increases level of fluvoxamine

Lithium: rare reports of delirium with high- and low-potency neuroleptics

Opiates: hypotension

Hints & Tips:
- Injectable form available.
- Liquid form available.
- Midpotency typical neuroleptics lie midway between high- and low-potency agents with regard to EPS, hypotension, and sedation. They may, thus, be useful when it is desirable to avoid either extreme.
- All neuroleptics may lower seizure threshold.
- Use with caution in patients with prior side effects to high-potency antipsychotics (EPS)

Mesoridazine

Trade Name:	Serentil
Chemical Class:	Piperidine phenothiazine derivative
"Off-Label" Indications:	Mania
	Other psychotic symptoms
Dosage:	Typical: 100 to 150 mg/day with bulk of dose at bedtime to minimize daytime sedation.

High range: 200 to 400 mg/day with bulk of dose at bedtime to minimize daytime sedation

Geriatric: 10 to 50 mg/day

Intramuscular form: 25 to 50 mg/dose

Titration Schedule:	Start 50 to 100 mg twice daily and increase every 1 to 2 days as indicated.
Taper/Switch Schedule:	25% per week. May initiate other agents.
Laboratory Monitoring:	N/A
Side Effects:	CNS: somnolence (+++), **neuroleptic malignant syndrome** (+), EPS (+), **tardive dyskinesia** (++ with use over years)

CV: **QT prolongation** (+) (has FDA **Black Box warning**), tachycardia (+)

EENT: **macular degeneration** at doses of greater than 400 mg/day (+)

GI: constipation (++), increased appetite (++)

GU: urinary retention (++), menstrual irregularities (++), gynecomastia, lactation (++)

HEME: leukopenia (+)
METAB: weight gain (++)
Skin: photosensitivity

Overdose Toxicity:	Hypotension, stupor, arrhythmias
Pregnancy and Lactation:	Category C: breast milk excretion unclear
Contraindications:	QTc interval ≥ 500 msec
Common Drug Interactions:	Barbiturates: decrease mesoridazine levels

Beta-blockers: increase mesoridazine levels
and increase beta-blocker levels
Carbamazepine: decreases mesoridazine levels
Fluvoxamine: increases level of mesoridazine
and increases level of fluvoxamine
Lithium: rare reports of delirium with high-
and low-potency neuroleptics
Nonsedating antihistamines: elongated QT
interval, may cause cardiac arrhythmias
with QTc of greater than 500 msec
Opiates: hypotension

Hints & Tips:

- Injectable form available.
- Liquid form available.
- Mesoridazine is the active metabolite of thioridazine.
- With FDA Black Box warning and dose limitation due to macular degeneration risk, confers no advantages over chlorpromazine when a low-potency typical agent is desired.
- Low-potency typical neuroleptics have lower rates of EPS but higher rates of sedation and hypotension than high-potency agents.
- May be preferable to use a low-potency neuroleptic than to combine a high-potency agent plus an anti-EPS agent plus a benzodiazepine for sedation.
- All neuroleptics may lower seizure threshold.

Molindone

Trade Name:	Moban
Chemical Class:	Dihydroinolone derivative
Therapeutic/Clinical Class:	Typical antipsychotic (medium potency)
"On-Label" Indications:	Schizophrenia
"Off-Label" Indications:	Mania

Other psychotic symptoms

Dosage:	Typical: 50 to 100 mg twice daily, with single daily dosing at steady state for convenience

High range: 125 to 150 mg twice daily with
single daily dosing at steady state for
convenience
Geriatric: 10 to 25 mg twice daily

Titration Schedule:	Start 25 mg twice daily and increase every 1 to 2 days as indicated.

Taper/Switch Schedule:	25% per week. May initiate other agents.
Laboratory Monitoring:	N/A
Side Effects:	CNS: drowsiness (+), **neuroleptic malignant syndrome** (+), EPS (++), **tardive dyskinesia** (++ with use over years)
	CV: hypotension (+), tachycardia (+)
	EENT: blurred vision (+), dry eyes (+), dry mouth (+)
	GI: constipation (+), decreased appetite (++)
	GU: urinary retention (+), menstrual irregularities (++), gynecomastia (++), lactation (++)
	HEME: leukopenia (+)
	METAB: weight loss (+)
	Skin: photosensitivity (+)
Overdose Toxicity:	Stupor, EPS
Pregnancy and Lactation:	Category C: excreted into breast milk
Contraindications:	N/A
Common Drug Interactions:	Barbiturates: decrease molindone levels
	Beta-blockers: increase molindone levels and increase beta-blocker levels
	Carbamazepine: decreases molindone levels
	Fluoxetine: increases molindone levels
	Fluvoxamine: increases level of molindone and increases level of fluvoxamine
	Lithium: rare reports of delirium with high- and low-potency neuroleptics
	Opiates: hypotension
	Paroxetine: increases molindone levels

Hints & Tips:

- Liquid form available.
- Among neuroleptics, least likely to cause weight gain and may even be associated with weight loss.
- Midpotency typical neuroleptics lie midway between high- and low-potency agents with regard to EPS, hypotension, and sedation. They may, thus, be useful when it is desirable to avoid either extreme.
- All neuroleptics may lower seizure threshold.
- Use with caution in patients with prior side effects to high-potency antipsychotics (EPS).

Perphenazine

Trade Name:	Trilafon
Chemical Class:	Piperidine phenothiazine derivative
Therapeutic/Clinical Class:	Typical antipsychotic (medium potency)
"On-Label" Indications:	Schizophrenia
"Off-Label" Indications:	Mania
	Other psychotic symptoms
Dosage:	Typical: 2 to 16 mg twice daily, with single daily dosing at steady state for convenience

	High range: 16 mg three to four times daily with single daily dosing at steady state for convenience
	Geriatric: 2 to 4 mg twice daily
	Intramuscular form: 2 to 4 mg/dose
Titration Schedule:	2 to 4 mg twice daily and increase every 1 to 2 days as indicated
Taper/Switch Schedule:	25% per week. May initiate other agents.
Laboratory Monitoring:	N/A
Side Effects:	CNS: drowsiness (+), **neuroleptic malignant syndrome** (+), EPS (++), **tardive dyskinesia** (++ with use over years)

CV: hypotension (+), tachycardia (+)

EENT: blurred vision (+), dry eyes (+), dry mouth (+)

GI: constipation (+), increased appetite (++)

GU: urinary retention (+), menstrual irregularities (++), gynecomastia (++), lactation (++)

HEME: leukopenia (+)

METAB: weight gain (+)

Skin: photosensitivity (+)

Overdose Toxicity:	Stupor, EPS
Pregnancy and Lactation:	Category C: excreted in breast milk
Contraindications:	N/A
Common Drug Interactions:	Barbiturates: decrease perphenazine levels

Beta-blockers: increase perphenazine levels and increase beta-blocker levels

Carbamazepine: decreases perphenazine levels

Fluvoxamine: increases level of perphenazine and increases level of fluvoxamine

Lithium: rare reports of delirium with high- and low-potency neuroleptics

Opiates: hypotension

Hints & Tips:
- Injectable form available.
- Liquid form available.
- Midpotency typical neuroleptics lie midway between high- and low-potency agents with regard to EPS, hypotension, and sedation. They may thus be useful when it is desirable to avoid either extreme.
- All neuroleptics may lower seizure threshold.
- Use with caution in patients with prior side effects to high-potency antipsychotics (EPS).

Thioridazine

Trade Name:	Mellaril
Chemical Class:	Piperazine phenothiazine derivative
Therapeutic/Clinical Class:	Typical antipsychotic (low potency)
"Off-Label" Indications:	Mania

	Other psychotic symptoms
Dosage:	Typical: 100 to 600 mg/day with bulk of dose at bedtime to minimize daytime sedation
	High range: 800 mg/day maximum due to risk of macular degeneration
	Geriatric: 25 to 75 mg/day
Titration Schedule:	Start 50 to 100 mg twice daily and increase every 1 to 2 days as indicated.
Taper/Switch Schedule:	25% per week. May initiate other agents.
Laboratory Monitoring:	N/A
Side Effects:	CNS: somnolence (+++), **neuroleptic malignant syndrome** (+), EPS (+), **tardive dyskinesia** (++ with use over years)
	CV: **QT prolongation** (+) (has FDA Black Box warning), tachycardia (+++)
	EENT: **macular degeneration** at doses of greater than 800 mg/day (+)
	GI: constipation (++), increased appetite (++)
	GU: urinary retention (++), menstrual irregularities (++), gynecomastia, lactation (++)
	HEME: leukopenia (+)
	METAB: weight gain (++)
	Skin: photosensity
Overdose Toxicity:	Hypotension, stupor, arrhythmias
Pregnancy and Lactation:	Category C: breast milk excretion unclear
Contraindications:	QTc interval ≥ 500 msec
Common Drug Interactions:	Barbiturates: decrease thioridazine levels
	Beta-blockers: increase thioridazine levels and increase beta-blocker levels
	Carbamazepine: decreases thioridazine levels
	Fluvoxamine: increases level of thioridazine and increases level of fluvoxamine
	Lithium: rare reports of delirium with high- and low-potency neuroleptics
	Nonsedating antihistamines: elongated QT interval, may cause cardiac arrhythmias with QTc of greater than 500 msec
	Opiates: hypotension
Hints & Tips:	• Liquid form available
	• With FDA Black Box warning and dose limitation due to macular degeneration risk, confers no advantages over chlorpromazine when a low-potency typical agent is desired.
	• Low-potency typical neuroleptics have lower rates of EPS but higher rates of sedation and hypotension than high-potency agents.
	• May be preferable to use a low-potency neuroleptic than to combine a high-potency agent plus an anti-EPS agent plus a benzodiazepine for sedation.
	• All neuroleptics may lower seizure threshold.

Thiothixene

Common Trade Name:	Navane
Chemical Class:	Thioxanthene derivative
Therapeutic/Clinical Class:	Typical antipsychotic (medium potency)
"On-Label" Indications:	Schizophrenia
"Off-Label" Indications:	Mania
	Other psychotic symptoms
Dosage:	Typical: 5 to 15 mg twice daily, with single daily dosing at steady state for convenience
	High range: 20 to 30 mg twice daily with single daily dosing at steady state for convenience
	Geriatric: 1 to 3 mg twice daily
Titration Schedule:	Start 2 to 4 mg twice daily and increase every 1 to 2 days as indicated.
Taper/Switch Schedule:	25% per week. May initiate other agents.
Laboratory Monitoring:	N/A
Side Effects:	CNS: drowsiness (+), **neuroleptic malignant syndrome** (+), EPS (++), **tardive dyskinesia** (++ with use over years)
	CV: hypotension (+), tachycardia (+)
	EENT: blurred vision (+), dry eyes (+), dry mouth (+)
	GI: constipation (+), increased appetite (++)
	GU: urinary retention (+), menstrual irregularities (++), gynecomastia (++), lactation (++)
	HEME: leukopenia (+)
	METAB: weight gain (+)
	Skin: photosensitivity (+)
Overdose Toxicity:	Stupor, EPS
Pregnancy and Lactation:	Category C: excretion into breast milk unknown
Contraindications:	N/A
Common Drug Interactions:	Barbiturates: decrease thiothixene levels
	Beta-blockers: increase thiothixene levels and increase beta-blocker levels
	Carbamazepine: decreases thiothixene levels
	Fluvoxamine: increases level of thiothixene and increases level of fluvoxamine
	Lithium: rare reports of delirium with high- and low-potency neuroleptics
	Opiates: hypotension
Hints & Tips:	• Liquid form available.
	• Midpotency typical neuroleptics lie midway between high- and low-potency agents with regard to EPS, hypotension, and sedation. They may, thus, be useful when it is desirable to avoid either extreme.
	• May lower seizure threshold.
	• Use with caution in patients with prior side effects to high-potency antipsychotics (EPS).

Trifluoperazine

Trade Name:	Stelazine
Chemical Class:	Piperazine phenothiazine derivative
Therapeutic/Clinical Class:	Typical antipsychotic (medium potency)
"On-Label" Indications:	Schizophrenia
"Off-Label" Indications:	Mania
	Other psychotic symptoms
Dosage:	Typical: 5 to 10 mg twice daily, with single daily dosing at steady state for convenience
	High range: 20 to 30 mg twice daily with single daily dosing at steady state for convenience
	Geriatric: 1 to 2 mg twice daily
	Intramuscular form: 2 mg/dose
Titration Schedule:	2 to 4 mg twice daily and increase every 1 to 2 days as indicated
Taper/Switch Schedule:	25% per week. May initiate other agents.
Laboratory Monitoring:	N/A
Side Effects:	CNS: drowsiness (+), **neuroleptic malignant syndrome** (+), EPS (++), **tardive dyskinesia** (++ with use over years)
	CV: hypotension (+), tachycardia (+)
	EENT: blurred vision (+), dry eyes (+), dry mouth (+)
	GI: constipation (+), increased appetite (++)
	GU: urinary retention (+), menstrual irregularities (++), gynecomastia (++), lactation (++)
	HEME: leukopenia (+)
	METAB: weight gain (+)
	Skin: photosensitivity (+)
Overdose Toxicity:	Stupor, EPS
Pregnancy and Lactation:	Category C: excreted in breast milk
Contraindications:	N/A
Contraindications:	Barbiturates: decrease trifluoperazine levels
	Beta-blockers: increase trifluoperazine levels and increase beta-blocker levels
	Carbamazepine: decreases trifluoperazine levels
	Fluvoxamine: increases level of trifluoperazine and increases level of fluvoxamine
	Lithium: rare reports of delirium with high- and low-potency neuroleptics
	Opiates: hypotension
Hints & Tips:	• Injectable form available.
	• Midpotency typical neuroleptics lie midway between high- and low-potency agents with regard to EPS, hypotension, and sedation. They may, thus, be useful when it is desirable to avoid either extreme.
	• May lower seizure threshold.
	• Use with caution in patients with prior side effects to high-potency antipsychotics (EPS).

ATYPICAL NEUROLEPTICS

Introductory Notes

- Agents appear equally efficacious, although there are sufficient data to presume that clozapine is effective in refractory psychosis.
- Choose based on side effects desired and not desired (see Introductory Notes for typical Neuroleptics above and individual agent profiles).

Clozapine

Trade Name:	Clozaril
Chemical Class:	Dibenzodiazepine derivative
Therapeutic/Clinical Class:	Atypical antipsychotic
"On-Label" Indications:	Schizophrenia
"Off-Label" Disorders:	Psychosis in Parkinson disease
	Movement disorders due to basal ganglia dysfunction
	Other psychotic symptoms
Dosage:	Typical: 50 to 800 mg at bedtime or divided twice daily with bulk at bedtime
	High range: greater than 900 mg/day if serum levels warrant
	Geriatric: 25 to 100 mg/day
Titration Schedule:	Start 25 to 50 mg at bedtime and titrate 25 to 50 mg/day each 4 to 7 days.
Taper/Switch Schedule:	Over 1 to 2 weeks while initiating other therapy except carbamazepine
Laboratory Monitoring:	CBC every 1 to 2 weeks. Serum level for nonresponse despite high doses.
Side Effects:	CNS: somnolence (++), **seizures (+)**
	CV: tachycardia (+++)
	EENT: blurred vision (+), sialorrhea (++), dry mouth (++)
	GI: constipation (++)
	GU: abnormal ejaculation (++), urinary retention (++)
	HEME: **agranulocytosis (+),** neutropenia (++)
	Skin: photosensitivity (+)
	METAB: **weight gain of greater than 50 pounds possible (+++), diabetes type II (++),** hypertriglyceridemia
Overdose Toxicity:	Hypotension, stupor, neutropenia
Pregnancy and Lactation:	Category B: may be excreted in breast milk
Contraindications:	• Narrow-angle glaucoma
	• Myeloproliferative disorders
	• Neutropenia

- Epilepsy
- History of drug-induced agranulocytosis or severe granulocytopenia
- Cotreatment with carbamazepine or other drugs with myelosuppressive potential
- Uncontrolled diabetes
- Morbid obesity
- Severe hyperlipidemia

Common Drug Interactions: Erythromycin/clarithromycin: increases clozapine levels

Fluvoxamine: increases clozapine levels

Phenytoin: decreases clozapine levels

Valproate: decreases clozapine levels

Hints & Tips:

- Agranulocytosis is not dose-related and typically occurs within the first 3 to 6 months. Rapid decreases in neutrophil counts (>20% in 1 week) are particularly cause for concern.
- Neutropenia to 50% of baseline values is dose-related, not uncommon, and not associated with agranulocytosis.
- Efficacy extends to those unresponsive to standard antipsychotics.
- Because of agranulocytosis, typically reserved for:
  - Refractory psychosis
  - Psychosis with prominent movement disorders
  - Intolerance to other antipsychotics
- Some reports of reduction in preexisting tardive dyskinesia/dystonia.
- Must be given in context of structured treatment program that ensures weekly to biweekly monitoring of blood counts.
- Agranulocytosis notwithstanding, other side effects make use difficult for many.
- Triglyceride levels of greater than 700 mg/dl may cause sludging and microvascular compromise.

Olanzapine

Trade Name: Zyprexa

Chemical Class: Thiobenzodiazepine derivative

Therapeutic/Clinical Class: Atypical antipsychotic

"On-Label" Indications: Schizophrenia

Mania

"Off-Label" Indications: Other psychotic symptoms

Dosage: Typical: 5 to 20 mg at bedtime

High range: 25 to 40 mg at bedtime

Geriatric: 2.5 to 7.5 mg at bedtime

Titration Schedule:	5 mg twice daily and increase in 1 to 2 days as tolerated; convert to consumption at bedtime, dosing at steady state to minimize daytime sedation.
Taper/Switch Schedule:	Over 1 to 2 weeks while initiating other therapy
Laboratory Monitoring:	Weight, fasting blood sugar, triglycerides, cholesterol prior to initiating treatment, at 1 month, and every 6 months thereafter
Side Effects:	CNS: EPS (+), headache (+), dizziness (+), somnolence (+++), **neuroleptic malignant syndrome** (+), tardive dyskinesia (+)
	CV: edema (+), postural hypotension (+), tachycardia (+)
	GI: constipation (+), increased appetite (+++), abdominal pain (+)
	GU: menstrual irregularities (+)
	METAB: **weight gain of over 50 possible (+++), diabetes type II (++)**
Overdose Toxicity:	Stupor
Pregnancy and Lactation:	Category C: breast milk excretion unclear
Contraindications:	• Uncontrolled diabetes
	• Morbid obesity
	• Severe hyperlipidemia
Common Drug Interactions:	Carbamazepine: decreases olanzapine levels
	Cimetidine: increases olanzapine levels
	Fluvoxamine: increases olanzapine levels
Hints & Tips:	• Risk of weight gain, diabetes type II, and hyperlipidemia exceeds that from typical neuroleptics and can be disfiguring (obesity) and cause significant cardiovascular disease.
	• Triglyceride levels of greater than 700 mg/dl may cause sludging and microvascular compromise.
	• A diskette that dissolves on or under the tongue is available.
	• Incidence of tardive dyskinesia and acute EPS are lower than with typical neuroleptics, although risk does exist.

Quetiapine

Trade Name:	Seroquel
Chemical Class:	Dibenzodiazepine derivative
Therapeutic/Clinical Class:	Atypical antipsychotic
"On-Label" Indications:	Schizophrenia
"Off-Label" Indications:	Mania
	Other psychotic symptoms
Dosage:	Typical: 200 to 400 mg/day with bulk of dose at bedtime to minimize daytime sedation
	High range: 600 to 800 mg/day with bulk of dose at bedtime to minimize daytime sedation
	Geriatric: 50 to 100 mg/day

Titration Schedule:	Start 50 to 100 mg twice daily and titrate every 1 to 2 days as indicated
Taper/Switch Schedule:	Over 1 to 2 weeks while initiating other therapy
Laboratory Monitoring:	Weight, fasting blood sugar, triglycerides, cholesterol prior to initiating treatment, at 1 month, and every 6 months thereafter
Side Effects:	CNS: EPS (++), headache (+), dizziness (+), somnolence (++), **neuroleptic malignant syndrome** (+), tardive dyskinesia (+)
	CV: edema (+), postural hypotension (+), tachycardia (+)
	GI: constipation (+), increased appetite (+++), abdominal pain (+)
	GU: menstrual irregularities (+)
	METAB: **weight gain of over 50 pounds possible (+++), diabetes type II (++)**
Overdose Toxicity:	Stupor
Pregnancy and Lactation:	Category C: breast milk excretion unclear
Contraindications:	• Uncontrolled diabetes
	• Morbid obesity
	• Severe hyperlipidemia
Common Drug Interactions:	Carbamazepine: decreases quetiapine levels
	Cimetidine: increases quetiapine levels
Hints & Tips:	• Risk of weight gain, diabetes type II, and hyperlipidemia exceeds that from typical neuroleptics and can be disfiguring (obesity) and cause significant cardiovascular disease.
	• Triglyceride levels of greater than 700 mg/dl may cause sludging and microvascular compromise.
	• Incidence of tardive dyskinesia and acute EPS are lower than with typical neuroleptics, although risk does exist.

Risperidone

Trade Name:	Risperdal
Chemical Class:	Benzisoxazole derivative
Therapeutic/Clinical Class:	Antipsychotic
"On-Label" Indications:	Schizophrenia
"Off-Label" Indications:	Mania
	Other psychotic symptoms
Dosage:	Typical: 2 to 8 mg twice daily. Can be converted to single daily dose at steady state.
	High range: 8 to 10 mg twice daily. Can be converted to single daily dose at steady state.
	Geriatric: 0.25 to 1 mg once or twice daily
Titration Schedule:	Start 2 mg twice daily and increase every 1 to 2 days as indicated.

Taper/Switch Schedule:	Over 1 to 2 weeks while initiating other therapy except MAOIs
Laboratory Monitoring:	N/A
Side Effects:	CNS: drowsiness (+), **neuroleptic malignant syndrome** (+), EPS (++)
	CV: hypotension (+), tachycardia (+)
	EENT: blurred vision (+), dry eyes (+), dry mouth (+)
	GI: constipation (+), increased appetite (++)
	GU: urinary retention (+), menstrual irregularities (++), gynecomastia (+), lactation (+)
	HEME: leukopenia (+)
	METAB: weight gain (+)
Overdose Toxicity:	Stupor, EPS
Pregnancy and Lactation:	Category C: excreted in breast milk
Contraindications:	N/A
Common Drug Interactions:	Barbiturates: decrease risperidone levels
	Beta-blockers: increase risperidone levels and increase beta-blocker levels
	Carbamazepine: decreases risperidone levels
	Fluvoxamine: increases level of risperidone and increases level of fluvoxamine
	Lithium: rare reports of delirium with high- and low-potency neuroleptics
	Opiates: hypotension
Hints & Tips:	• With ziprasidone, least likely among atypical neuroleptics to cause weight gain, and does not have prominent QTc prolongation effects.
	• At higher doses (≥12 mg) behaves more like a typical neuroleptic, similar to haloperidol, in terms of extrapyramidal effects.

Ziprasidone

Trade Name:	Geodon
Chemical Class:	Dibenzodiazepine derivative
Therapeutic/Clinical Class:	Atypical antipsychotic
"On-Label" Indications:	Schizophrenia
"Off-Label" Indications:	Mania
	Other psychotic symptoms
Dosage:	Typical: 20–100 mg twice daily
	High range: N/A
	Geriatric: 10 to 20 mg twice daily
Titration Schedule:	20 mg twice daily and increase every 1 to 2 days as indicated
Taper/Switch Schedule:	Over 1 to 2 weeks while initiating other therapy
Laboratory Monitoring:	EKG at baseline, at 1 week, and at steady state to ensures QTc interval of less than 500 msec.
Side Effects:	CNS: drowsiness (+), **neuroleptic malignant syndrome** (+), EPS

CV: hypotension (+), tachycardia (+), **QT prolongation** (++)

GI: constipation (+), increased appetite (++)

GU: urinary retention (+)

HEME: leukopenia (+)

Overdose Toxicity:	**Arrhythmias**
Pregnancy and Lactation:	Category C: breast milk excretion unclear
Contraindications:	• Cardiac dysrhythmia
	• QTc interval of ≥ 500 msec
Common Drug Interactions:	Carbamazepine: decreases ziprasidone levels
	Diuretics: reduce potassium and increase arrhythmia risk
Hints & Tips:	• One of few neuroleptics, along with molindone, that does not cause weight gain.
	• Among atypical neuroleptics, along with risperidone, is least sedating and least likely to cause weight gain.
	• QT interval prolongation can lead to torsade de pointes, arrhythmia, and sudden death.
	• Beware of use with other drugs that prolong QT interval, e.g.:

- Anti-arrhythmics (class IA, III)
- Antihistamines (nonsedating)
- Neuroleptics (especially mesoridazine, thioridazine)
- Tricyclic antidepressants

BENZODIAZEPINES

Introductory Notes

- Agents are equally efficacious and should be chosen based on onset of action and half-life desired.
- Alprazolam may differ somewhat from others in having antidepressant effects.
- Benzodiazepines used as hypnotics have been studied only in short-term (about 2 week) trials.

Alprazolam

Trade Name:	Xanax
Chemical Class:	Benzodiazepine
Therapeutic/Clinical Class:	Anxiolytic
"On-Label" Indications:	Generalized anxiety disorder
	Panic disorder
"Off-Label" Indications:	Phobias
	Insomnia
	Major depressive disorder

Dosage:	Typical: 0.5 to 1 mg two to three times daily
	High range: 6 to 8 mg/day
	Geriatric: 0.25 to 0.5 mg two to three times daily
Titration Schedule:	Begin at typical dose and adjust over 2 weeks
Taper/Switch Schedule:	Over 1 to 2 weeks while initiating other therapy
Laboratory Monitoring:	N/A
Side Effects:	CNS: dizziness (+), confusion (+), sedation (+), ataxia and **falls (+), dependence (++)**
	CV: hypotension (+)
	EENT: blurred vision (+)
	GI: constipation (+), diarrhea (+)
	GU: erectile dysfunction (+)
Overdose Toxicity:	Stupor, **especially with alcohol or other sedatives**
Pregnancy and Lactation:	Category D: excreted into breast milk
Contraindications:	• Cirrhosis
	• Cholestasis
	• Active substance use disorders
Common Drug Interactions:	Beta-blockers: increase alprazolam levels
	Carbamazepine: decreases alprazolam levels
	Cimetidine: increases alprazolam levels
	Erythromycin/clarithromycin: increases alprazolam levels
	Fluoxetine: increases alprazolam levels
	Fluvoxamine: increases alprazolam levels
	Ketoconazole: increases alprazolam levels
	Nefazodone: increases alprazolam levels
	Omeprazole: increases alprazolam levels
	Paroxetine: increases alprazolam levels
	Phenytoin: decreases alprazolam levels
Hints & Tips:	• Pharmacokinetic profile (hours):
	• Time to peak level: 1 to 2
	• Half-life: 11 to 15
	• Unique among benzodiazepines, has demonstrated antidepressant effects at 1 to 2 mg three times daily.
	• Also unique among benzodiazepines, has been reported to induce irritability in individuals with manic-depressive disorder.
	• Use caution with elderly (hip fractures, confusion) or those with history of drug abuse.

Chlordiazepoxide

Trade Name:	Librium
Chemical Class:	Benzodiazepine
Therapeutic/Clinical Class:	Anxiolytic
"On-Label" Indications:	Generalized anxiety disorder
"Off-Label" Indications:	Panic disorder
	Alcohol detoxification
	Phobias

Dosage:	Typical: 10 to 25 mg twice daily
	High range: 50 to 75 mg two to three times daily
	Geriatric: 5 to 10 mg twice daily
Titration Schedule:	Begin at typical dose and adjust over 2 weeks
Taper/Switch Schedule:	Over 1 to 2 weeks while initiating other therapy
Laboratory Monitoring:	N/A
Side Effects:	CNS: dizziness (+), confusion (+), sedation (+), ataxia and **falls (+), dependence (++)**
	CV: hypotension (+)
	EENT: blurred vision (+)
	GI: constipation (+), diarrhea (+)
	GU: erectile dysfunction (+)
Overdose Toxicity:	See alprazolam
Pregnancy and Lactation:	Category D, excreted into breast milk
Contraindications:	• Cirrhosis
	• Cholestasis
	• Active substance use disorders
Common Drug Interactions:	Beta-blockers: increase chlordiazepoxide levels
	Carbamazepine: decreases chlordiazepoxide levels
	Cimetidine: increases chlordiazepoxide levels
	Erythromycin/clarithromycin: increases chlordiazepoxide levels
	Fluoxetine: increases chlordiazepoxide levels
	Fluvoxamine: increases chlordiazepoxide levels
	Ketoconazole: increases chlordiazepoxide levels
	Omeprazole: increases chlordiazepoxide levels
	Paroxetine: increases chlordiazepoxide levels
	Phenytoin: decreases chlordiazepoxide levels
Hints & Tips:	• Pharmacokinetic profile (hours):
	• Time to peak level: 1 to 4
	• Half-life: 24 to 96 (with active metabolites)
	• Injectable form poorly absorbed.
	• Use caution with elderly (hip fractures, confusion) or those with history of drug abuse.
	• See Introduction for note on dosing in renal compromise.
	• Because of long half-life, standard for uncomplicated alcohol detoxification (see **Appendix 2**)

Clonazepam

Trade Name:	Klonopin
Chemical Class:	Benzodiazepine
Therapeutic/Clinical Class:	Anxiolytic, anticonvulsant
"On-Label" Indications:	Panic disorder
"Off-Label" Indications:	Generalized anxiety disorder
	Phobias
	Restless legs syndrome
	Seizures
Dosage:	Typical: 0.5 to 1.5 mg twice daily

319

	High range: 2 mg two to three times daily
	Geriatric: 0.25 to 0.5 mg twice daily
Titration Schedule:	Begin at typical dose and adjust over 2 weeks.
Taper/Switch Schedule:	Over 1 to 2 weeks while initiating other therapy
Laboratory Monitoring:	N/A
Side Effects:	CNS: dizziness (+), confusion (+), sedation (+), ataxia and **falls (+), dependence (+ +)**

CV: hypotension (+)
EENT: blurred vision (+)
GI: constipation (+), diarrhea (+)
GU: erectile dysfunction (+)

Overdose Toxicity:	See alprazolam
Pregnancy and Lactation:	Category D: excreted into breast milk
Contraindications:	• Cirrhosis
	• Cholestasis
	• Active substance use disorders
Common Drug Interactions:	Fluoxetine: increases clonazepam levels
	Fluvoxamine: increases clonazepam levels
Hints & Tips:	• Pharmacokinetic profile (hours):

  • Time to peak level: 1 to 2
  • Half-life: 18 to 48
• Restless legs dosing 1 to 2 mg at bedtime
• Use caution with elderly (hip fractures, confusion) or those with history of drug abuse.

Diazepam

Common Trade Name:	Valium
Chemical Class:	Benzodiazepine
Therapeutic/Clinical Class:	Anxiolytic, anticonvulsant
"On-Label" Indications:	Generalized anxiety disorder
	Insomnia
"Off-Label" Indications:	Alcohol withdrawal
	Epilepsy
	Panic disorder
	Delirium tremens
Dosage:	Typical: 2 to 5 mg twice daily
	High range: 10 to 15 mg two to three times daily
	Geriatric: 2 mg twice daily
	Intravenous form: 2 to 5 mg/dose
Titration Schedule:	Begin at typical dose and adjust over 2 weeks.
Taper/Switch Schedule:	Over 1 to 2 weeks while initiating other therapy
Laboratory Monitoring:	N/A
Side Effects:	CNS: dizziness (+), confusion (+), sedation (+), ataxia and **falls (+), dependence (+ +)**

CV: hypotension (+)
EENT: blurred vision (+)
GI: constipation (+), diarrhea (+)
GU: erectile dysfunction (+)

Overdose Toxicity:	See alprazolam
Pregnancy and Lactation:	Category D: excreted into breast milk
Contraindications:	• Cirrhosis
	• Cholestasis
	• Active substance use disorders
Common Drug Interactions:	Beta-blockers: increase diazepam levels
	Carbamazepine: decreases diazepam levels
	Cimetidine: increases diazepam levels
	Erythromycin/clarithromycin: increases diazepam levels
	Fluoxetine: increases diazepam levels
	Fluvoxamine: increases diazepam levels
	Ketoconazole: increases diazepam levels
	Nefazodone: increases diazepam levels
	Omeprazole: increases diazepam levels
	Paroxetine: increases diazepam levels
	Phenytoin: decreases diazepam levels
Hints & Tips:	• Pharmacokinetic profile (hours):
	• Time to peak level: 0.5 to 2
	• Half-life: 18 to 96 (with active metabolites)
	• Parenteral form available for intravenous use, but not well absorbed if given intramuscularly.
	• Use caution with elderly (hip fractures, confusion) or those with history of drug abuse.

Lorazepam

Trade Name:	Ativan
Chemical Class:	Benzodiazepine
Therapeutic/Clinical Class:	Anxiolytic, anticonvulsant
"On-Label" Indications:	Generalized anxiety disorder
"Off-Label" Indications:	Insomnia
Dosage:	Typical: 0.5 to 1.5 mg twice daily
	High range: 2 mg two to three times daily
	Geriatric: 0.25 to 0.5 mg twice daily
	Intramuscular form: 0.5 to 1.0 mg/dose
Titration Schedule:	Begin at typical dose and adjust over 2 weeks
Taper/Switch Schedule:	Over 1 to 2 weeks while initiating other therapy
Laboratory Monitoring:	N/A
Side Effects:	CNS: dizziness (+), confusion (+), sedation (+), ataxia and **falls (+)**, **dependence (++)**
	CV: hypotension (+)
	EENT: blurred vision (+)
	GI: constipation (+), diarrhea (+)
	GU: erectile dysfunction (+)
Overdose Toxicity:	See alprazolam
Pregnancy and Lactation:	Category D: excreted into breast milk
Contraindications:	• Active substance use disorders
Common Drug Interactions:	N/A

Hints & Tips:
- Pharmacokinetic profile (hours):
  - Time to peak level: 1 to 6
  - Half-life: 10 to 20
- Best intramuscular absorption among benzodiazepines.
- No active hepatic metabolites, so may be used if cirrhosis or other cholestasis
- Use for alcohol detoxification if cirrhosis or cholestasis (see **Appendix 2**).
- Use caution with elderly (hip fractures, confusion) or those with history of drug abuse.

Oxazepam

Trade Name:	Serax
Chemical Class:	Benzodiazepine
Therapeutic/Clinical Class:	Anxiolytic
"On-Label" Indications:	Generalized anxiety disorder
"Off-Label" Indications:	Alcohol detoxification
Dosage:	Typical: 10 to 15 mg three times daily
	High range: to 20 mg three to four times daily
	Geriatric: 10 mg two to three times daily
Titration Schedule:	Begin at typical dose and adjust over 2 weeks
Taper/Switch Schedule:	Over 1 to 2 weeks while initiating other therapy
Laboratory Monitoring:	N/A
Side Effects:	CNS: dizziness (+), confusion (+), sedation (+), ataxia and **falls (+), dependence (++)**
	CV: hypotension (+)
	EENT: blurred vision (+)
	GI: constipation (+), diarrhea (+)
	GU: erectile dysfunction (+)
Overdose Toxicity:	See alprazolam
Pregnancy and Lactation:	Category D: excreted into breast milk
Contraindications:	• Cirrhosis
	• Cholestasis
	• Active substance use disorders
Common Drug Interactions:	N/A

Hints & Tips:
- Pharmacokinetic profile (hours):
  - Time to peak level: 2 to 4
  - Half-life: 4 to 18
- No active hepatic metabolite, so may be used if cirrhosis or other cholestasis.
- Longest onset of action, so is devoid of "buzz" that may accompany other benzodiazepines. Therefore, benzodiazepine of choice if one must be used in an individual at risk for substance use disorder.
- Use caution with elderly (hip fractures, confusion) or those with history of drug abuse.

Temazepam

Trade Name:	Restoril
Chemical Class:	Benzodiazepine
Therapeutic/Clinical Class:	Hypnotic
"On-Label" Indications:	Insomnia
"Off-Label" Indications:	N/A
Dosage:	Typical: 15 mg at bedtime
	High range: 30 to 45 mg at bedtime
	Geriatric: 15 mg at bedtime
Titration Schedule:	Begin at typical dose and adjust over 2 weeks
Taper/Switch Schedule:	If chronic, daily treatment: over 1 to 2 weeks while initiating nonbenzodiazepine therapy
Laboratory Monitoring:	N/A
Side Effects:	CNS: dizziness (+), confusion (+), sedation (+), ataxia and **falls (+), dependence (++)**
	CV: hypotension (+)
	EENT: blurred vision (+)
	GI: constipation (+), diarrhea (+)
	GU: erectile dysfunction (+)
Overdose Toxicity:	See alprazolam
Pregnancy and Lactation:	Category D: excreted into breast milk
Contraindications:	• Cirrhosis
	• Cholestasis
	• Active substance use disorders
Common Drug Interactions:	Cimetidine: increases temazepan levels
	Disulfiram: increases temazepan levels
Hints & Tips:	• Pharmacokinetic profile (hours):
	• Time to peak level: 1 to 2
	• Half-life: 8 to 18
	• Use caution with elderly (hip fractures, confusion) or those with history of drug abuse.
	• Typically used only as a hypnotic.
	• Tolerance may develop if given nightly; recommend maximum 3 to 4 times per week.

Triazolam

Trade Name:	Halcion
Chemical Class:	Benzodiazepine
Therapeutic/Clinical Class:	Hypnotic
"On-Label" Indications:	Insomnia
"Off-Label" Indications:	N/A
Dosage:	Typical: 0.25 to 0.50 mg at bedtime
	High range: 0.75 to 1.0 mg at bedtime
	Geriatric: 0.125 to 0.25 mg at bedtime
Titration Schedule:	Begin at typical dose and adjust over 2 weeks.
Taper/Switch Schedule:	If chronic, daily treatment: over 1 to 2 weeks while initiating nonbenzodiazepine therapy
Laboratory Monitoring:	N/A
Side Effects:	CNS: dizziness (+), confusion (+), sedation (+), ataxia and **falls (+), dependence (++)**
	CV: hypotension (+)

	EENT: blurred vision (+)
	GI: constipation (+), diarrhea (+)
	GU: erectile dysfunction (+)
Overdose Toxicity:	See alprazolam
Pregnancy and Lactation:	Category D: excreted into breast milk
Contraindications:	• Cirrhosis
	• Cholestasis
	• Active substance use disorders
Common Drug Interactions:	Beta-blockers: increase triazolam levels
	Carbamazepine: decreases triazolam levels
	Cimetidine: increases triazolam levels
	Erythromycin/clarithromycin: increases triazolam levels
	Fluoxetine: increases triazolam levels
	Fluvoxamine: increases triazolam levels
	Ketoconazole: increases triazolam levels
	Omeprazole: increases triazolam levels
	Nefazodone: increases triazolam levels
	Paroxetine: increases triazolam levels
	Phenytoin: decreases triazolam levels
Hints & Tips:	• Pharmacokinetic profile (hours):
	• Time to peak level: 0.5 to 1
	• Half-life: 2 to 6
	• Typically used only as a hypnotic.
	• Tolerance may develop if given nightly; recommend maximum 3 to 4 times per week.
	• Perhaps because of very short half-life, has been used for phase-shifting during jet lag, but also has been associated with confusional episodes during sleep periods.
	• Use caution with elderly (hip fractures, confusion) or those with history of drug abuse.

NONBENZODIAZEPINE HYPNOTICS

Introductory Notes

- Agents appear equally efficacious.
- Like benzodiazepines, they are GABAergic, and have abuse potential and tolerance to hypnotic effects.
- Efficacy trials are all short-term (about 2 weeks).

Zaleplon

Trade Name:	Sonata
Chemical Class:	Pyrazolopyrimidine
Therapeutic/Clinical Class:	Nonbenzodiazepine hypnotic

"On-Label" Indications:	Insomnia, short-term treatment
"Off-Label" Indications:	N/A
Dosage:	Typical: 5 to 10 mg at bedtime
	High range: N/A
	Geriatric: 5 mg at bedtime
Titration Schedule:	Begin at 5 or 10 mg/day night
Taper/Switch Schedule:	If chronic, daily treatment: over 1 to 2 weeks while initiating non-GABAergic therapy
Laboratory Monitoring:	N/A
Side Effects:	CNS: **dependence/abuse** (+), paresthesias (+), rebound insomnia (++), **ataxia** (+), hangover (+)
	GU: Incontinence (+)
	MS: muscle pain (+)
Overdose Toxicity:	See alprazolam
Pregnancy and Lactation:	Category C
Contraindications:	• Active substance use disorders
	• End-stage lung disease
	• Cirrhosis
Common Drug Interactions:	Carbamazepine: decreases zaleplon levels
	Cimetidine: increases zaleplon levels
Hints & Tips:	• Abuse potential as for benzodiazepines
	• Less anxiolytic effect than benzodiazepines
	• Tolerance may develop if given nightly; recommended dosing 3 to 4 times per week

Zolpidem

Trade Name:	Ambien
Chemical Class:	Imidazopyridine derivative
Therapeutic/Clinical Class:	Nonbenzodiazepine hypnotic
"On-Label" Indications:	Insomnia, short-term treatment
"Off-Label" Indications:	N/A
Dosage:	Typical: 5 to 10 mg at bedtime
	High range: N/A
	Geriatric: 5 mg at bedtime
Titration Schedule:	Begin at 5 to 10 mg/night
Taper/Switch Schedule:	If chronic, daily treatment: over 1 to 2 weeks while initiating non-GABAergic therapy
Laboratory Monitoring:	N/A
Side Effects:	CNS: dependence/abuse (+) headache (+), drowsiness (+) **ataxia** (+), hangover (+)
	CV: palpitations (+)
	GU: incontinence (+)
Overdose Toxicity:	See alprazolam
Pregnancy and Lactation:	Category B: excreted into breast milk in small amounts
Contraindications:	• Active substance use disorders
	• End-stage lung disease
	• Cirrhosis

Common Drug Interactions:	Carbamazepine: decreases zolpidem levels
Hints & Tips:	• Abuse potential as for benzodiazepines.
	• Less anxiolytic effect than benzodiazepines.
	• Tolerance may develop if given nightly; recommended dosing is 3 to 4 times per week.

OTHER AGENTS USED IN ANXIETY DISORDERS

Introductory Notes

- This heterogeneous group includes several agents with established or putative effects in various anxiety disorders and perhaps some others:
  - Buspirone: FDA approved for generalized anxiety disorder
  - Clonidine: FDA-approved antihypertensive with:
    - Some utility for hyperautonomic symptoms of PTSD
    - Symptomatic relief in opiate detoxification
  - Gabapentin: Safe medication FDA-approved anticonvulsant used widely for many off-label indications *without* a great deal of efficacy data:
    - Anxiety symptoms
    - Mood stabilization in manic-depressive disorder
    - Neuropathic pain
  - Prazosin: FDA-approved antihypertensive with some utility for sleep symptoms of PTSD

Buspirone

Common Trade Name:	BuSpar
Chemical Class:	Azaspirodecanedione
Therapeutic/Clinical Class:	Anxiolytic
"On-Label" Indications:	Generalized anxiety disorder
"Off-Label" Indications:	PTSD
	Some reports of efficacy for tardive dyskinesia in very high doses (120–180 mg/day)
Dosage:	Typical: 15 mg twice daily
	High range: 30 to 45 mg twice daily
	Geriatric: 5 to 10 mg twice daily
Titration Schedule:	Start at 10 to 15 mg twice daily. Increase to 30 mg b.i.d. if no response at 2 to 3 weeks.
Taper/Switch Schedule:	Reduce by 25% every 2 to 7 days
Laboratory Monitoring:	N/A
Side Effects:	CNS: dizziness (+), fatigue (+), tremor (+), agitation (+)
	CV: palpitations (+), tachycardia (+), hypertension (+)
	GI: constipation (+), diarrhea (+), nausea (+)
	GU: hesitancy (+), frequency (+)

Overdose Toxicity:	Stupor
Pregnancy and Lactation:	Category B: use caution in nursing mothers.
Contraindications:	N/A
Common Drug Interactions:	Carbamazepine: decreases buspirone levels
	Cimetidine: increases buspirone levels
	Nefazodone: increases buspirone levels
	Phenytoin: decreases buspirone levels
Hints & Tips:	• See Introduction note for use in renal compromise.
	• Nonaddictive anxiolytic.
	• Requires 2 to 6 weeks for full therapeutic effect.
	• Commonly used for cognitive symptoms in PTSD.

Clonidine

Trade Name:	Catapres
Chemical Class:	α_2 agonist
Therapeutic/Clinical Class:	Antihypertensive
"On-Label" Indications:	Hypertension
"Off-Label" Indications:	PTSD
	Opiate detoxification
Dosage:	Typical: 0.1 mg twice daily to 0.1 mg four times daily (opiate detoxification)
	0.1 mg twice daily to 0.3 mg three times daily (PTSD)
	High dose: maximum dose approximately 2.4 mg/day
	Geriatric: N/A
Titration Schedule:	Start 0.05 to 0.1 mg twice daily following blood pressure. Can be increased each day by 0.1 to 0.3 mg/day. Initial dose can result in paradoxic hypertension.
Taper/Switch Schedule:	25% every 4 days, watching for rebound hypertension
Laboratory Monitoring:	Blood pressure prior to starting and as indicated during titration.
Side Effects:	CNS: **dizziness** (+++), sedation (+), headache (++)
	CV: **hypotension** (+++), bradycardia (+), tachycardia (++), rebound hypertension (+)
	GI: constipation (++), liver transaminase elevations (+)
	MS: cramps (+)
Overdose Toxicity:	**Hypotension**
Pregnancy and Lactation:	Category C: secreted into breast milk
Contraindications:	• Hypotension, bradycardia, recent myocardial infarction
Common Drug Interactions:	Beta-blockers: when clonidine is discontinued may result in rebound hypertension

327

Insulin: blocks peripheral hypoglycemic
symptoms

Hints & Tips:
- PTSD applications not well supported by controlled trial data, but may have damping effect on hypervigilance and autonomic hyperarousal.
- Frequently used for symptomatic relief (jitteriness, autonomic symptoms) during opiate withdrawal (see **Appendix 4**).
- In case of sedative side effects, may be given primarily at bedtime

Gabapentin

Trade Name:	Neurontin
Chemical Class:	Cyclohexanacetic acid derivative
Therapeutic/Clinical Class:	Anticonvulsant
"On-Label" Indications:	Seizures
"Off-Label" Indications:	Anxiety
	Neuropathic pain
	Possible adjuvant mood stabilizer in manic-depressive disorder
Dosage:	Typical: 300 to 600 mg three times daily
	High range: Up to 900 mg five times daily
	Geriatric: 100 to 300 mg three times daily
Titration Schedule:	Begin 100 to 300 mg three times daily and increase by 300 to 600 mg/day every 2 to 3 days.
Taper/Switch Schedule:	Reduce by 25% every 2 to 7 days
Laboratory Monitoring:	N/A
Side Effects:	CNS: dizziness (+), somnolence (++), ataxia (+)
	CV: hypotension (+)
	EENT: diplopia (+)
	GI: dry mouth (+)
	GU: impotence (+)
	MS: myalgia (+), twitching (+)
	Skin: flushing (+)
Overdose Toxicity:	Sedation (saturable active transport from gut minimizes overdose toxicity)
Pregnancy and Lactation:	Category C
Contraindications:	N/A
Common Drug Interactions:	Antacids: decrease gabapentin levels

Hints & Tips:
- See Introduction note on use in renal compromise.
- Intestinal absorption is via active amino acid transport.
- Transport is saturable: give no more than 900 mg/dose.
- Though safe and well tolerated, efficacy for psychiatric conditions is questionable. One controlled trial showed worse than placebo in mania, but uncontrolled data suggest adjuvant role for some.

Prazosin

Trade Name:	Minipress
Chemical Class:	α_1 antagonist
Therapeutic/Clinical Class:	Antihypertensive
"On-Label" Indications:	Hypertension
"Off-Label" Indications:	PTSD (especially sleep disturbances, nightmares)
Dosage:	Typical: 2 to 10 mg at bedtime
	High dose: maximum dose 5 mg in the early evening and 10 mg at bedtime
	Geriatric: 1 to 2 mg at bedtime
Titration Schedule:	Start 1 mg at bedtime for 1 to 2 days following blood pressure. Increase by 1 to 2 mg every 4 to 5 days. Initial dose can result in marked hypotension.
Taper/Switch Schedule:	25% every 4 days
Laboratory Monitoring:	Blood pressure prior to starting and as indicated during titration.
Side Effects:	CNS: **dizziness** (+++), sedation (++), headache (++)
	EENT: blurred vision (+), tinnitus (+)
	CV: **hypotension** (+++), tachycardia (++)
	GI: diarrhea (++), constipation (++)
	MS: cramps (+)
Overdose Toxicity:	**Hypotension**
Pregnancy and Lactation:	Category C: breast milk secretion unclear
Contraindications:	• Hypotension, bradycardia, recent myocardial infarction
Common Drug Interactions:	NSAIDs: inhibit antihypertensive response to prazosin
	Verapamil: increases prazosin levels
Hints & Tips:	• PTSD applications not well supported by controlled trial data, but appears to have beneficial effects on sleep disruption and nightmares possibly by normalizing REM and stage 1, stage 2 sleep.

COGNITIVE ENHANCERS

Introductory Notes

- Agents are fairly equivalent in effects but differ in side effect profile.
- FDA-approved for Alzheimer-type dementia but not vascular dementia.
- However, in the real world of clinical work, dementia is often mixed and, absent contraindications, the clinician would not be faulted in erring on the side of treatment.

Donepezil

Trade Name:	Aricept
Chemical Class:	Acetylcholinesterase inhibitors
Therapeutic/Clinical Class:	Cognitive enhancer
"On-Label" Indications:	Mild to moderate dementia of the Alzheimer type
"Off-Label" Indications:	N/A
Dosage:	Typical: N/A
	High range: N/A
	Geriatric: 5 to 10 mg daily
Titration Schedule:	5 mg orally daily; increase to 10 mg at bedtime after 4 to 6 weeks if no response
Taper/Switch Schedule:	25% per week for taper or while adding other cognitive enhancer at same rate
Laboratory Monitoring:	N/A
Side Effects:	CNS: abnormal dreams (+), dizziness (+), fatigue (+), headache (+), insomnia (+), somnolence (+)
	CV: **bradycardia** (++)
	GI: anorexia (++), diarrhea (+)
	GU: frequent urination (+)
	HEME: bruising (+)
	MS: cramps (+)
Overdose Toxicity:	**Hypotension, bradycardia,** stupor
Pregnancy and Lactation:	Category C: excretion in breast milk unknown
Contraindications:	N/A
Common Drug Interactions:	Fluvoxamine: increases fluvoxamine levels
Hints & Tips:	• Better effects at 10 mg/day

Galantamine

Trade Name:	Reminyl
Chemical Class:	Acetylcholinesterase inhibitors
Therapeutic/Clinical Class:	Cognitive enhancer
"On-Label" Indications:	Mild to moderate dementia of the Alzheimer type
"Off-Label" Indications:	N/A
Dosage:	Typical: N/A
	High range: N/A
	Geriatric: 8 to 12 mg twice daily
Titration Schedule:	4 mg twice daily and increase by 4 mg every 4 weeks
Taper/Switch Schedule:	25% per week for taper or while adding other cognitive enhancer at same rate
Laboratory Monitoring:	N/A
Side Effects:	CNS: headache (+), drowsiness (+), tremor (+), dizziness (+)
	CV: **bradycardia** (++)
	GI: anorexia and weight loss (+), nausea (++), vomiting (+)

Overdose Toxicity:	**Hypotension, bradycardia,** stupor
Pregnancy and Lactation:	Category B: excretion into breast milk unknown
Contraindications:	N/A
Common Drug Interactions:	Amitriptyline: increases galantamine levels
	Cimetidine: increases galantamine levels
	Fluoxetine: increases galantamine levels
	Ketoconazole: increases galantamine levels
	Paroxetine: increases galantamine levels
	Quinidine: increases galantamine levels
Hints & Tips:	• Available in liquid form.
	• Slows progression and may lead to minor improvement.
	• Take twice daily with meals.

Rivastigmine

Trade Name:	Exelon
Chemical Class:	Acetylcholinesterase inhibitors
Therapeutic/Clinical Class:	Cognitive enhancer
"On-Label" Indications:	Mild to moderate dementia of the Alzheimer type
"Off-Label" Indications:	N/A
Dosage:	Typical: N/A
	High range: N/A
	Geriatric: 1.5 to 6 mg twice daily
Titration Schedule:	1.5 mg twice daily and increase by 1.5 mg every 4 weeks
Taper/Switch Schedule:	25% per week for taper or while adding other cognitive enhancer at same rate
Laboratory Monitoring:	N/A
Side Effects:	CNS: headache (+), drowsiness (+), weakness (+), tremor (+)
	CV: **bradycardia** (++)
	EENT: tinnitus (+)
	GI: anorexia and weight loss (+), diarrhea (+), nausea (++), vomiting (+)
Overdose Toxicity:	**Hypotension, bradycardia,** stupor
Pregnancy and Lactation:	Category B: excretion into breast milk is unknown
Contraindications:	N/A
Common Drug Interactions:	N/A
Hints & Tips:	• Available in liquid form.
	• Slows progression and may lead to minor improvements.
	• Unclear whether advantage over older cognitive enhancers.
	• Take twice daily with meals.

Tacrine

Trade Name:	Cognex
Chemical Class:	Acetylcholinesterase inhibitors

Therapeutic/Clinical Class:	Cognitive enhancer
"On-Label" Indications:	Mild to moderate dementia of the Alzheimer type
"Off-Label" Indications:	N/A
Dosage:	Typical: N/A
	High range: N/A
	Geriatric: 30 to 40 mg four times daily
Titration Schedule:	10 mg orally four times daily for 4 weeks, then 20 mg four times daily for 4 weeks; increase at 4-week intervals
Taper/Switch Schedule:	25% per week for taper or while adding other cognitive enhancer at same rate
Laboratory Monitoring:	N/A
Side Effects:	CNS: agitation (+), ataxia (+), depression (+), dizziness (+)
	CV: **bradycardia** (++), hypertension (+)
	GI: **hepatotoxicity** (+), anorexia (+), diarrhea (+), vomiting (+)
	GU: frequency (+), incontinence (+)
Overdose Toxicity:	**Hypotension, bradycardia,** stupor
Pregnancy and Lactation:	Category C: excretion into breast milk unknown
Contraindications:	• Liver disease
Common Drug Interactions:	Cimetidine: increases tacrine levels
	Theophylline: increases theophylline levels
Hints & Tips:	• Because of hepatotoxicity and GI side effects, try other cognitive enhancers first.

STIMULANTS

Introductory Notes:

- Methylphenidate tends to be first-line treatment, with amphetamine combinations (e.g., Adderall) and pemoline second-line. For amphetamine dosing, see Attention Deficit Disorders in **Section III.**
- Stimulants are occasionally used for major depressive episodes refractory to other medications, although nowadays there are now so many antidepressants available that this practice is fading.

Methylphenidate

Common Trade Name:	Ritalin
Chemical Class:	Piperidine derivative of amphetamine
Therapeutic/Clinical Class:	Stimulant
"On-Label" Indications:	Attention deficit disorder with or without hyperactivity
	Narcolepsy

"Off-Label" Indications:	Major depressive disorder
	Bipolar depressive episodes
Dosage:	Typical: 10 to 20 mg two to three times daily dosed in the morning, at noon, and at midafternoon to prevent insomnia
	High range: 60 to 80 mg/day
	Geriatric: N/A
Titration Schedule:	Begin 10 mg twice daily and increase weekly.
Taper/Switch Schedule:	Over 1 to 2 weeks while initiating other therapy except MAOIs
Laboratory Monitoring:	N/A
Side Effects:	CNS: agitation/mania (++), insomnia (++)
	CV: palpitations (+), tachycardia (+) **dysrhythmias** (+)
	GI: anorexia (+), dry mouth (+)
Overdose Toxicity:	Tachycardia, hypertension, agitation, psychosis
Pregnancy and Lactation:	Category C
Contraindications:	• Active substance use disorders
	• Use of MAOIs within 2 weeks
	• Glaucoma
	• Tourette syndrome
Common Drug Interactions:	**MAOIs: hypertensive crisis**
	Phenytoin: increases phenytoin levels
	Tricyclics: increases tricyclic levels
Hints & Tips:	• Extended-release form available, but typically still requires twice daily dosing (morning and noon).
	• For t.i.d. dosing, give no later than midafternoon to prevent insomnia.
	• Tachyphylaxis may occur.
	• First-line treatment for attention deficit disorders.

Pemoline

Common Trade Name:	Cylert
Chemical Class:	Oxazolidine derivative of amphetamine
Therapeutic/Clinical Class:	Stimulant
"On-Label" Indications:	Attention deficit disorder with or without hyperactivity
"Off-Label" Indications:	Narcolepsy
	Major depressive disorder
	Bipolar depressive episodes
Dosage:	Typical: 37.5 mg two to three times daily dosed in the morning, at noon, and at midafternoon to minimize insomnia
	High range: to 150 mg/day
	Geriatric: N/A
Titration Schedule:	37.5 mg in the morning and increased biweekly

Taper/Switch Schedule:	Over 1 to 2 weeks while initiating other therapy except MAOIs
Laboratory Monitoring:	N/A
Side Effects:	CNS: agitation/mania (++), insomnia (++)
	CV: palpitations (+), tachycardia (+) **dysrhythmias** (+)
	GI: anorexia (+), dry mouth (+)
Overdose Toxicity:	Tachycardia, hypertension, agitation, psychosis
Pregnancy and Lactation:	Category C
Contraindications:	• Active substance use disorders
	• Use of MAOIs within 2 weeks
	• Glaucoma
	• Tourette syndrome
Common Drug Interactions:	**MAOIs: hypertensive crisis**
	Phenytoin: increases phenytoin levels
	Tricyclics: increase tricyclic levels
Hints & Tips:	• Second-line treatment for attention deficit disorders after methylphenidate.
	• For t.i.d. dosing, give no later than mid-afternoon to prevent insomnia.
	• Tachyphylaxis may occur.

Therapeutic Devices Used in Psychiatry

ELECTROCONVULSIVE THERAPY

Procedure

Electric current sufficient to produce seizure is passed through frontal lobes by means of surface electrodes placed either over the nondominant hemisphere or bilaterally. Individual receiving ECT is placed under sedation and neuromuscular blockade to prevent physical seizure. Typical course of ECT is 6 to 12 treatments given three times per week as an inpatient or outpatient. Maintenance ECT typically is given once monthly.

Indications

- Major depressive disorder (especially with psychotic features)
- Manic-depressive disorder (depressed, manic, or mixed episode)
- Refractory psychosis
- Catatonia
  Note: Solid and extensive efficacy data exist for depressive episodes. Some studies indicate higher treatment response rates than for antidepressants. First-line treatment of choice for psychotic depressions; anguished, agitated depressions; and depressions with severe suicidality.

Side Effects

- Periprocedural amnesia. Not infrequent that individuals have little recollection of the entire period during which ECT was administered.
- Some complain of memory deficits long term, but these are too subtle to be corroborated by objective testing or disentangled from primary effects of psychiatric disorder. A risk especially in the elderly.
- May cause manic switches, yet also treats mania.

BRIGHT VISIBLE SPECTRUM LIGHT

Procedure

Individuals sit in front of fluorescent tube light box with diffuser at sufficient distance to receive 2,500 to 10,000 lux (a measure of intensity), depending on procedure. They typically read, watch television, or do other quiet activities but remain at the indicated distance from the light box. Duration is 30 to 120 minutes depending on intensity. Timing is typically in the morning for treatment of depression or for phase-delayed sleep cycle. See also **Appendix 7.**

Indications

* Major depressive disorder with seasonal pattern ("winter depression")
* Subsyndromal depressive symptoms with winter occurrence
* Circadian sleep-phase disorders
  Note: Solid and extensive efficacy data exist for pure winter depressions (i.e., with symptoms *only* in the fall-winter and no depression during spring-summer). Has been used with some success, although with fewer data, in depressive syndromes that is not strictly seasonal. Reasonable evidence exists for shifting sleep-wake cycle in circadian sleep-phase disorders.

Side Effects

Although light boxes are available to lay persons from many mail order and other sources and are not FDA-regulated, they do have side effects:
* (Hypo)mania
* Insomnia
* Jitteriness
* Anxiety
* Erythema

RESEARCH INTERVENTIONS

Two devices are under active investigation at the time of this writing. They are available only at select centers and typically under the rubric of experimental treatment protocols:
* **Transcranial magnetic stimulation:** High-intensity magnetic waves applied to surface of skull. Under exploration primarily for treatment of depression.
* **Vagal nerve stimulation:** Electrical stimulation of vagus nerve. Under exploration primarily for treatment of refractory depression.

APPENDIX 1

Cognitive Screening Instruments

MINI-MENTAL STATE EXAMINATION (MMSE)

As we were preparing this Field Guide, we were stunned to be denied permission to provide the Mini-Mental State Exam for your use. Although the MMSE is widely available on templated forms in many hospitals and clinics and is in wide usage in research, the owner of the copyright, Psychological Assessment Resources, has unfortunately chosen to keep this useful tool out of the public domain. Obviously, this is a money-making venture.

The MMSE has been published in a peer-reviewed journal. The reference is: Folstein MF, et al. "Mini-Mental State:" a practical method for grading the cognitive state of patients for the clinician. *J Psychiatr Res* 1975;12:189–198.

If you wish to officially use the MMSE, you may contact PAR at 800-331-8378 or pdrexler@parinc.com. You will pay them for this privilege.

Alternatively, many other well-validated resources exist for cognitive assessment. The clinician will wish to consult the section in **Key References** on "Instruments for Psychiatric Assessment" for alternatives. The VA Measurement Excellence Initiative Web site cited there will provide easy and free access to the information needed to choose alternate and free assessment instruments depending on your needs and resources.

EXECUTIVE FUNCTION SCREENING

(Based on the EXIT Interview from Royall D, Mahurin R, Gray K. Bedside assessment of executive cognitive impairment: the EXIT Interview. *J Am Geriatr Soc* 1992;40:1221–1226, reprinted with permission.)

This selection of items, adapted from Royall's EXIT (which we call the TEXAS, Telephone EXecutive Assessment Scale), has been used by our group to screen for executive cognitive dysfunction (see **Module 8, Panel 11**). In our experience, **a total score of 4 or more** is suspicious for executive deficits sufficient to impact negatively on illness management and warrant further evaluation and perhaps management. (Bauer M, McBride L, Shea N, et al. Screening for executive cognitive dysfunction in bipolar disorder [Abstract]. *Biol Psych* 1994;35:79A).

<u>1. Number-Letter Task</u>

"I'd like you to say some numbers and letters for me like this: 1-A, 2-B, 3-What would come next?" "C."

"Now you try it starting from the number 1. Keep going until I tell you to stop."
1-A, 2-B, 3-C, 4-D, 5-E   [Stop the subject]
Score: 0 = No errors
                   1 = Completes task with prompting or repeat instructions
                   2 = Doesn't complete task

<u>2. Word Fluency</u>

"I am going to give you a letter. You will have 1 minute to name as many words as you can think of that begin with that letter. For example, with the letter 'P' you could say, 'People, pot, plant . . .' and so on. Do you have any questions? Your letter is 'A.' Are you ready? Go."

Score: 0 = 10 or more words
1 = 5 to 9 words
2 = fewer than 5 words

3. Anomalous Sentence Repetition

"Listen very carefully and repeat these sentences exactly."
[Read the following sentences in a neutral tone]
"I pledge allegiance to this flag."
"Mary fed a little lamb."
"A stitch in time saves lives."
"Tinkle, tinkle little star."
"A B C D U F G."
Score: 0 = No errors
1 = Fails to make one or more changes
2 = Continues with one or more expressions automatically (e.g., "Mary had a little lamb whose fleece was white as snow . . .") or disinhibited behavior.

4. Memory/Distraction Task

"Remember these three words: *book, tree, house.*"
[Subject repeats words until all three are registered]
"Remember them—I'll ask you to repeat them for me later. Now spell *cat* for me. Now spell it backward. Now tell me those three words you learned."
Score: 0 = Subject names all three words correctly
1 = Any errors except as below, or unable to remember all
2 = Names "cat" as one of the words (perseveration)

5. Serial Order Reversal Task

Ask subject to recite the months of the year.
"Now start with January and say them all in reverse order."
Score: 0 = No errors at least through September
1 = Requires repeat directions but gets through September
2 = Cannot get through September

APPENDIX 2

Alcohol and Benzodiazepine Detoxification Procedure: The Clinical Institute Withdrawal Assessment (CIWA) Protocol

1. The CIWA Assessment is administered every 6 hours until no benzodiazepine is required for 24 hours, or according to clinician judgment.
2. A nurse, nursing assistant, or similarly trained staff person administers the Assessment.
3. The score on each of the items is summed and translated into a benzodiazepine dose (see below), which is administered to the individual orally.
4. Symptomatic treatment for nausea, vomiting, or diarrhea should also be provided.
5. Detoxification is typically finished in 2 to 4 days.

The CIWA Assessment

1.	Pulse	80 to 90 beats/min	= 1
		over 90 beats/min	= 2
2.	Blood pressure	150/90 to 180/90 mm Hg	= 2
		≥ 180/90 mm Hg	= 3
3.	Nausea/vomiting	Mild nausea with dry heaves	= 1
		Constant nausea with vomiting	= 2
4.	Tremors	Palpable to fingertip only	= 1
		Moderate and visible with extended arms	= 2
		Severe even with arms at side	= 3
5.	Anxiety/agitation	Mildly anxious, increased activity	= 1
		Moderately anxious with psychomotor agitation	= 2
		Severely anxious or near panic	= 3
6.	Confusion	Uncertain about date or whereabouts	= 1
		Disoriented to time, place, surrounding events	= 2
		Completely disoriented to time, place, person	= 3
7.	Perspiration	Barely perceptible with moist palms	= 1
		Drenching sweats	= 2

TOTAL = _____

Total Score	Chlordiazepoxide Dose
0 to 3	None
4 to 5	25 mg
6 to 7	50 mg
8 to 9	75 mg
≥ 10	100 mg (but see notes 3 and 4)

Notes

1. For severe withdrawal, the CIWA Assessment interval can be reduced to every 4 hours or even every 2 hours. There is no danger of overdosing because the physical assessment will drive the amount of benzodiazepine administered.
2. For individuals with cirrhosis or cholestasis due to alcoholic or other acute hepatitis, active metabolites of chlordiazepoxide can accumulate and cause confusion or respiratory suppression. Therefore, with total bilirubin levels

above the normal range, substitute lorazepam, which has no active metabolites. Chlordiazepoxide 25 mg is equivalent to lorazepam 1 mg.

3. Scores of more than 10, or visual or tactile hallucinations, are suspicious for impending delirium tremens ("the DTs"), and DTs must be managed with aggressive parenteral benzodiazepines and hydration. Chlordiazepoxide 25 mg orally is equivalent to diazepam 5 mg or 1 mg lorazepam intravenously. CIWA Assessment can be administered every 1 hour after a loading dose of 20 mg diazepam (4 mg lorazepam) intravenously. Monitor fluid and electrolyte balance carefully and have respiratory support available. Treatment on a medical floor or in an intensive care unit is indicated

4. For established delirium tremens, assume the individual is delirious due to severe deficiency of GABA effect (or whatever alcohol and benzodiazepines provide in this state)—that is, "the tank is empty." Up to 50 to 60 mg/hour intravenous diazepam (10 to 12 mg/hour lorazepam) for several hours may be required to normalize hyper-autonomic signs and mentation, followed by institution of the CIWA every 1 hour using parenteral benzodiazepines. Clearly, respiratory support and fluid and electrolyte monitoring in an intensive care unit is required.

5. The same protocol can be used for benzodiazepine dependence.

Barbiturate Detoxification and the Pentobarbital Challenge Test

PURPOSE

To establish the starting dose for detoxification from barbiturates and related compounds (e.g., glutethimide, meprobamate/carisoprodol).

Note: Benzodiazepines will *not* cover barbiturate withdrawal, but barbiturates will cover benzodiazepine and alcohol withdrawal. Therefore, if the patient is barbiturate dependent, barbiturate detoxification must be used.

PROCEDURES

1. Administer 200 mg pentobarbital orally (secobarbital may be substituted at same dosage).
2. Evaluate at 60 minutes postdose. Clinical status at 60 minutes will determine daily dose of pentobarbital required to prevent withdrawal (see Table).
3. Convert to longer-acting phenobarbital: 100 mg pentobarbital/secobarbital = 30 mg phenobarbital.
4. Administer phenobarbital with total daily dose divided three times daily.
5. Maintain initial dose for 48 hours.
6. Taper at 30 mg phenobarbital/day until discontinued.
7. Dosages are approximate—adjust upward/downward based on history and clinical course.

Clinical Status at 60 min Postdose	Required Daily Pentobarbital Dose	Conversion to Daily Phenobarbital Dose	Phenobarbital t.i.d. Dose (in 30-mg increments)
Asleep	Zero	—	—
Obvious intoxication: slurred speech, ataxia, sedation	400–600 mg/day	120–180 mg/day	30–60 mg
Nystagmus only	600–800 mg/day	180–240 mg/day	60–90 mg
No barbiturate effects[a]	>800 mg/day	>240 mg/day	90+ mg

[a]Some protocols continue dosing 100 mg pentobarbital every 2 hours until signs of intoxication occur up to a total dose of 500 mg pentobarbital, then multiply the dose received by 4, and then convert that dose to phenobarbital equivalents as above. For example, 500 mg × 4 = 2,000 mg/day pentobarbital converts to 600 mg/day phenobarbital, or 200 mg t.i.d. However, beginning dose of 90 mg t.i.d. with observation and up-titration if necessary will cover most situations.

APPENDIX 4

Opiate Detoxification Procedures

GENERAL OPIATE DETOXIFICATION

1. Clonidine 0.1 mg test dose to ascertain blood pressure stability.
2. Clonidine 0.1 mg four to six times per day as needed for withdrawal symptoms, monitoring blood pressure to prevent hypotension.
3. Treat nausea, diarrhea, vomiting symptomatically.
4. Treat until withdrawal symptoms remit:
   a. Approximately 2 to 5 days for heroin, morphine, oxycodone
   b. Approximately 10 to 21 days for methadone

DETOXIFICATION FROM METHADONE USING METHADONE

1. Reduce dose by 5 to 10 mg/day until 10 mg daily dose.
2. Then reduce dose 2 mg/day until none.
3. Provide nonpharmacologic support as indicated during detoxification.

Note:
1. Subjective feeling of "not being right" without physiologic withdrawal symptoms can persist for several weeks for heroin, several months for methadone. This warrants support but not continued pharmacologic treatment.
2. Buprenorphine, a mixed agonist-antagonist, is used for detoxification in some centers.

APPENDIX 5

Stimulant Detoxification Procedures

1. There are no specific procedures for detoxification from cocaine, amphetamines, or other stimulants.
2. Neuroleptics should be used for psychosis (e.g., from amphetamines).
3. Expect depressive symptoms, sometimes severe, and be ready to address issues of suicidality due either to pharmacologic effects of withdrawal or psychosocial complications or both.

APPENDIX 6

Nicotine Detoxification Procedures

Note: All nicotine detoxification studies have assessed replacement pharmacotherapy in the context of an ongoing behavioral management psychosocial intervention.

1. Gum: 2- to 4-mg sticks every hour as needed for up to 3 months.
2. Patch:
   21 mg/day for 2 to 6 weeks, then
   14 mg/day patch for 2 weeks, then
   7 mg/day patch for 2 weeks, then discontinue (total approximately 6–12 weeks)
3. Nasal spray: 1 mg/spray as needed up to 30 times per day for up to 12 weeks
4. Inhaler: As needed for up to 12 weeks
5. Bupropion 150 to 300 mg/day for up to 6 weeks

APPENDIX 7
Biopsychosocial Approach to Sleep Complaints

FRONT-LINE: BEHAVIORAL INTERVENTIONS

Insomnia

Remove Inciting Factors (**see Module 11**)
Daytime Routine
- Regular wake time with alarm if necessary
- No caffeine (coffee, tea, soda)
- Moderate exercise during the day, daily
- No naps
- No alcohol—especially if hypnotics are prescribed

Bedtime Routine
- Avoid large meals for 4 hours before bedtime.
- After-dinner exercise helps some, hinders others: experiment.
- Bedroom only for sleep and sex: no TV, reading, etc.
- No nicotine for 4 hours before bedtime or through the night.
- Relaxation tapes, 5 to 15 minutes of deep breathing exercises, or meditation
  - Before bed
  - For nocturnal awakenings
- Sleep restriction
  - Stay in bed at most 15 minutes longer than current subjective sleep time.
  - Increase time in bed as sleep increases.
  - Example:
    - Estimated sleep 11:00 p.m. to 4:00 a.m.
    - To bed 11:00 p.m., up at 4:15 a.m.
    - Adjust bedtime earlier next night if necessary.

Phase Shifting

Behavioral
- Human circadian period is slightly longer than 24 hours.
- Therefore, if possible, plan work schedule to shift later rather than earlier:
  - Nights to days to afternoons to nights.
  - Not nights to afternoons to days to nights.
  - The longer on a single schedule the better (e.g., months rather than days).
- For non–shift-work problems and if possible to arrange 2 weeks with minimal role responsibilities, adjust bedtime by shifting schedule *later,* even if desire is for an earlier bedtime.
  - Example:
    - Sleep onset 2:00 a.m. and wake time 10:00 a.m.
    - Target: sleep onset 11:00 p.m. and wake time 7:00 a.m.
    - Go to bed at 2:30 a.m. first night, 3:00 a.m. second night, etc., until bedtime at 11:00 p.m..

Bright Light Therapy (see also Therapeutic Devices in Section IV)
- Bright visible spectrum light box at 2,500 lux for 30 to 120 minutes:
  - 6:00 a.m. to shift sleep onset earlier
  - 8:00 p.m. to shift sleep onset later

Note: Light boxes are available from many providers. **However,** bright visible spectrum light has side effects:

- (Hypo)mania in predisposed individuals
- Insomnia
- Jitteriness/anxiety
- Erythema (sunburn possible with ultraviolet rays)

SECOND-LINE TREATMENT: SUGGESTED PHARMACOLOGIC STRATEGIES FOR INSOMNIA

General Guidelines

- Remove inciting factors first.
- Use behavioral strategies first.
- Use behavioral strategies concurrently with medications.
- Lower expectations: "I can't make you sleep like a baby."
- Avoid nightly hypnotic use: 4 to 5 nights/week maximum to avoid:
  - Tachyphylaxis
  - Behavioral dependence
- Avoid chronic use: no hypnotic has proven efficacy > 2 weeks.
- Rotate agents from different classes if necessary.
- Use nonabusable medications if substance abuse is a concern.
- Kill two birds with one stone whenever possible:
  - Rather than stimulating antidepressant plus hypnotic:
    - Sedating antidepressant (e.g., trazodone, mirtazapine, tertiary amine tricyclic)
    - Same with neuroleptics (e.g., olanzapine, quetiapine, chlorpromazine)

Medication Options

Agents With Abuse Potential

- Benzodiazepines: Use quick-onset, short half-life agents, such as:
  - Temazepam
  - Triazolam
- Chloral hydrate
- Zolpidem
- Zaleplon

Agents Not Typically Abused (with Typical Hypnotic Doses)

- Diphenhydramine 25 to 75 mg
  - Over-the-counter
  - Active component of many tablets/capsules/elixirs
- Doxepin 25 to 150 mg
- Hydroxyzine 10 to 25 mg
- Trazodone 25 to 150 mg

Not Recommended

Antipsychotics (atypical or typical) without psychosis
Barbiturates
Carisoprodol/meprobamate
Opiates

APPENDIX 8

Abnormal Involuntary Movements Scale (AIMS)

PREPARATORY PROCEDURES

1. Ask the individual whether there is anything in mouth (i.e., gum, candy, etc.) and if there is, to remove it.
2. Ask the individual about the current condition of his or her teeth. Ask if individual wears dentures. Do teeth or dentures bother the individual now?
3. Ask whether the individual notices any movements in mouth, face, hands, or feet. If yes, ask to describe and to what extent they currently bother individual or interfere with activities.

EXAMINATION PROCEDURES

Note: Because individual may suppress movements that are attended to, look at entire body for movements during each procedure.

1. Have individual sit in chair with hands on knees, legs slightly apart, and feet flat on floor.
2. Ask individual to sit with hands hanging unsupported. If male, between legs, if female and wearing a dress, hanging over knees.
3. Ask individual to open mouth. Do this twice.
4. Ask individual to protrude tongue. Do this twice.
5. Ask individual to tap thumb, with each finger, as rapidly as possible for 10 to 15 seconds, separately with right hand, then with left hand.
6. Flex and extend individual's left and right arms one at a time. Note any rigidity separately.
7. Ask individual to stand up and observe in profile.
8. Ask individual to extend both arms outstretched in front with palms down.
9. Have individual walk a few paces, turn, and walk back to chair. Do this twice.

Note: For movement ratings, score highest severity observed. Rate movements that occur upon activation one value less than those observed spontaneously.

0 = None   1 = Minimal   2 = Mild   3 = Moderate   4 = Severe

Facial and Oral Movements (Dentures Removed)

1. Muscles of facial expression   _____
   Movements of forehead, eyebrows, periorbital area, cheeks; include frowning, blinking, smiling, grimacing

2. Lips and perioral area   _____
   Puckering, pouting, smacking

3. Jaw   _____
   Biting, clenching, chewing, mouth opening, lateral movements

4. Tongue   _____
   Rate only increase in movement both in and out of mouth, not inability to sustain movement

Extremity Movements

5. Upper (arms, wrists, fingers)   _____
Include choreic movements (rapid, objectively, purposeless, irregular, spontaneous) and/or athetoid movements (slow, irregular, complex, serpentine). Do not include tremor (repetitive, regular, rhythmic)

6. Lower (legs, knees, ankles, toes)   _____
Lateral knee movement, foot tapping, heel dropping, foot squirming, inversion and eversion of foot

Trunk Movements

7. Neck, shoulders, hips   _____
Rocking, twisting, squirming, pelvic gyrations.
Total score of items 1 through 7   _____

Global Judgments (rate 0 to 4)

8. Global severity of abnormal movements   _____
9. Incapacitation due to abnormal movements   _____
10. Individual's awareness of abnormal movements   _____
(Rate only individual's report.)

Dental Status

11.	Current problems with teeth and/or dentures:	No	Yes
12.	Does individual usually wear dentures:	No	Yes

APPENDIX 9

Guide to Opiate Selection for Chronic Pain

Generic	Brand/Combination	Time to Peak Serum Level	Serum Half-Life ($t_{1/2}$)	Approximate Equianalgesic Dosage and Schedule	Comments
Morphine[a]	MS Contin (sustained release)	30–60 min immediate release	2–4 h (immediate release)	10–30 mg every 3–4 h (oral); 5–20 mg every 3–4 h (rectal); 30–60 mg every 8–12 h (sustained release)	Starting dose 5–10 mg every 3–4 h. Sustained release preferable for chronic pain use. Available for rectal administration.
Codeine	Tylenol #2–#4[b]	30–60 min	2–4 h	120–150 every 3–4 h	Weak agonist, much constipation, nausea; little to recommend use.
Fentanyl	Duragesic (patch)	N/A	17 h (after removal)	25–50 μg/h patch	Available in 25, 50, 75 μg/h patches; provides steady-state serum levels; more difficult to abuse than pills.
Hydrocodone	Vicodin[b]	80 min	4 h	30 mg every 4–6 h	Only available in combinations in the United States.
Hydromorphone	Dilaudid	45 min	3–4 h	4–8 mg every 3–4 h (orally); 3–6 mg every 3–4 h (rectally)	Short duration of action; available for rectal administration.
Meperidine	Demerol	30–60 min	3–4 h	300 mg every 2–3 h	Weak agonist, much constipation, nausea; little to recommend use; lethality with MAOIs.
Methadone	Dolophine	30–60 min	15–40 h	20 mg every 6–8 h (for pain; opiate dependence maintenance dosing is typically 30–120 mg every day); 30 mg every 3–4 h (immediate release)	Very difficult, protracted withdrawal.
Oxycodone	Percocet/Percodan,[b] Tylox,[b] Oxycontin (sustained release)	30–60 min (non-sustained release)	3–4 h (immediate release)	30–60 mg every 8–12 h (sustained release)	Oxycontin has high street value (used via bite-and-dissolve sublingually).
Oxymorphone	Numorphan	30–60 min	2–3 h	5 mg every 3–4 h (rectally)	Rectal administration.
Pentazocine	Talwin	15–60 min	4–5 h	150 mg every 3–4 h	Partial agonist; little to recommend use.
Prophyxyphene	Darvon, Darvocet[b]	30–60 min	4–6 h	130 every 3–4 h	Weak agonist, nausea, constipation; little to recommend use.

[a]Equianalgesic dosing based on 10 to 30 mg morphine every 3–4 h.

[b]Denotes combination with acetaminophen. Little utility to using combinations. Alternate recommendation: Opiate + NSAID for additional antiinflammatory effect. See Module 13.

Some Self-Help Resources for Individuals Being Treated and Their Significant Others

VARIOUS DIAGNOSES

Gamian Europe
Web site *www.gamian-europe.com*
Promotes the understanding of mental illness and the treatments available. Information available in multiple languages.

National Alliance for the Mentally Ill (NAMI)
Colonial Place Three
2107 Wilson Blvd., Suite 300
Arlington, VA 22201
Phone (703) 524-7600
NAMI Helpline (800) 950-NAMI(6264)
Web site *www.nami.org*
Provides support to people affected by serious mental illness.

National Mental Health Association (NMHA)
1021 Prince Street
Alexandria, VA 22314-2971
Phone (703) 684-7722
Information center (800) 969-NMHA
E-mail *infoctr@nmha.oprg*
Web site *www.nmha.org*
Education organization for mental health and mental illness.

National Partnership for Workplace Mental Health
American Psychiatric Association
1400 K St. NW
Washington, DC 20005
E-mail *info@workplacementalhealth.org*
Web site *www.workplacementalhealth.org*
Serves as a source of information, resources, training, and understanding to enable employers and employees to succeed in the face of disaster, trauma, terror, and uncertain economic times.

ANXIETY DISORDERS

Anxiety Disorders Association of America (ADAA)
8730 Georgia Avenue, Suite 600
Silver Spring, MD 20910
Phone (240) 485-1001
Web site *www.adaa.org*
Provides resources for people who suffer from anxiety disorders.

National Center for PTSD (NCPTSD)
Web site *www.ncptsd.org*

Mission is to advance the clinical care and social welfare of America's veterans through research, education, and training in the science, diagnosis, and treatment of PTSD and stress-related disorders.

Obsessive-Compulsive Foundation (OCF)
337 Notch Hill Road
North Branford, CT 06471
Phone (203) 315-2190
E-mail *info@ocfoundation.org*
Web site *www.ocfoundation.org*
Educates the public and professional communities about obsessive-compulsive disorder.

ATTENTION DEFICIT DISORDERS

Children and Adults with Attention-Deficit/Hyperactivity Disorder (CHADD)
8181 Professional Place, Suite 201
Landover, MD 20785
National Call Center (800) 233-4050
Business (301) 306-7070
E-mail *national@chadd.org*
Web site *www.chadd.org*
Provides information for children and adults with attention-deficit/ hyperactivity disorder.

COGNITIVE DISORDERS

Alzheimer's Association
919 North Michigan Avenue, Suite 1100
Chicago, IL 60611-1676
Phone (800) 272-3900
312-335-8700
Web site *www.alz.org*
Provides information about Alzheimer disease and related cognitive disorders.

GAMBLING

Gamblers Anonymous
P.O. Box 17173
Los Angeles, CA 90017
Phone: (213) 386-8789
E-mail *isomain@gamblersanonymous.org*
Web site *www.gamblersanonymous.org*
Fellowship of men and women who share their experience, strength, and hope with each other that they may solve their common problem and help others to recover from a gambling problem.

Gambling
Phone (877) 9-GAMBLE
This toll-free number is available 24 hours a day and will provide help with problem gambling.

MOOD DISORDERS

Child and Adolescent Bipolar Foundation (CABF)
1187 Wilmette Avenue, PMB 331
Wilmette, IL 60091
Phone (847) 256-8525
(847) 920-9498
Web site *www.bpkids.org*
Provides information about children and adolescents with bipolar illness.

Depression and Bipolar Support Alliance (DBSA), formally known as the National Depressive and Manic-Depressive Association (NDMDA)
730 North Franklin Street, Suite 501
Chicago, IL 60610-7204
Phone (800) 826-3632
Web site *www.absalliance.org*
Provides support for people with depression and bipolar disorders.

EATING DISORDERS AND DISORDERS OF APPEARANCE

National Eating Disorders Association
603 Stewart Street, Suite 803
Seattle, WA 98101
Phone (206) 382-3587
Web site *Nationaleatingdisorders.org*
For individuals and their families affected by anorexia, bulimia, and other forms of "body dissatisfaction."

PAIN

American Pain Society
201 N. Charles Street, Suite 710
Baltimore, MD 21201-4111
Phone (888) 615-7246
Web site *www.painfoundation.org*
Serves people with pain through information, advocacy, and support. Their mission is to improve the quality of life for people with pain by raising public awareness, providing practical information, promoting research, and advocating to remove barriers and increase access to effective pain management.

SUBSTANCE USE DISORDERS

Recovery Resources Online
Web site *www.soberrecovery.com*
Links to online resources for substance dependence of all types.

Al-Anon and Alateen
1600 Corporate Landing Parkway
Virginia Beach, VA 23454-5617
Phone (888) 4AL-ANON
Web site *www.al-anon.org*
For family members and teens affected by substance dependence.

Alcoholics Anonymous
AA General Service Office
475 Riverside Drive
New York, NY 10015
Phone (212) 870-3400
Web site *www.alcoholics-anonymous.org*
Self-help groups for alcohol abuse and dependence using the 12-step approach.
Includes worldwide chapter contact information and links to local sites with locations and schedules.

Cocaine Anonymous
CAWSO
3740 Overland Avenue, Suite C
Los Angeles, CA 90034
PO Box 2000
Los Angeles, CA 90049-8000
Phone (310) 559-5833
Web site *www.ca.org*
Self-help groups for cocaine abuse and dependence using the 12-step approach.
Includes worldwide chapter contact information and links to local sites with locations and schedules.

Narcotics Anonymous
P.O. Box 9999
Van Nuys, CA 91409
Phone (818) 773-9999
Web site *www.na.org*
Self-help groups for narcotic abuse and dependence using the 12-step approach.
Includes worldwide chapter contact information and links to local sites with locations and schedules.

SUICIDE

American Association of Suicidology
4201 Connecticut Avenue, NW, Suite 408
Washington, DC 20008
National Hopeline Network 1-800-SUICIDE
Phone (202) 237-2280
E-mail *info@suicidology.org*

Web site *www.suicidology.org*
Dedicated to the understanding and prevention of suicide.

Suicide Prevention Action Network of USA (SPAN USA)
5034 Odins Way
Marietta, GA 3008
Phone (888) 649-1366
Web site *www.spanusa.org*
Dedicated to the creation and implementation of effective National Suicide Prevention Strategies.

APPENDIX 11

Psychotropic Drug Equivalency Tables

Note: The purpose of this appendix is not to provide exact milligram-for-milligram equivalencies, especially not across classes (e.g., TCAs to SSRIs). Rather, they provide a general guide to the clinician, and may be of use when switching agents within a class (e.g., escitalopram to paroxetine). Cross-titration for agents from different classes (e.g., SSRIs to TCAs) is typically necessary, as it is for agents, within a class that have very different side effect profiles (e.g., perphenazine to chlorpromazine).

Antidepressant Dose Equivalencies

Drug Name				
Generic	Sample Brand	Dose		
Imipramine	Tofranil	100–199 mg	200–299 mg	300+ mg
Tricyclic				
Amitriptyline	Elavil	100–199	200–299	300+
Amoxapine	Asendin	100–149	150–449	450+
Clomipramine	Anafranil	75–99	100–249	250+
Desipramine	Norpramine	50–124	125–249	250+
Doxepin	Sinequan	100–199	200–299	300+
Nortriptyline	Aventyl	50–74	75–149	150+
Protriptyline	Vivactil	10–24	25–49	50+
Trimipramine	Surmontil	50–74	75–299	300+
Selective serotonin reuptake inhibitors				
Citalopram	Cylexa	10–19	20–59	60+
Escitalopram	Lexapro	5–9	10–29	30+
Fluoxetine	Prozac	10–19	20–59	60+
Paroxetine	Paxil	10–19	20–59	60+
Sertraline	Zoloft	25–49	50–199	200+
Monoamine oxidase inhibitors				
Phenelzine	Nardil	15–29	30–89	90+
Tranylcypromine	Parnate	10–19	20–59	60+
Other				
Bupropion	Wellbutrin	100–199	200–399	400+
Maprotiline	Ludiomil	50–74	75–199	200+
Nefazodone	Serzone	100–299	300–599	600+
Mirtazepine	Remeron	15–29	30–44	45+
Trazodone	Deseryl	100–149	150–449	450+
Venlafaxine	Effexor	75–149	150–299	300+

Benzodiazepine Dose Equivalencies

Generic	Sample Brand	Dose
Diazepam	Valium	10 mg
Alprazolam	Xanax	2
Chlordiazepoxide	Librium	50
Clonazapam	Klonopin	2
Clorazepate	Tranxene	15
Flurazepam	Dalmane	30
Halazepam	Paxipam	40
Lorazepam	Ativan	2
Oxazepam	Serax	30
Prazepam	Centrax	20
Temazepan	Restoril	30
Triazolam	Halcion	0.5

Typical Neuroleptic Dose Equivalencies

Generic	Sample Brand	Dose
Chlorpromazine	Thorazine	100 mg
Acetophenazine	Tindal	20
Chlorprothixene	Taractan	100
Droperidol	Inapsine	2
Fluphenazine	Prolixin/Permitil	2
Haloperidol	Haldol	2
Loxapine	Loxitane/Daxolin	10
Mesoridazine	Serentil	50
Molidone	Moban	10
Perphenazine	Trilafon	10
Pimozide	Orap	2
Thioridazine	Mellaril	100
Thiothixene	Navane	4
Trifluoperazine	Stelazine	5
Fluphenazine depot	25 mg every 3 wk = 1,000 mg chlorpromazine	
Haloperidol depot	100 mg every 4 wk = 500 mg chlorpromazine	

Atypical Neuroleptic Dose Equivalencies

Generic	Sample Brand	
Risperidone	Risperdal	2 mg
Clozapine	Clozaril	100
Olanzapine	Zyprexa	2
Quetiapine	Seroquel	100
Ziprazadone	Geodon	20

Cytochrome P-450 Effects for Major Psychotropic Medications

NOTES ON USAGE OF THIS TABLE

Recall from the Introduction to **Section IV** that drug interactions may be of two types: *pharmacokinetic* and *pharmacodynamic.* Pharmacokinetic interactions refer to the handling of the drug throughout the body (e.g., absorption, protein binding, metabolism) (including enzymatic breakdown via the P-450 and other systems, and oxidation and glucuronidation), and excretion. Pharmacodynamic interactions refer to effects at receptors. The role of P-450 enzyme interactions is to affect only one aspect of the pharmacokinetics of the involved substances. Nonetheless, the effects of P-450 enzyme interactions can be quite marked and clinically relevant.

Multiple sources were consulted to construct this table. If there was disagreement between sources, the cautious approach was taken and the characteristic listed. Several inhibition or induction effects were noted by multiple sources as particularly potent. These are noted in **bold italics.** Note, however, that this listing reflects both *in vivo* and *in vitro* data, unlike the drug-drug interaction notes in each medication entry in **Section IV.** Thus, some of these P-450 interactions (and those of other compilations) are of more theoretical than clinical concern.

Therefore, the best use of this table is to raise a warning flag that drugs may interact. The clinician is, thus, advised that the situation may require either preemptive moves (e.g., reducing the dose of one of the drugs) or closer monitoring for the "bioassay" of side effects.

	Substrate for	Inhibits	Induces
Antidepressants			
Tricyclics			
Amitriptyline	1A2, 2C9, 2C19, 2D6, 3A4		
Clomipramine	1A2, 2C19, 2D6, 3A4	2D6	
Desipramine	1A2, 2D6, 2C19	2D6	
Imipramine	1A2, 2C19, 2D6, 3A4		
Nortriptyline	2D6		
Protriptyline	2D6		
Serotonin Reuptake Inhibitors			
Citalopram	1A2, 2C9, 2C19, 3A4	2D6, 3A4	
Fluoxetine	2C9, *2D6*, 3A4	2C9, 2C19, *2D6*, 3A4	
Fluvoxamine	2D6	1A2, *2C9*, *2C19*, 2D6, 3A4	
Paroxetine	2D6, 3A4	2C9, 2C19, *2D6*, 3A4	
Sertraline	2D6, 3A4	2C9, 2D6, 3A4	
MAO inhibitors			
Phenelzine			
Tranylcypromine		2C19	
Other antidepressants			
Mirtazepine	1A2, 2D6, 3A4		
Nefazodone	3A4	3A4	
Trazodone	2D6, 3A4		
Venlafaxine	2D6, 3A4		
Adjuvant mood medications			
Triiodothyronine			
Thyroxine			
Antimanics and putative mood stabilizers			
Carbamazepine	3A4		1A2, 2C9, 2C19, *3A4*
Lamotrigine			
Lithium	—	—	—
Oxcarbazepine			*3A4*
Topiramate		2C19	
Valproate	3A4	2D6, 3A4	2C9, 2C19
Verapamil	1A2, 3A4	3A4	
Neuroleptics			
Atypical			
Clozapine	1A2, 2D6, 3A4		
Olanzapine	1A2		
Quetiapine	2D6, 3A4		
Risperidone	2D6		
Ziprasadone			
Typical			
Chlorpromazine	2D6	2D6	
Fluphenazine			
Haloperidol	1A2, 2D6, 3A4	2D6	
Loxapine			
Mesoridazine	2D6		
Molindone			
Perphenazine	2D6	2D6	
Thioridazine	2D6	2D6	
Thiothixene			
Trifluoperazine	2D6		
Benzodiazepines			
Alprazolam	3A4		
Chlordiazepoxide			
Clonazepam			
Diazepam	2C9, 2C19, 3A4		
Oxazepam			

(Continued)

	Substrate for	Inhibits	Induces
Temazepam			
Triazolam	3A4		
Nonbenzodiazepine hypnotics			
Zaleplon	3A4		
Zolpidem	3A4		
Cognitive enhancers			
Donepezil	2D6		
Galantamine			
Rivastigmine			
Tacrine	1A2, 2D6	1A2	
Stimulants			
Methylphenidate	2D6		
Pemoline	2D6		
Other psychotropics			
Buspirone	2B6, 3A4		
Clonidine			
Gabapentin	—		
Prazosin		—	—
Commonly encountered nonpsychotropic medications			
Analgesics			
NSAIDs	2C9		
Antiasthmatics			
Zafirlukast		2C9	
Antibiotics			
Macrolide antibiotics (except azithromycin)		3A4	
Anticonvulsants			
Phenobarbital			*2B6*
Phenytoin	2C19		*2B6*
Antidiabetics			
Tolbutamide	2D6		
Antihistamines		2D6	
Chlorpheniramine			
Antihypertensives			
Beta-blockers (lipophilic)	2D6		
Antineoplastics			
Cyclosporin	3A4		
Antiretrovirals			
HIV protease inhibitors	3A4	2D6, 3A4	
Efavirenz and nevirapine	3A4		3A4
Nelfinavir	2C19, 3A4		
Hormones			
Oral contraceptives	*3A4*		
Psychoactive compounds, miscellaneous			
St. John's wort			3A4
Tobacco smoke			
Nicotine[a]			1A1, 1A2, 2E1
Statins			
HMG CoA reductase inhibitors (except pravastatin)	3A4		
Ulcer medications			
Cimetidine		*1A2, 2C19*	
Proton pump inhibitors	2C19	2C19	

[a]Nicotine also induces polycyclic aromatic hydroxylases and enzymes of oxydation/glucuronidation. These effects are frequently responsible for a net reduction in serum levels of many psychotropic medications in nicotine users.

On the other hand, if a medication does not appear in this table to have interactions, it does not mean the combination has a clean bill of health. To cite an obvious example: The combination of diazepam and trazodone will clearly lead to increased sedation—but because of additive sedative properties in the brain, and not because of P-450 interactions in the liver.

Additionally, this table does not differentiate between major effects and minor effects. Moreover, all bets are off when three or more psychotropics are combined, as is, unfortunately, often necessary. Finally, not all medications have been well characterized regarding their P-450 effects; this is particularly true for lesser used (e.g., molindone) and newer (e.g., galantamine) medications. Thus, absence of data does not necessarily mean the absence of effect (which is listed as "—").

APPENDIX 13

Dietary and Pharmacologic Substances Causing Adverse Interactions with Monoamine Oxidase Inhibitor (MAOI) Antidepressants

Foodstuffs high in tyramine
    Beverages
        Dark Beer
        Red Wine
    Cheese
        Almost all except cream, cottage, ricotta
    Meats
        Organ meats (e.g., liver, sweetbreads)
        Fermented meats (e.g., sausages)
        Smoked meats
    Fruits
        Raspberries
    Vegetables
        Broad beans
    Fish
        Any pickled fish
    Other
        Soups containing forbidden foods
        Soy sauce
    Foods with any signs of spoilage (when in doubt, toss it out!)
Most commonly encountered medications[a]
    Over-the-counter
        Pseudophedrine
        Phenylpropanolamine
    Prescription only
        Meperidine
        Epinephrine
        Local anesthetics that contain epinephrine
        Levodopa
        Amphetamines and stimulants
        Methylphenidate
        Isoproteronol
        Antidepressants

[a]No medications should be taken without the express permission of the prescribing physician. Note that over-the-counter remedies often include forbidden medications. Great care must be taken in reading ingredient labels to avoid adverse interactions. This is especially true of cold medications.

APPENDIX 14

Alternative and Complementary Agents Used for Psychiatric Symptoms

Many alternative and complementary treatments have been used for hundreds or even thousands of years (by the 1894 edition of Potter's *Materia Medica* cited in the Preface, kava-kava had just been listed as a "New Remedy," joining the already established valerian and hops). We consider them "alternative," or more sympathetically, "complementary," from the perspective of the scientifically based, allopathic tradition dominant in today's industrialized cultures.

The purpose of this appendix is not to provide the clinician with a guide to the use of complementary treatments, as for the major psychotropic agents and psychotherapeutic modalities provided in **Section IV.** Rather, the table below lists the most commonly encountered alternative and complementary agents used for treatment of psychiatric symptoms, why they are used, and the potential issues and problems that may arise in cotreating individuals with agents from both the dominant scientifically based and the complementary cultures.

For more detailed information, including efficacy data, the clinician may refer to the **Pharmacologic Treatment Resources (Alternative and Complementary)** section in **Key References.** References are provided from both the dominant and the alternative/complementary perspectives. Note that there are some reasonable, though not unequivocal, scientific data supporting the use of several of these medications, including:

- Ginkgo biloba: Alzheimer dementia and vascular dementia
- Melatonin: insomnia and circadian phase shifting
- Omega-3 fatty acids: rapid cycling manic-depressive disorder
- S-adenosyl methionine: depressive disorders
- St. John's wort: depressive disorders
- Vitamin E: tardive dyskinesia, memory impairment in the elderly
- Yohimbine: impotence (FDA-approved)
- Kava: anxiety

Substance	Use	Potential Issues
Black cohash	Premenstrual symptoms	—
Chamomile	Anxiety, insomnia	—
Ephedra/ ma huang	Fatigue, depression, "herbal Ecstacy"	Tachycardia; hypertension; tremors; additive adrenergic effects with tricyclics; mania; potential hypertensive crisis with MAOIs; banned by NCAA and U.S. Olympic Committee
Ginkgo biloba	Dementia, impotence, memory decline	Reports of interaction with anticoagulants; headaches; nausea
Ginseng	Memory decline, depression, impotence	Tachycardia; hypertension; tremors; unclear potential for MAOI, tricyclic interactions
Hops	Insomhia	Additive sedative effects to those of psychotropics
Kava	Anxiety, impotence, insomnia recreational (alcohol-like) effects	Additive sedative effects to those of psychotropics
Melatonin	Insomnia	Additive sedative effects to those of psychotropics
Omega-3 fatty acids	Mood, anxiety symptoms	
S-adenosyl methionine	Depression	Possible arrhythmias
St. John's wort (hypericum perforatum)	Depression	Induction of P450 enzyme 3A4 (see **Appendix 12** for potential psychotropic effects); potential hypertensive crisis with MAOIs
Valerian	Anxiety, insomnia, muscle relaxant, premenstrual symptoms	Additive sedative effects to those of psychotropics; dystonia; hepatitis
Vitamin B_6 (pyridoxine)	Premenstrual symptoms	Increased liver transaminases; sensory neuropathy; reduced antiparkinsonian effects of levodopa; reduced phenytoin levels
Vitamin E, mega-dose	Dementia, impotence, memory deficits	Hypervitaminosis (for any fat soluble vitamin, A, D, E, K)
Yohimbine (in herbal preparations)	Impotence (FDA-approved as pills manufactured by pharmaceutical corporations)	Tachycardia, hypertension, tremors; potential hypertensive crisis with MAOIs

An Annotated Bibliography for Additional Clinically Relevant Information

BIOPSYCHOSOCIAL ASSESSMENT AND TREATMENT MODEL

Engel GL. The need for a new medical model: a challenge for biomedicine. *Science* 1977;196:129–196.
Engel GL. The biopsychosocial model and the education of health professionals. *Ann NY Acad Sci* 1978;310:169–187.
  • Classic articles by the master.

COLLABORATIVE PRACTICE TREATMENT MODEL

Bauer MS, McBride L. *The life goals program: structured group psychotherapy for bipolar disorder,* 2nd edition. New York: Springer, 2003.
  • Book illustrating collaborative practice and psychoeducation strategies specifically for bipolar disorder, specifically in group format. Easily adaptable strategies for a collaborative approach to other serious mental illnesses.
Von Korff M, Gruman J, Schaefer J, et al. Collaborative management of chronic illness. *Ann Intern Med* 1997;127:1097–1102.
Wagner EH, Austin BT, Von Korff M. Organizing care for patients with chronic illness. *Milbank Q* 1996;74:511–544.
  • Conceptual overviews and reviews of the wide applicability of collaborative practice approaches to chronic medical illnesses.

COMPETENCE

Grisso T, Appelbaum PS. *Assessing competence to consent to treatment. A guide for physicians and professionals.* New York: Oxford University Press, 1998.
  • Competence assessment, its theoretical/legal/philosophical basis, and instrument for clinical use by leaders in the field.
Slavney PR. *Psychiatric dimensions of medical practice. What the primary care physician should know about delirium, demoralization, suicidal thinking, and competence to refuse medical advice.* Baltimore: Johns Hopkins University Press, 1998.
  • Extremely good, concise discussion of competence issues, along with a number of other thorny issues faced by nonpsychiatric physicians. Mental health clinicians will also benefit from insights throughout.

CULTURAL ISSUES IN DIAGNOSIS

Mezzich JE, Kleinman A, Fabrega H, et al., eds. *Culture and psychiatric diagnosis. A DSM-IV perspective.* Washington, DC: American Psychiatric Press, 1996.
  • Addresses important diagnostic issues when dealing with individuals from outside of the Western/industrialized culture dominant in medicine and mental health practice.

Okpaku SO, ed. *Clinical methods in transcultural psychiatry.* Washington, DC: American Psychiatric Press, 1998.
- Chapters cover a variety of issues regarding the needs of individuals from specific racial and ethnic backgrounds in treatment, as well as a substantial amount of scientific data.

EVIDENCE-BASED MEDICINE: DECISION SCIENCES

Hennekens CH, Buring JE. *Epidemiology in medicine.* Philadelphia: Lippincott Williams & Wilkins (formerly by Little Brown), 1987 and Fletcher RH, Fletcher SW, Wagner EH. *Clinical epidemiology: the essentials,* 3rd ed. Baltimore, MD: Williams & Wilkins, 1996.
- Solid general epidemiology texts with straightforward chapters on test characteristics.

Sox SC, Blatt MA, Higgins MC, et al. *Medical decision making.* Boston: Butterworths, 1988.

Weinstein MC, Fineberg HV. *Clinical decision analysis.*Philadelphia: WB Saunders, 1980.
- Older, but classic texts covering basics, derivation, and applications of decision analytic tools and concepts, including test characteristics.

EVIDENCE-BASED MEDICINE: TREATMENTS

The Cochrane Collaboration Library (*www.update-software.com*).
- Rigorous, state-of-the-art syntheses of available controlled trial data for many mental health, medical, and surgical conditions. Frequently updated. Expensive but many academic institutions have subscriptions. Abstracts are available to all without subscription.

EVIDENCE-BASED MENTAL HEALTH

BMJ Group. *Clinical evidence: mental health.* London: BMJ Group, 2002.
- A recent compilation of mental health evidence for various treatments, reprinted from *Clinical Evidence,* Issue 7, 2002.

Maj M, Sartorius N. *World Psychiatric Association series: evidence and experience in psychiatry.* New York: Wiley, 1999 and ongoing.
- Comprehensive series of evidence-based texts covering major psychiatric disorders. Includes not only pharmacologic and psychotherapeutic treatment but also data on epidemiology, course, outcome, and costs. Novel format wherein a comprehensive review is written by an expert in the field, followed by multiple, short commentaries and elaborations by other experts. Volumes to date include: Dementia, Depressive Disorders, Bipolar Disorder, Obsessive-Compulsive Disorder, and Schizophrenia. Series is continuing.

Roth A, Fonagy P. *What works for whom? A critical review of psychotherapy research.* New York: Guilford, 1996.
- Evidence-based review of psychotherapy outcome studies organized by disorder. Invaluable, though getting dated. Companion volume exists for treatment of children and adolescents.

366

GENERAL PSYCHIATRY TEXTS

American Psychiatric Association. *Diagnostic and statistical manual of mental disorders,* 4th edition text revision (DSM-IV-TR). Washington, DC: American Psychiatric Press, 2000.
- Beyond the criteria, a treasure trove of descriptive information compiled by workgroups of experts in each field. The 1994 DSM-IV was updated to reflect more recent information in this "TR" edition. The criteria did not change between these two versions. Available in smaller spiral-bound pocket guides that include only the criteria without the text.

Sadock BJ, Sadock VA. *Pocket handbook of clinical psychiatry,* 3rd ed. Philadelphia: Lippincott Williams & Wilkins, 2001.
- Best almost-pocket-sized handbook of psychiatry. Based on popular full-size text.

Tasman A, Kay J, Lieberman JA. *Psychiatry,* 2nd ed. Philadelphia: WB Saunders, 2003.
- Comprehensive two-volume text with helpful spin-off products (e.g., self-testing review booklet).

INSTRUMENTS FOR PSYCHIATRIC ASSESSMENT

American Psychiatric Association. *Handbook of psychiatric measures.* Washington, DC: American Psychiatric Press, 2000.
- Comprehensive, reviewed by experts. Standard review format. Includes psychometric data, practical administration issues, how to get instrument. Many instruments available on enclosed CD. Pricey but fills an important niche.

Measurement Excellence Initiative. *www.MeasurmentExperts.org.*
- Comprehensive web-based site sponsored by the Department of Veterans Affairs Health Services Research and Development Program at Houston. Similar degree of expert review as the American Psychiatric Association source. Standard review format. Includes psychometric data, practical administration issues, how to get instrument. Covers all major health-care areas, not just mental health. Free.

PAIN MANAGEMENT

Ballantyne J, Fishman SM, Abdi S. *The Massachusetts General Hospital handbook of pain management.* Boston: Little, Brown, 2002.

McCaffery M, Pasero C. *Pain: clinical manual,* 2nd ed. Boston: CV Mosby, 1999.
- Both are excellent and comprehensive sources of pain management information, based on both research and the authors' accumulated extensive clinical experience.

PERSONALITY DISORDERS

Black DW. *Bad boys, bad men: confronting antisocial personality disorder.* New York: Oxford University, 2000.
- A scholarly, but readable and clinically useful book by a long-term expert in an often neglected, yet fascinating, area.

367

Gunderson JG. *Borderline personality disorder. A clinical guide.* Washington, DC: American Psychiatric Press, 2001.
- Comprehensive, incorporating both reams of empirical data and a wealth of clinical experience. Covers all relevant topics from neurobiology to treatment. Addresses issues of other cluster B disorders as well.

Williams L. A "classic" case of borderline personality disorder. *Psychiatr Serv* 1998;49:173–174.
- Two-page first-person account of what it is like to have borderline personality disorder. Required reading.

PHARMACOLOGIC TREATMENT RESOURCES: ALTERNATIVE AND COMPLEMENTARY

Muskin PR, ed. *Complementary and alternative medicine and psychiatry.* Review of psychiatry. Vol. 19. Washington, DC: American Psychiatric Press, 2000.
- Comprehensive compendium of herbal, manipulation, and meditation-related therapies relevant to psychiatry. Both scientifically comprehensive and clinically relevant.

Pressman A, Buff S. *The complete idiot's guide to alternative medicine.* New York: Alpha/Macmillan, 1999.
- Cited here not just to demonstrate the incredible reach of the "Complete Idiot's Guide" series, but also to illustrate the type of information the individuals we treat are likely to come upon. Comprehensive, unabashedly enthusiastic (e.g., Why take diazepam to calm tension and anxiety ". . . when there are so many herbs that do the same thing, safely and without side effects?")

Wong AH, Smith M, Boon HS. Herbal remedies in psychiatric practice. *Arch Gen Psych* 1998;55:1033–1044.
- Scholarly, comprehensive, yet concise reference in a first-rate scientific journal.

PHARMACOLOGIC TREATMENT RESOURCES: GENERAL

American Society of Health System Pharmacists. *American Hospital Formulary Services ("red book").* Bethesda, MD: American Society of Health System Pharmacists, 2002.
- A comprehensive compendium of drug information.

Cozza KL, Armstrong SC. *The cytochrome P450 system. Drug interaction principles for medical practice.* Washington, DC: American Psychiatric Press, 2001.
- Exhaustive, and at times exhausting, but compact book summarizing all known P-450-based drug interactions relevant to psychiatric treatment. Includes both psychotropic and nonpsychotropic medications.

Ellsworth AJ, Witt DM, Duigdale DC, et al. *2001–2002 Medical drug reference.* Philadelphia: CV Mosby, 2001.
- Comprehensive and up-to-date, but succinct and easy to use, general drug reference guide. Good coverage of psychotropics, drug interactions.

Swann SK, Bennett WM. Use of drugs in patients with renal failure. In: Schrier RW, ed. *Diseases of the kidney and urinary tract.* Philadelphia: Lippincott Williams & Wilkins, 2001:3139–3186.
- Remarkably complete guide to principles of drug dosing in individuals with renal compromise, including tables with specific dosing recommendations for specific agents. Chapter contains 581 references.

Web-Based and Personal Digital Assistant (PDA) Programs

- *www.medscape.com* (web-based): Comprehensive, up-to-date, good printable patient information.
- *www.epocrates.com* (PDA): Frequently updated, good psychotropic coverage, emphasizes currency and breadth perhaps at expense of depth. Over-calls drug interactions. Basic version free, subscription version pricey.
- *www.mosby.com* (PDA): PDA-downloadable for a price. More depth than epocrates.com, but less frequently updated and psychotropic coverage is spotty.
- *www.drug-interactions.com* (web-based): Reasonably frequently updated table of P-450 drug interactions, with supporting primary source material. Includes both psychotropic and nonpsychotropic medications.

PHARMACOLOGIC TREATMENT RESOURCES: PSYCHOPHARMACOLOGY

Kaplan GB, Hammer RP, eds. *Brain circuitry and signaling in psychiatry: basic science and clinical implications.* Washington, DC: American Psychiatric Press, 2002.
- State-of-the-art discussion of neurobiologic basis of major psychiatric disorders by experts in the field.

Schatzberg AF, Cole JO, DeBattista C. *Manual of clinical psychopharmacology,* 4th ed. Washington, DC: American Psychiatric Press, 2002.
- Comprehensive, clinically oriented almost pocket-sized manual.

Stahl SM. Essential psychopharmacology. *Neuroscientific basis and practical applications,* 2nd ed. New York: Cambridge University Press, 2000.
- Basic science text with ample clinical relevance. Most basic mechanisms of drugs, many putative mechanisms for disorders. Copious, creative, entertaining (but sometimes too cutesy) illustrations.

PREVALENCE OF PSYCHIATRIC DISORDERS

Segal SP, Hardiman ER, Hodges JQ. Characteristics of new clients at self-help and community mental health agencies in geographic proximity. *Psych Serv* 2002;53:1145–1152.
- Another of the very few sources that contains data regarding prevalence of psychiatric diagnoses in a nonselective mental health outpatient setting, this one in a public community mental health setting; compares rates with those of nonclinical self-help settings.

Tsuang MT, Tohen M, Zahner GEP. *Textbook in psychiatric epidemiology,* 2nd ed. Baltimore: Wiley, 2002.
- Comprehensive but pricey text just updated covering concepts, methods, and most relevant existing community-based data.

Zimmerman M, Mattia JI. Principal and additional DSM-IV disorders for which outpatients seek treatment. *Psych Serv* 2000;51:1299–1304.
- One of the few sources for prevalence data in outpatient mental health clinics, this one private and academically affiliated. Based on standardized assessments that also reveal "hidden" secondary comorbid diagnoses.

PSYCHOTHERAPY: BEHAVIORAL AND COGNITIVE

Barlow DH. *Anxiety and its disorders: the nature and treatment of anxiety and panic.* New York: Guilford, 2001.
- Recent and comprehensive book on cognitive-behavioral approaches to understanding and treating anxiety disorders.

Beck AT, Rush AJ, Emery G, et al. *Cognitive therapy of depression.* New York: Guilford, 1989.
- Older, but classic, text on cognitive-behavioral approaches to depression. Still serves as the basis for "variations on the theme" for other cognitive-behavioral treatments for mood disorders.

Lewinsohn PM, Antonuccio DO, Steinmetz JL. *The Coping with Depression Course: a psychoeducational intervention for unipolar depression.* Eugene, OR: Castalia Publishing, 1984.
- Older reference, but represents the more behaviorally oriented branch of treatment for depression.

PSYCHOTHERAPY: GENERAL

(See also Evidence-Based Medicine Mental Health)

Rollnick S, Mason P, Butler C. *Health and behavior change: a guide for practitioners.* London: Churchill Livingston, 1999.
- Practical, clinician-oriented guide to motivational interviewing techniques that breaks down into explicit components the intuitive impression that clinicians have of individuals' readiness to change health behaviors, and provides clinically useful strategies with which to address same.

PSYCHOTHERAPY: PSYCHOANALYTIC

Davanloo H. *Short-term dynamic psychotherapy.* New York: Jason Aronson, 1995.

Luborsky L. *Principles of psychoanalytic psychotherapy.* New York: Basic Books, 2000.
- Manual-based psychotherapy based on psychoanalytic principles. Not ultra-short-term but well studied and structured in delivery.

Sifneos PE. *Short-term dynamic psychotherapy: evaluation and technique,* 2nd ed. New York: Kluwer Academic, 1987.
- Two of the most well-known and established ultra-short-term psychoanalytic psychotherapies.

SEXUAL DISORDERS

Wincze JP, Carey M. *Sexual dysfunction: a guide for assessment and treatment.* New York: Guilford, 1991.

Rosen RC, Leiblum SR. *Erectile disorders: assessment and treatment.* New York: Guilford, 1992.
- Two solid books that general clinicians will find useful for everyday practice.

SUBSTANCE USE DISORDERS

American Society of Addiction Medicine (ASAM). *ASAM PPC-2R: ASAM patient placement criteria for the treatment of substance-related disorders,* 2nd ed, revised. Chevy Chase, MD: American Society of Addiction Medicine, 2001.

- Explicit criteria for assigning individuals with substance use disorders to specific levels of intensity of treatment based on clinical findings. In wide usage, guiding both clinician behavior and reimbursement practices.

Lowinson JH, Ruiz P, Millman RB, et al. *Substance abuse: a comprehensive textbook,* 3rd ed. Baltimore: Williams & Wilkins, 1997.

- A comprehensive text on virtually all aspects of substance use disorders. Worthwhile, though pricey.

TARDIVE DYSKINESIA/DYSTONIA

Adityanjee, Aderibigbe YA, Jampala VC, et al. The current status of tardive dystonia. *Biol Psych* 1999;45:715–730.

- The most comprehensive recent review on the chronic, disfiguring, painful syndrome of tardive dystonia, including description, course, possible mechanisms, and treatment.

Gardos G, Cole JO. The evaluation and treatment of neuroleptic-induced movement disorders. *Harv Rev Psych* 1995;3:130–139.

- Older, but comprehensive review of tardive dyskinesia, dystonia, and akathisia.

SUBJECT INDEX

A

Abnormal involuntary movements scale, 347–348
Abuse
  amphetamine, 190, 194–195
  cocaine, 190, 194–195
  drug, 190–191
  hallucinogens, 190, 194–195
  opiates, 190–192, 194–195
  substance, 49
Acetazolamide, 20
Acetophenazine, 357
Acute stress disorder, 187–189
Acyclovir, 70
Adjustment disorder
  comorbidities, 205
  course of, 205
  definition of, 18, 32
  DSM criteria, 204
  features of, 205
  prevalence of, 205
  treatment of, 205–206
Adrenergic agents, 26
Affect, 6
Agnosia, 75, 77
Agoraphobia
  comorbidities, 179
  course of, 179
  DSM criteria, 177–178
  panic disorder with, 35, 176
  prevalence of, 178–179
  treatment of, 180
Akathisia
  assessment of, 151
  definition of, 144–145
  management of, 152
  risk factors, 151
Akinesia, 144
Alcohol
  abuse of, 190–191, 194–195, 259
  dependence on, 190–191
  detoxification procedure, 339–340

disorders associated with, 20, 26, 34, 70
self-help resources, 353
sexual problems, 105
sleep problems, 97
withdrawal symptoms, 53
Alpha methyldopa, 20
Alprazolam, 317–318, 356
Alliance building, 13
Alprostadil, 112
Alternative and complementary agents, 363–364
Alzheimer dementia, 80, 206
Amantadine, 150
Ambien (*See* Zolpidem)
Amitriptyline, 262–264, 355
Amnesia
  description of, 38, 80
  dissociative, 234–236
Amoxapine, 355
Amphetamines
  abuse of, 190, 194–195
  disorders associated with, 20, 26, 34
Anabolic steroids, 20, 26, 70, 97
Anafranil (*See* Clomipramine)
Angiotensin-converting enzyme inhibitors, 70
Anorexia nervosa, 86, 220–221
  (*See also* Eating disorders)
  psychotherapy for, 260
Antiasthmatics, 97
Anticholinergics, 70
Anticonvulsants, 105
Antidepressants
  anxiety caused by, 34
  bupropion, 283–284, 355
  cytochrome P-450 effects, 359
  description of, 70, 262
  equivalency tables, 355
  mania caused by, 26
  mirtazapine, 284–285, 355
  monoamine oxidase inhibitors
    (*See* Monoamine oxidase inhibitors)

373

Antidepressants (*contd.*)
    nefazodone, 285–286, 355
    selective serotonin reuptake
        inhibitors (*See* Selective
        serotonin reuptake
        inhibitors)
    sleep problems, 97
    trazodone, 227, 286–287, 346,
        355
    tricyclic (*See* Tricyclic
        antidepressants)
    venlafaxine, 287–288, 355
Antihistamines, 70, 227
Antihypertensives, 70
Antiinflammatory agents, 70
Antineoplastic agents, 70
Antipsychotics, 300–311 (*See
    also Neuroleptics,
    individual agents*)
Antisocial personality disorder
    clinical features of, 240–241
    course of, 242
    DSM criteria, 237–238
    prevalence of, 242
Anxiety disorders
    acute stress disorder, 187–189
    differential diagnosis, 28
    generalized anxiety disorder
        (*See* Generalized anxiety
        disorder)
    medical illnesses that cause, 34
    medications that cause, 34
    obsessive-compulsive disorder
        (*See* Obsessive-
        compulsive disorder)
    paroxysmal episodes with, 33
    phobias (*See* Phobia)
    posttraumatic stress disorder
        (*See* Posttraumatic stress
        disorder)
    psychotherapy for, 258
    screening for, 29
    self-help resources, 350–351
    sleep symptoms in, 96
    trauma-associated, 31
Anxiolytics, 190, 194–195

Aphasia, 75, 77
Appearance disorders
    focus of concern determina-
        tions, 87–88
    screening for, 87
    self-help resources, 352
Apraxia, 75, 77
Aricept (*See* Donepezil)
Asendin (*See* Amoxapine)
Aspirin, 119
Assaultiveness
    assessment of, 57–58
    debriefing, 66
    differential diagnosis, 56
    ideation, 56
    intent, 59–60
    management of, 62
    risk factors, 61
Assessment, psychiatric
    principles of, 1–2, 15, 160
    tasks of, 1, 15, 160, 245
Asterixis, 144
Atenolol, 148
Athetosis, 144
Ativan (*See* Lorazepam)
Attention-deficit/hyperactivity
    disorder, 208–210, 351
Atypical depression, 22–23
Atypical neuroleptics, 312–317,
    355, 357
Autonomy, 140
Aventyl (*See* Nortriptyline)
Avoidant personality disorder
    clinical features of, 240–241
    course of, 242
    DSM criteria, 239
    prevalence of, 242
Axial, 144

B

Baclofen, 97, 157
Barbiturates
    detoxification, 341
    disorders caused by, 20, 34, 70
    sexual problems, 105
    sleep problems, 97
    withdrawal symptoms, 53

Beneficence, 140
Benzodiazepines
  alprazolam, 317–318, 356
  chlordiazepoxide, 318–319,
      356
  clonazepam, 319–320, 356
  cytochrome P-450 effects,
      359–360
  description of, 317
  diazepam, 320–321
  disorders caused by, 20, 34, 70
  dose equivalencies, 356
  lorazepam, 72, 152, 321–322,
      356
  oxazepam, 322, 356
  sexual problems, 105
  sleep problems, 97
  temazepam, 323, 356
  triazolam, 323–324, 356
  withdrawal symptoms, 53
Benztropine, 150, 154
Bereavement, 18
Beta-blockers, 105
Bibliography, 365–371
Binging, 88, 221–222
Biopsychosocial assessment
  advantages of, 1
  assaultiveness, 58
  components of, 4, 365
  core clinical tasks, 1
  cost-benefit ratio, 2
  costs of, 3
  dementia, 74
  mental status examination, 6
  personality disorders,
      approach to, 243–244
  principles of, 1–3, 365
  reasons for, 3, 365
  social history, 5
  suicidality, 58
Bipolar disorder (*See* Manic-
      depressive disorder)
Black cohosh, 364
Body dysmorphic disorder, 90,
      218–220

Borderline personality disorder
  clinical features of, 240–241
  course of, 242
  DSM criteria, 238
  prevalence of, 242
Breathing-related sleep disorder
  clinical features of, 225
  course of, 226
  description of, 98
  DSM criteria, 224
  prevalence of, 225
Brief reactive psychosis, 43
Bromocriptine, 73, 234
Bronchodilators, 26
Bulimia nervosa, 86, 221–223
      (*See also* Eating disorders)
  psychotherapy for, 261
Buprenorphine, 192
Bupropion, 283–284, 355
Buspirone (BuSpar), 156, 251,
      326–327

C

Caffeine, 34, 97
Calan (*See* Verapamil)
Calcium carbonate, 234
Calcium channel blockers, 20, 70
Cannabis, 190, 194–195
Carbamazepine, 288–290
Carisoprodol, 97, 105
Catalepsy, 71
Cataplexy, 92
Catapres (*See* Clonidine)
Catatonia
  definition of, 41
  diagnosis of, 71
  management of, 72
Central sleep apnea, 98
Centrax (*See* Prazepam)
Chamomile, 364
Chief complaint, 13
Chlordiazepoxide, 251, 318–319,
      356
Chlorpromazine, 301–302
Chlorprothixene, 357
Chorea, 144

Chronic depression, 22
Cimetidine, 20, 70, 97, 105
Circadian rhythm sleep disorder
  clinical features of, 224
  description of, 92
  prevalence of, 226
Circumstantiality, 40
Citalopram, 273–274, 355
Clang associations, 40
Clinical Institute Withdrawal
      Assessment protocol,
      339–340
Clomipramine, 264–265, 355
Clonazepam, 319–320, 356
Clonidine
  characteristics of, 327–328
  description of, 20
  disorders associated with, 97,
      105, 152, 156
Clorazepate, 356
Clozapine (Clozaril), 312–313,
      357
Cocaine
  abuse of, 190, 194–195
  disorders associated with, 20,
      26, 34
  maintenance therapy, 192
  self-help resources, 353
Codeine, 70, 349
Cognex (See Tacrine)
Cognitive disorders
  biopsychosocial assessment of,
      75
  caregiver impact assessments,
      79
  characterizing of, 76
  comorbidities, 82
  dementia (See Dementia)
  functional impact assessments,
      78
  reversible/modifiable causes
      of, 81
  screening instruments, 337
  self-help resources, 350–351
  sleep symptoms in, 96

Cognitive enhancers
  cytochrome P-450 effects, 360
  description of, 329
  donepezil, 330
  galantamine, 330–331
  rivastigmine, 331
  tacrine, 331–332
Cognitive screening instruments,
      337–338
Cogwheeling, 144
Collaborative practice model,
      245, 253–256, 365
Competency
  abilities, 139–141
  assessment of, 138
  decision making, 137
  definition of, 136
  differential diagnosis, 136
  eliciting information, 141
  psychiatric symptoms that
      affect, 136
  rational manipulation of infor-
      mation, 140
Complementary and alternative
      agents, 363–364
Concentration problems, 84–85
Concreteness, 40
Confidentiality, 65
Continuous quality improve-
      ment, 66
Contract for safety, 64
Conversion disorder, 126,
      215–216
Corticosteroids, 20, 26, 70, 97
Countertransference, 133,
      241–244
COX-2 inhibitors, 119
CQI (See Quality improvement,
      continuous)
Cyclobenzaprine, 70
Cyclothymia, 27, 173–174
Cylert (See Pemoline)
Cylexa (See Citalopram)
Cytochrome P-450, 249,
      358–360
Cytomel (See Triiodothyronine)

D

Dalmane (*See* Flurazepam)
Danazol, 234
Dantrolene, 73
Darvocet (*See* Propoxyphene)
Darvon (*See* Propoxyphene)
Decision sciences, 8–9, 14
Decongestants, 26, 34, 97
Delirium
    catatonia (*See* Catatonia)
    dementia vs., 68, 74
    differential diagnosis, 67, 68
    DSM system definition of, 67
    medical conditions that cause, 69
    medications that cause, 70
    psychosis vs., 68
    sleep symptoms in, 96
Delirium tremens, 53
Delusion(s)
    definition of, 39
    paranoid, 42
Delusional disorder, 203–204
Dementia
    Alzheimer, 80, 206
    biopsychosocial assessment of, 74
    caregiver impact assessments, 79
    comorbidities, 82, 207
    co-occurring symptoms, 78
    course of, 207
    criteria for, 77
    definition of, 75
    delirium vs., 68
    differential diagnosis, 74
    DSM criteria, 206
    frontotemporal, 80
    functional impact assessments, 78
    Lewy body, 80
    medical causes of, 80
    Parkinson, 80
    prevalence of, 207
    psychosis vs., 68
    sleep symptoms in, 96
    traumatic brain injury-induced, 80
    treatment of, 207–208
    types of, 80
    vascular, 80, 206
Dementia praecox, 198
Demerol (*See* Meperidine)
Depakene (*See* Valproate)
Depakote (*See* Valproate)
Dependent personality disorder
    clinical features of, 240–241
    DSM criteria, 239
    prevalence of, 242
Depersonalization disorder, 234–236
Depersonalization/derealization, 38, 234–236
Depression (*See also* Major depressive disorder; Major depressive episode)
    atypical, 22–23
    bereavement vs., 18
    catatonic, 22
    chronic, 22
    differential diagnosis, 17
    medical illnesses that cause, 19
    medications that cause, 20
    melancholic, 22–23
    mnemonic, diagnostic, 20
    postpartum, 22
    psychotic, 22
    screening for, 17–18
    seasonal pattern, 22
    stress differential diagnosis, 18
Depressive episode (*See* Major depressive episode)
Derailment, 40
Desipramine, 265–267, 355
Desyrel (*See* Trazodone)
Detoxification
    alcohol, 339–340
    barbiturate, 341
    definition of, 193
    methadone, 342
    nicotine, 344

Detoxification (*contd.*)
opiates, 342
stimulant, 343
Devises, putative psychoactive,
335–336
Diazepam, 152, 157, 320–321
Diet medications, 34
Digoxin, 105
Dilaudid (*See* Hydromorphone)
Diphenhydramine, 97, 150, 227,
346
Dissociation, 38
Dissociative amnesia, 234–236
Dissociative disorders, 234–236
Dissociative fugue, 234–236
Dissociative identity disorder,
234–236
Disulfiram, 26, 70
Diuretics, 97
Divalproex (*See* Valproate)
Dolophine (*See* Methadone)
Donepezil, 330
Dopamine agonists, 97
Dopaminergic agents, 26, 70
Doxepin, 267–268, 346, 355
Droperidol, 357
Drug abuse, 190–191
Drug dependence, 190–191
DSM
criteria, 161 (*See also specific
disorder, DSM criteria*)
description of, 7
strengths of and weaknesses
of, 134–135, 160–161
Duragesic (*See* Fentanyl)
Duty to warn, 65, 110
Dyskinesia, 144
Dyspareunia, 106, 228, 230
Dyssomnias (*See also specific
disorder*)
description of, 98
DSM criteria, 224
Dysthymia, 23, 167–169
psychotherapy for, 257
Dystonia
acute

assessment of, 149
characteristics of, 148–149
definition of, 144
differential diagnosis, 144
incidence of, 149
management of, 150
prevalence of, 149
risk factors, 149
tardive
assessment of, 155
management of, 157

E

Eating disorders
anorexia nervosa, 86,
220–221, 260
binging assessments, 88
bulimia nervosa, 86, 221–223,
261
differential diagnosis, 86
focus of concern, determining,
87–88
laboratory findings, 89
physical examination, 89
physical status evaluation, 88
psychotherapy for, 260–261
review of system findings, 89
screening for, 87
self-help resources, 352
sleep symptoms in, 96
Echolalia, 40
Ecstasy, 194–195
ECT (*See* Electroconvulsive
therapy)
Educational resources, 350–354
Effexor (*See* Venlafaxine)
Elavil (*See* Amitriptyline)
Electroconvulsive therapy
(ECT), 335–336
Embarrassment
in individuals being interviewed, 11
in clinicians, 66
Ephedra, 364
Equivalency tables, 249, 355–357
Ergotamines, 70

Escitalopram oxalate, 274–275, 355
Eskalith (*See* Lithium)
Estrogens, 20, 34, 105
Evidence-based interviewing
  alliance building, 13
  background, 8–9, 14
  chief complaint, 13
  description of, 7
  example of, 10
  questions, 11
  review of systems used in, 12
  strategies for, 9
  structuring of, 12–13
Executive function
  deficits of, 74–75, 83
  screening of, 337–338
Exelon (*See* Rivastigmine)
Exhibitionism, 107, 229, 231
Expressive aphasia, 77
Extrapyramidal symptoms, 143, 145

F

Factitious disorder, 127–128, 217–218
Female orgasmic disorder, 106, 228, 230
Fentanyl, 349
Fetishism, 107, 229, 231
Flashbacks, 31, 38
Flight of ideas, 40
Fluoroquinolones, 70
Fluoxetine, 275–276, 355
Fluphenazine, 302–303, 357
Flurazepam, 356
Fluvoxamine, 276–278
Frontotemporal dementia, 80
Frotteurism, 107, 229, 231
Fugue
  description of, 38
  dissociative, 234–236

G

Gabapentin, 251, 328
Galantamine, 330–331

Gambling
  pathological, 54, 196–197, 260, 351–352
  psychotherapy for, 260
Gender identity disorder, 108, 229, 231
Generalized anxiety disorder
  comorbidities, 181–182
  course of, 181
  description of, 33, 96
  DSM criteria, 180
  features of, 180–181
  mnemonic, diagnostic, 33
  prevalence of, 181
  psychotherapy for, 258
  treatment of, 182, 258
Geodon (*See* Ziprasidone)
Gestures, suicidal, 59
Ginkgo biloba, 364
Ginseng, 364
Glomerular filtration rate, 250
Glutethimide, 70

H

Halazepam, 356
Halcion (*See* Triazolam)
Hallucinations, 36–38, 92
Hallucinogens
  abuse of, 190, 194–195
  description of, 34, 70
Haloperidol (Haldol), 303–304, 357
Hepatic failure, 249–251
Histrionic personality disorder
  clinical features of, 240–241
  DSM criteria, 238–239
  prevalence of, 242
HMG-CoA reductase inhibitors, 20, 34
Hops, 364
Hydrochlorothiazide, 105
Hydrocodone, 349
Hydromorphone, 349
Hydroxyzine, 227, 346
Hyperarousal, 31

Hypersomnia, primary
  course of, 226
  DSM criteria, 224
  prevalence of, 225
Hypnagogic/hypnopompic hallu-
    cinations, 37, 92
Hypnotics
  description of, 190, 194–195
  zaleplon, 324–325
  zolpidem, 325–326
Hypoactive sexual desire dis-
    order, 106, 228, 230
Hypochondriasis, 128, 214–215
Hypokinesia, 145
Hypomania
  definition of, 24
  DSM criteria, 169
  mania vs., 26
  mnemonic, diagnostic, 25
  signs and symptoms of, 25
  sleep symptoms in, 96

I

Ideas of reference, 39
Identity, 38
Illusions, 38
Imaging work-up tables (See
    also medical disorder
    panels in individual
    modules)
  delirium, 69
  dementia, 80–81
Imipramine, 268–270
Impulsivity, 84–85
Inapsine (See Droperidol)
Indomethacin, 70
Inhalants, 190, 194–195
Insomnia, primary
  biopsychosocial approach, 345
  course of, 225–226
  description of, 98
  DSM criteria, 224
  pharmacologic treatment of,
    346
  prevalence of, 225
  treatment of, 227, 346

Interferon, 20, 70
Interviewing, principles of, 1–14
Involuntary commitment, 63–64
Irritability, 84–85
Isoniazid, 26, 70
Isotretinoin cream, 20

J

Judgment, inference of, 6

K

Kava, 364
Klonopin (See Clonazepam)
Kohlman Evaluation of Living
    Skills (KELS examina-
    tion), 83

L

LAAM, 192
Laboratory work-up tables (See
    also medical disorder
    panels in individual
    modules)
  delirium, 69, 73
  dementia, 81
  eating disorders, 89
Lamictal (See Lamotrigine)
Lamotrigine, 172, 290–291
Legal issues
  competency, 136–141
  contract for safety, 65
  duty to warn, 65, 110
  involuntary commitment, 63
  Tarasoff decisions, 65
"Lethal catatonia," 73
Lethality, 60
Levodopa, 26
Levothyroxine, 297–298
Lewy body dementia, 80
Lexapro (See Escitalopram
    oxalate)
Librium (See Chlordiazepoxide)
Lidocaine, 70
Life narrative, 13–14
Light
  bright visible spectrum light,
    336, 345–346

Liothyronine, 298–299
Lithane (See Lithium)
Lithium, 105, 251, 291–293
Lithobid (See Lithium)
Loose associations, 40
Lorazepam, 72, 152, 321–322, 356
Loxapine (Loxitane), 304–305, 357
Ludiomil (See Maprotiline)
Luvox (See Fluvoxamine)

M

Magnesium, 234
Ma huang, 364
Major depressive disorder (See also Depression)
    comorbidities, 166
    description of, 20, 82
    DSM criteria, 164
    features of, 164–165
    gender issues, 165
    prevalence of, 165–166
    psychotherapy for, 257
    sleep symptoms in, 96
    treatment of, 166–167
Major depressive episode
    in manic-depressive disorder, 169–173
    subtypes, 22–23
    vs. major depressive disorder, 21, 164
Male erectile disorder, 106, 228, 230
Malingering, 127–128, 217–218
Mania
    definition of, 24
    differential diagnosis, 24
    DSM criteria, 170
    hypomania vs., 26
    medical conditions that cause, 27
    medications that cause, 26–27
    mnemonic, diagnostic, 25
    mood in, 24–25
    screen for, 21, 24–25

signs and symptoms of, 25
    subsyndromal, 27
Manic-depressive disorder
    comorbidities, 171
    course of, 171
    DSM criteria, 169–170
    features of, 170
    prevalence of, 171
    psychotherapy for, 257
    treatment of, 171–173, 257
Maprotiline, 355
Medications, organization of in text (See also specific medication)
    contraindications, 248
    dosage of, 246
    drug interactions, 248
    equivalency tables, 355–357
    hepatic failure dosing, 249–251
    laboratory monitoring, 247
    on- and off-label indications, 246
    overdose toxicity, 248
    pregnancy and lactation classes, 247
    renal failure dosing, 249–251
    side effects, 247
    taper/switch schedule, 247
    titration schedule, 247
Melancholic depression, 22–23
Melatonin, 364
Mellaril (See Thioridazine)
Memory disorders
    dementia (See Dementia)
    executive function deficits, 74–75, 83
Mental status examination, 6
Meperidine, 70, 349
Mesoridazine, 305–306, 357
Methadone, 192, 342, 349
Methyldopa, 70, 105
Methylphenidate, 332–333
Metoclopramide, 34
Metronidazole, 34

Mini-Mental State Examination, 76, 337
Minipress (*See* Prazosin)
Mirtazapine, 284–285, 355
Mnemonic, diagnostic
  depression, 20
  generalized anxiety disorder, 33
  (hypo)mania, 25
  panic disorder, 35
  suicide, major risk factors, 62
Modafinil, 227
Molindone (Moban), 306–307, 357
Monoamine oxidase inhibitors
  cytochrome P-450 effects, 359
  description of, 105, 280
  equivalency tables, 355
  food interactions, 362
  interactions with, 362
  phenelzine, 280–281
  tranylcypromine, 282–283, 355
Mood
  definition of, 6
  in mania, 24–25
Mood disorders
  cyclothymia, 27, 173–174
  differential diagnosis, 17
  dysthymia, 23, 167–169
  major depressive disorder
    (*See* Major depressive disorder)
  self-help resources, 352
Mood stabilizers
  carbamazepine, 288–290
  cytochrome P-450 effects, 359
  description of, 288
  lamotrigine, 290–291
  lithium, 291–293
  oxcarbazepine, 293–294
  topiramate, 294
  valproate, 295–296
  verapamil, 296–297
Morphine, 349
MS Contin (*See* Morphine)

Münchausen's syndrome, 127
Mutism, 40
Myoclonus, 145

N

Naltrexone, 192
Narcissistic personality disorder
  clinical features of, 240–241
  DSM criteria, 238
  prevalence of, 242
Narcolepsy
  clinical features of, 225
  course of, 226
  description of, 98
  DSM criteria, 224
  prevalence of, 225
Nardil (*See* Phenelzine)
Navane (*See* Thiothixene)
Nefazodone, 285–286, 355
Neologisms, 40
Neuroleptic(s)
  atypical, 312–317, 357
  chlorpromazine, 301–302
  clozapine, 312–313, 357
  cytochrome P-450 effects, 359
  description of, 20, 300
  disorders associated with, 70, 105, 200–201
  dose equivalencies, 357
  fluphenazine, 302–303, 357
  haloperidol, 303–304, 357
  loxapine, 304–305, 357
  mesoridazine, 305–306, 357
  molindone, 306–307, 357
  olanzapine, 313–314, 357
  perphenazine, 307–308, 357
  quetiapine, 314–315, 357
  risperidone, 315–316
  thioridazine, 308–309, 357
  thiothixene, 310, 357
  trifluoperazine, 311, 357
  ziprasidone, 316–317
Neuroleptic malignant syndrome, 73
Neuroleptic-associated movement disorders, 148–149

Neurontin (*See* Gabapentin)
Neurosis, 103, 132, 134–135
Nicotine
    description of, 53, 97
    detoxification, 344
    disorders associated with, 97,
        190, 194–195
Nightmare disorder
    clinical features of, 225
    description of, 99
    DSM criteria, 224
    prevalence of, 225, 226
Nocturna myoclonus, 99
Nonsteroidal antiinflammatory
        drugs, 119
Norpramin (*See* Desipramine)
Nortriptyline, 270–271, 355
Numorphan (*See* Oxymorphone)

O

Obesity hypoventilation syn-
        drome, 98
Obsessive-compulsive disorder,
        33, 182–184
    psychotherapy for, 258
Obsessive-compulsive personal-
        ity disorder
    clinical features of, 240–241
    DSM criteria, 239–240
    prevalence of, 242
Obstructive sleep apnea, 98, 227
Olanzapine, 313–314, 357
Omega-3 fatty acids, 364
Open-ended questioning (*See*
        Questions, open-ended)
Opiates
    abuse of, 190–192, 194–195
    detoxification, 342
    disorders associated with, 34,
        70
    maintenance therapy, 192
    pain treated using, 121, 349
    sexual problems, 105
    sleep problems, 97
    withdrawal symptoms, 53
Oral contraceptives, 20, 234

Orap (*See* Pimozide)
Orgasmic disorders, 106
Overvalued ideas, 39
Oxazepam, 322, 356
Oxcarbazepine, 293–294
Oxycodone, 349
Oxycontin (*See* Oxycodone)
Oxymorphone, 349

P

Pain
    assessment of, 115
    clinician's guide to, 114
    differential diagnosis, 113
    evaluation of, 129
    mechanical, 116
    neuropathic, 116
    psychiatric disorders that pro-
        duce or worsen, 113
    queries for assessing, 115
    self-help resources, 352
    sexual, 228
    subjective perception of, 123
    treatment of
        adjuvant, 120, 122
        analgesic agents, 119, 122
        antiinflammatory agents,
            119, 122
        "house of pain" approach,
            117–122
        nonpharmacologic, 118, 122
        opiates, 121, 349
        planning of, 116
Pain disorder, 212–213
Pamelor (*See* Nortriptyline)
Panic attack, 174–175
Panic disorder
    with agoraphobia, 35, 176
    comorbidities, 176
    course of, 176
    description of, 35, 96
    DSM criteria, 175
    features of, 175
    mnemonic, diagnostic, 35
    prevalence of, 175–176
    psychotherapy for, 258

383

Panic disorder (*contd.*)
  treatment of, 176–177, 258
  without agoraphobia, 176
Paranoid delusions, 42
Paranoid personality disorder
  clinical features of, 240–241
  DSM criteria, 237
  prevalence of, 242
Paraphilias, 107, 228–229, 231
Paraphrenia, 198
Parasomnias (*See also specific disorder*)
  description of, 92, 99
  DSM criteria, 224
Parkinson dementia, 80
Parkinsonism
  assessment of, 153
  definition of, 144–145
  management of, 154
  risk factors, 154
Parnate (*See* Tranylcypromine)
Paroxetine, 251, 278–279, 355
Pathological gambling, 54, 196–197, 260, 351–352
Paxil (*See* Paroxetine)
Paxipam (*See* Halazepam)
Pedophilia, 107, 229, 231
Pemoline, 333–334
Pentazocine, 349
Pentobarbital challenge test, 341
Percocet (*See* Oxycodone)
Percodan (*See* Oxycodone)
Periodic limb movements in sleep, 99, 227
Perphenazine, 307–308, 357
Perseveration, 40
Personal problems
  assessment of, 131
  differential diagnosis, 130
  primary, 132
  psychiatric disorders presenting as, 132
Personality disorders (*See also specific personality disorder*)

Biopsychosocial approach to, 243–244
  clinical features of, 240–241
  comorbidities, 243
  course of, 242
  description of, 133
  DSM criteria, 236–240
  prevalence of, 242
  psychotherapy for, 261
  treatment of, 243–244
Pharmacodynamics, 248
Pharmacokinetics, 248
Phencyclidine, 190, 194–195
Phenelzine, 280–281, 355
Phobia
  agoraphobia
    comorbidities, 179
    course of, 179
    DSM criteria, 177–178
    panic disorder with, 35, 176
    prevalence of, 178–179
    treatment of, 180
  features of, 178
  social
    comorbidities, 179
    course of, 179
    definition of, 35
    DSM criteria, 177
    prevalence of, 178
    treatment of, 180
  specific
    comorbidities, 179
    course of, 179
    definition of, 35
    DSM criteria, 177
    prevalence of, 178
    treatment of, 180
  treatment of, 179–180
Pickwickian syndrome, 98
Pill-rolling tremor, 145
Pimozide, 357
Postpartum depression, 22
Posttraumatic stress disorder
  comorbidities, 186
  course of, 186
  description of, 32, 96

DSM criteria, 184–185
features of, 185
prevalence of, 185–186
psychotherapy for, 258
treatment of, 186–187
Poverty of content, 40
Prazepam, 356
Prazosin, 329
Predictive value, positive and negative, 8, 14
Premature ejaculation, 106, 228, 230
Premenstrual dysphoric disorder, 232–234
Pressured speech, 40
Prevalence, 14, 162–163
Primary hypersomnia, 98
Procainamide, 70
Progesterone, 105, 234
Prolixin (*See* Fluphenazine)
Propoxyphene, 349
Propranolol, 148, 156
Protriptyline, 271–273, 355
Prozac (*See* Fluoxetine)
Pseudodementia, 82
Pseudoparkinsonism, 145
Psychosis
brief reactive, 43
data gathering for assessments, 41
delirium vs., 68
dementia vs., 68
differential diagnosis, 36
disorders associated with, 37
interviewing probes for, 42
medical illnesses that cause, 44
medications that cause, 44
perceptual disorders, 38
screening for, 10
sleep symptoms in, 96
stress differential diagnosis, 43
symptoms of, 36
thought patterns, 40
without clear precipitant, 44
Psychotherapy
formal

definition of, 252
dementia, 208
dysthymia, 168
eating disorders, 260–261
gambling, 260
generalized anxiety disorder, 182, 258
major depressive disorder, 166, 257
manic-depressive disorder, 172
obsessive-compulsive disorder, 184
overview of, 257
panic disorder, 258
phobias, 258
posttraumatic stress disorder, 187
schizoaffective disorder, 202
schizophrenia, 260
somatization disorder, 260
substance use disorders, 259
supportive
collaborative disease management agenda, 255
components of, 254
definition of, 252
overview of, 253
problem-solving agenda, 256
Psychotic depression, 22
Psychotropic-induced movement disorders
categorizing of, 146
differential diagnosis, 144
Purging, 88
Pyridoxine, 364

Q

Quality improvement, continuous (CQI), 66
Questions
high-sensitivity, 9
high-specificity, 9
open-ended

Questions (*contd.*)
  alternatives to, 8–10
  costs and benefits of, 7
  social valence of, 11
Quetiapine, 314–315, 357

R

Rabbit syndrome, 145
Ranitidine, 20, 70
Receptive aphasia, 77
Recurrence of symptoms, differential diagnosis of, 158–159
Relationship problems
  assessment of, 131
  differential diagnosis, 130
  primary, 132
  psychiatric disorders presenting as, 132
Religious values, 39
REM sleep behavior disorder, 99
Remeron (*See* Mirtazapine)
Reminyl (*See* Galantamine)
Renal failure, 249–251
Reserpine, 156
Restless legs syndrome, 227
Restoril (*See* Temazepam)
Review of systems, 12
Rifampin, 70
Risperidone (Risperdal), 315–316
Ritalin (*See* Methylphenidate)
Rivastigmine, 331

S

S-Adenosyl methionine (SAMe), 364
Sarafem (*See* Fluoxetine)
Schizoaffective disorder, 201–202
Schizoid personality disorder
  clinical features of, 240–241
  DSM criteria, 237
  prevalence of, 242
Schizophrenia
  comorbidities, 200

course of, 200
disorganized, 198
DSM criteria, 197–198
features of, 198–199
paranoid, 198
prevalence of, 199
psychotherapy for, 260
residual, 198
treatment of, 200–201
undifferentiated, 198
Schizotypal personality disorder
  clinical features of, 240–241
  DSM criteria, 237
  prevalence of, 242
Screening for diagnoses (*See
  also individual
  diagnoses*), 8–9, 12, 14
Sedatives, 190, 194–195
Selective serotonin reuptake
  inhibitors
  citalopram, 273–274, 355
  cytochrome P-450 effects, 359
  description of, 273
  equivalency tables, 355
  escitalopram oxalate, 274–275, 355
  fluoxetine, 275–276, 355
  fluvoxamine, 276–278
  paroxetine, 251, 278–279, 355
  sertraline, 279–280, 355
Self-help groups, 350–354
Sensitivity, 8–9
Serax (*See* Oxazepam)
Serentil (*See* Mesoridazine)
Seroquel (*See* Quetiapine)
Serotonin reuptake inhibitors, 105, 167, 233 (*See* Mirtazepine, Tricyclic antidepressants, Venlafaxine)
Sertraline, 279–280, 355
Serzone (*See* Nefazodone)
Sexual aids, 111
Sexual arousal disorders, 106, 228, 230
Sexual aversion disorder, 106, 228

Sexual disorders
  categories of, 100–101
  clinical features of, 229–230
  differential diagnosis, 100
  DSM criteria, 228–229
  gender identity disorder, 108, 229
  medical illnesses that present as, 104
  medications that cause, 105
  medications to treat, 109, 111–112
  pain during sexual activity, 228
  paraphilias, 107, 228–229
  primary
    description of, 107
    facilitation strategies for, 111
    treatment planning for, 110–112
  psychotherapy for, 261
  screening for, 102
  sexual drive
    description of, 103
    primary, 103, 106
    secondary, 103
  treatment planning for, 109
Sexual masochism, 107, 229, 231
Sexual response, 101
Sexual sadism, 107, 229, 231
Shame (See Embarrassment)
Sildenafil, 111, 112
Sinequan (See Doxepin)
Sleep
  in older adults, 94
  stages of, 92
Sleep apnea, 98
Sleep disorders (See also specific disorder)
  biopsychosocial approach, 345–346
  breathing-related (See Breathing-related sleep disorder)
  characteristics of, 93
  circadian rhythm (See Circadian rhythm sleep disorder)
  classification of, 91
  differential diagnosis, 91
  dyssomnias (See Dyssomnias)
  medical conditions associated with, 95
  medications associated with, 97
  parasomnias (See Parasomnias)
  primary, 98–99
  symptom probes, 93
  terminology associated with, 92
  treatment of, 227–228
Sleep paralysis, 92
Sleep terror disorder
  clinical features of, 225
  description of, 99
  DSM criteria, 224
  prevalence of, 225, 226
Sleep–wake schedule disorder, 98
Sleepwalking disorder
  clinical features of, 225
  description of, 99
  DSM criteria, 224
  prevalence of, 225, 226
Social history, 5
Social phobia
  comorbidities, 179
  course of, 179
  definition of, 35
  DSM criteria, 177
  prevalence of, 178
  treatment of, 180
Social valence of interview questions, 11
Somatization disorder, 128, 210–212
  psychotherapy for, 260
Somatoform disorders
  differential diagnosis, 123
  hypochondriasis, 214–215
Sonata (See Zaleplon)

Specific phobia
  comorbidities, 179
  course of, 179
  definition of, 35
  DSM criteria, 177
  prevalence of, 178
  treatment of, 180
Specificity, 8–9
Speech, characterizing, 40
St. John's wort, 364
Stelazine (*See* Trifluoperazine)
Stigma (*See* Embarrassment)
Stimulants
  cytochrome P-450 effects, 360
  description of, 20, 26, 332
  detoxification, 343
  methylphenidate, 332–333
  pemoline, 333–334
  sleep problems, 97
  withdrawal symptoms, 53
Stress
  depression and, 18
  psychosis and, 43
Stress disorder
  acute, 187–189
  posttraumatic (*See* Posttraumatic stress disorder)
Substance use disorders (*See also specific drug*)
  abuse vs. dependence, 49
  complications of, 48
  current phase of, 48
  detoxification protocols, 339–344
  differential diagnosis, 45
  DSM criteria, 189
  extent of, 47
  features of, 189–190
  prevalence of, 190–191
  psychiatric comorbidities, 51–52
  psychotherapy for, 259
  screening for, 46
  self-help resources, 353
  sleep symptoms in, 96

  social sequelae, 50
  tasks in characterizing, 46
  treatment of, 193–195, 259
  withdrawal syndromes, 53
Subsyndromal depression, 23
Subsyndromal mania, 27
Suicidality/suicide
  acts
    examples of, 60
    management of, 62–63
  assessment of, 57–58
  confidentiality, 65
  "contract for safety," 64
  debriefing, 66
  differential diagnosis, 56
  "gestures," 59, 241
  ideation, 56
  intent, 59–60
  involuntary commitment, 63–64
  lethality assessments, 60
  mnemonic for major risk factors, 62
  risk factors, 61–62
  self-help resources, 353–354
Sumatriptan, 34
Surmontil (*See* Trimipramine)
Symptom-driven assessment, organization and principles of, 15–16
Synthroid (*See* Levothyroxine)

T

Tacrine, 331–332
Talwin (*See* Pentazocine)
Tangentiality, 40
Taractan (*See* Chlorprothixene)
Tarasoff decisions, 65
Tardive dyskinesia
  assessment of, 155–156
  definition of, 144–145
  management of, 156
Tardive dystonia (*See* Dystonia, tardive)
Tegretol (*See* Carbamazepine)

Temazepam, 323, 356
Theophylline, 26
Thioridazine, 308–309, 357
Thiothixene, 310, 357
Thorazine (*See* Chlorpromazine)
Thought blocking, 40
Thought disorder, 36, 39–40
Thought insertion, 40
Thought patterns, 40
Thought withdrawal, 40
Thyroxine, 297–298
Tic disorders, 145
Tindal (*See* Acetophenazine)
Tofranil (*See* Imipramine)
Tolerance, 48
Topiramate (Topamax), 70, 294
Transcranial magnetic stimulation, 336
Transvestic fetishism, 107, 229, 231
Tranxene (*See* Clorazepate)
Tranylcypromine, 282–283, 355
Trauma
    anxiety disorders, 31–32
    screening for, 30–31
    types of, 30
Traumatic brain injury, 80
Trazodone, 227, 286–287, 346, 355
Treatment
    Alliance (*See* Alliance-building)
    cost-benefit comparisons, 2
    electroconvulsive therapy, 335–336
    medications (*See* Medications; *specific medication*)
    overview of, 245–246
    psychotherapy (*See* Psychotherapy)
    self-help resources, 350–354
Tremor
    definition and types of, 145
    management of, 148
    psychotropic medications-induced, 144, 147

Triazolam, 323–324, 356
Tricyclic antidepressants
    amitriptyline, 262–264, 355
    clomipramine, 264–265, 355
    cytochrome P-450 effects, 359
    description of, 262
    desipramine, 265–267, 355
    disorders associated with, 105, 120
    doxepin, 267–268, 346, 355
    equivalency tables, 355
    imipramine, 268–270
    nortriptyline, 270–271, 355
    protriptyline, 271–273, 355
Trifluoperazine, 311, 357
Triiodothyronine, 298–299
Trilafon (*See* Perphenazine)
Trileptal (*See* Oxcarbazepine)
Trimipramine, 355
Triphenhexidyl, 150, 154
Tylox (*See* Oxycodone)

U

Unexplained physical complaints
    differential diagnosis, 123
    disorders that present with, 125
    vagal nerve stimulation, 336

V

Vaginismus, 106, 228
Valerian, 364
Valium (*See* Diazepam)
Valproate, 295–296
Vascular dementia, 80
Venlafaxine, 287–288, 355
Verapamil, 296–297
Vicodin (*See* Hydrocodone)
Vitamin B_6, 364
Vitamin E, 156, 233, 364
Vivactil (*See* Protriptyline)
Voyeurism, 107, 229

W

Wellbutrin (*See* Bupropion)

Withdrawal
  definition of, 48
  syndromes, 53
Word salad, 40

X

Xanax (*See* Alprazolam)

Y

Yohimbine, 364

Z

Zaleplon, 324–325
Zeitgeber, 92
Ziprasidone, 316–317, 357
Zoloft (*See* Sertraline)
Zolpidem, 325–326
Zyban (*See* Bupropion)
Zyprexa (*See* Olanzapine)